MW01036463

UNDERSTANDING PAIN

Also by Naheed Ali

Understanding Lung Cancer:
An Introduction for Patients and Caregivers

Understanding Celiac Disease:
An Introduction for Patients and Caregivers

Understanding Fibromyalgia:
An Introduction for Patients and Caregivers

Understanding Chronic Fatigue Syndrome:
An Introduction for Patients and Caregivers

Understanding Alzheimer's:
An Introduction for Patients and Caregivers

Understanding Parkinson's Disease:
An Introduction for Patients and Caregivers

Arthritis and You:
A Comprehensive Digest for Patients and Caregivers

Diabetes and You:
A Comprehensive, Holistic Approach

The Obesity Reality:
A Comprehensive Approach to a Growing Problem

UNDERSTANDING PAIN

An Introduction for Patients and Caregivers

Naheed Ali and Moshe Lewis

ROWMAN & LITTLEFIELD
Lanham • Boulder • New York • London

Published by Rowman & Littlefield
A wholly owned subsidiary of The Rowman & Littlefield Publishing Group,
Inc.
4501 Forbes Boulevard, Suite 200, Lanham, Maryland 20706
www.rowman.com

Unit A, Whitacre Mews, 26-34 Stannary Street, London SE11 4AB

British Library Cataloguing in Publication Information Available

Library of Congress Cataloging-in-Publication Data

Ali, Naheed, 1981– , author.
Understanding pain : an introduction for patients and caregivers / Naheed Ali and Moshe Lewis.
p. ; cm.
Includes bibliographical references and index.
ISBN 978-1-4422-3360-7 (cloth : alk. paper)—ISBN 978-1-4422-3361-4 (electronic)
I. Lewis, Moshe, 1968– , author. II. Title. [DNLM: 1. Pain—Popular Works. 2. Age Factors—
Popular Works. 3. Attitude to Health—Popular Works. 4. Pain Management—Popular Works. WL
704]
RB127
616'.0472—dc23
2014042262

Printed in the United States of America

Understanding Pain is dedicated to our readers, to people in pain, and to all who provided encouragement and support for this work.

CONTENTS

PREFACE

When someone is suffering from an injury, an illness, or severe mental or emotional distress, he or she is basically feeling pain. A widely agreed-upon definition of pain is that pain is an unpleasant sensory and emotional feeling associated with potential or real tissue damage, or is explained in terms of this damage.[1] Three facets of this definition must be well understood. First, pain is a physical and emotional experience that isn't always entirely in the body or in the mind. Second, the pain is in response to actual or potential tissue damage, so there may or may not be abnormal lab or radiography reports in spite of the presence of real pain. Third, pain is described in terms of such damage. This final component is aligned with an often-recommended definition of pain: Pain is whatever an individual suffering from it claims it is, surfacing whenever he says it does.[2]

So why does pain exist? According to many theories, the true function of pain is to persuade the individual who experiences it to withdraw from harmful situations and to prevent such experiences from occurring in the future.[3] When it comes to injuries, pain may help prevent further harm. A child who touches a hot stove pulls his hand away before a serious burn occurs. Pain that is (1) sudden and of any intensity, (2) anticipated *or* unpredictable, or (3) of a duration of less than six months is said to be acute. Chronic pain, however, is constant and recurring without anticipation and prediction and lasts greater than just a few months. We need to know about pain, its management and assessment, because complications may occur when we experience it, since the body produces a stress response in which harmful substances are released from injured tissue. These include breakdown of tissue, increased metabolic rate, impaired immune function, and negative emotions. This goes to show that pain also prevents one from participating in self-care activities. Unfortunately, pain can also bring forth feelings of helplessness and hopelessness. Pain management options allow one to maintain some control.

The caregiving team's responsibility is to teach the pain patient about the goals of pain management and why it's an important part of care. When a team member disregards the patient's report of pain, the patient will usually have a sense of not being believed. The patient may compensate by either underreporting pain—or, less commonly—anxiously overreporting. He or she may try to hide the pain for fear of being thought of as a complainer or drug seeker. Moreover, pain is more than a symptom; it can be a high-priority problem in itself. When in excess, it presents both physiological and psychological dangers to health and recovery. Severe pain is viewed as an emergency situation deserving prompt attention from formal caregivers such as physicians.[4]

Pain is the most common reason patients seek medical advice. Taking care of patients in pain is challenging, and it requires a systematic approach to assessment and treatment. Pain management requires careful assessment of the patient's condition while taking into consideration the ethical principles that affect patient care. Accurate assessment of pain is essential to effective treatment. Without this, it's not possible to intervene in a way that meets the patient's needs. Effective management can help reach goals by (1) enhancing comfort, (2) minimizing side effects of medications and complications related to inadequate control, and (3) reducing the length of hospital stay.

An unfamiliar environment such as a busy hospital lobby, with its noises, lights, and activity, can compound the effects of pain. In addition, a person who is without family or a support network may perceive pain as severe, whereas a person who has supportive people around may perceive much less pain. Some prefer to withdraw when they're in pain, whereas others prefer the distraction of people and activity around them. Family caregivers can be a significant support for a person in pain. With the increase in outpatient and home care, families are assuming a greater responsibility for medical pain management. Moreover, education related to the assessment and management of pain can positively affect the perceived quality of life for both the clients and their caregivers.[5] Expectations of significant others can affect a person's perception of (and responses to) pain, and sometimes, it may also be the presence of support people that changes a client's reaction to pain.

After reading through this book, the reader should understand that experiences with pain may also vary depending on the age group. An infant may respond to pain with increased sensitivity, avoiding pain by turning away or physically resisting. This can be compared with a toddler or a preschooler who already has the ability to describe pain and its location. The toddler might respond by crying or with anger because pain appears as a threat to his security. A school-age child may try to be more resilient when facing pain but should be provided with support and nurturing from the caregiver. An adolescent could be slow to acknowledge or recognize pain because "giving in" may be considered weak. When an adult experiences pain, he or she might exhibit gender-based behaviors learned as a child. An adult may ignore pain because to admit it could mean weakness or failure.

On the other hand, the elderly may perceive pain as part of the aging process. Studies have shown that chronic pain affects 25–50 percent of older pain clients living in the community and 45–80 percent of those in nursing homes.[6] Senior citizens constitute the largest group of individuals seeking health care services. While the prevalence of pain in the elderly population is generally higher due to both acute and chronic medical conditions, the pain threshold doesn't appear to change with aging, although the effect of analgesics may increase due to physiologic changes related to drug metabolism and *excretion* (getting rid of waste).[7] Sometimes, they may withhold complaints of pain because of fear of (1) treatment, (2) any lifestyle changes that may be involved, or (3) becoming dependent. The person may consider it unacceptable to admit or show pain and describe it differently, such as an "ache," "hurt," or "discomfort."

Although pain is a universal experience, the nature of such an experience is unique to the individual, based, in part, on the type of pain experienced, the psychosocial context or meaning, and the response needed. Before advancing any further, the reader should know that emotional or spiritual distress and the fear related to dependence on family caregivers may alter the patient's perception or reporting of pain. Some patients may feel pain more intensely because of the influence of fear, and others may underreport if they are trying to protect family members in some way or another. That said, it's important to learn as much as possible about pain and its management to effectively advocate for pain sufferers, assist with patient education, and provide appropriate resources for caregivers. Although it's not the authors' intension to make this book difficult to read, the reader should understand that certain concepts related to pain must be presented at the advanced reading level to provide the comprehensive overview of pain that this book seeks to provide. A glossary of terms has been provided as an aid to the reader's better understanding of these concepts. Moreover, the reader may notice redundancies throughout the book; it is hoped that occasionally repeating some material in different words will allow those who are unfamiliar with the topics to properly digest the presented material more easily.

I

Groundwork

I

INTRODUCTION TO PAIN

Everyone experiences pain once in a while; it might be because of headaches, sore throats, wounds, injuries, burns, or other reasons. Pain is the key reason why people search for medical assistance, since it's the major and most typical symptom of almost all existing illnesses. Although pain is usually uncomfortable and undesirable to feel, it serves as an indication that something—possibly overall health—isn't right. Therefore, the individual must never disregard pain. If possible, the person should immediately consult a physician once a considerable amount of pain is experienced, in order to know the principal cause of the suffering. If such pain is ignored, there is a very good possibility that the condition causing the pain could lead to a serious problem or illness that might be difficult to address.

Pain is an unpleasant physical sensation occasioned by actual or probable damaged tissues.[1] One thing to learn about pain is that it is subjective. This means that the intensity of pain an individual feels is not necessarily the same as another might feel, even though they have the same illness. In addition, the individual experiencing the pain is the only one who can correctly define and describe the pain that he or she is feeling. Pain is not only a sensation or outcome of physical consciousness; it also involves perception, which is the subjective consciousness of discomfort.[2] It is *perception* that provides information regarding where the pain is, its intensity, as well as a little about its nature.[3] The variety of conscious and unconscious reactions to both perception and sensation, including the emotional reaction, add further definition to the general concept of pain.[4]

ORIGINS OF TERMINOLOGY

Why and When the Term *Dolorology* Was Coined

The term *dolorology* was derived from the Latin word *dolor*, meaning "pain," along with the Greek word *logos*, which means "study."[5] The term was coined by a neurosurgeon, Dr. C. Norman Shealy, who found that his usual methods were not alleviating the suffering of his patients. He began to work with an electrical engineer to devise "a low-voltage electrical unit that could short-circuit pain by preventing the pain sensation from traveling up the spinal cord to the brain."[6] Their research resulted in the *transcutaneous electrical nerve simulator* (TENS), which is now used to control both acute and chronic pain. Shealy was the first physician to specialize in and dedicate himself to, the management of pain. He basically devised the term *dolorology* for his new medical specialty.[7]

Explanation of Dolorology

Dolorology is, broadly, "a medical specialty concerned with the study and treatment of pain."[8] It includes a shift in the medical conceptualization of pain as a symptom of disease to chronic pain as an independent clinical entity.[9] People who specialize in management or treatment of pain, also called "pain therapists," are sometimes referred to as dolorologists.[10]

   Dolorology, being the study of pain, involves pain management. "The treatment of pain is guided by the history of the pain, its intensity, duration, aggravating and relieving conditions, and structures involved in causing the pain."[11] So pain management involves accurately determining the source of the pain—that is, the cause of the stimulation of the nerves in that part of the body.

TRUE MEANINGS OF PAIN

Straightforward Definition

All people feel pain, but all pains are not the same. Pain is an uncomfortable sensory feeling along with emotion(s) linked to actual or potential damaged tissues. Nevertheless, pain is actually a sign that can't always be objectively measured. The caregiver can't observe an affected person and know specifically what is affected and what the pain feels like. The meaning of the pain is therefore, inevitably dependent on the individual experiencing it.[12]

Most people try to stay away from pain. On the other hand, some hold the notion that "suffering is good for you" or perhaps the pain is justified because "they brought it upon themselves." In the past, the presence of pain was sometimes believed to be an intrusion by evil spirits or a punishment for sins. For those who don't have a particular religious belief, pain can nonetheless be viewed as a positive means for self-growth or even self-evaluation. Surprisingly enough, some individuals can relate to sexual pleasure with particular kinds of pain.[13]

Chronic Pain Might Be a Disease Itself

Chronic pain is certainly an ailment, and because it has so many medical causes and consequences, experts are contemplating whether it should be classified as a disease. Chronic pain results when the root of the pain can't be handled anymore. It is persistent and frequently incapacitating. This sort of pain is frequently associated with a long-term or life-threatening disorder. A person experiencing long-term soreness could possibly be frustrated, withdrawn, and worn out.[14] Chronic pain is a condition initiated by real harm wherein the pain has survived so long (half a year or longer) that it has itself become an ailment. Typically, there is no foreseen end. Such a pain intrudes directly into the patient's existence. There is usually an intense mental adjustment for this "new lifestyle" and patients who depend on strong pain-eliminating treatments have often unfortunately fallen into a cycle of ache, major depression, and a lack of exercise. There are three types of chronic pain:

1. *Limited*: wherever the actual physical pathology is; here it might be identified in cases of cancer or slow-curing injuries, including burns or even damaged muscle tissue.
2. *Intermittent*: the affected individual has times when he's completely free from pain. Examples are: headache, such as migraine, and back pain.
3. *Prolonged or "chronic benign pain"*: This usually happens daily, and examples include middle-back pain or arthritis pain.

Sometimes, sensation associated with an injury or even disease never entirely vanishes. Such is the case with severe, repetitive headaches and other pains appearing without reason and then recurring or perhaps never disappearing. Several surgical treatments that patients resort to simply make the situation much worse, as does the unnecessary use of over-the-counter (OTC) medication.

Chronic pain can be recognized immediately. It could be a "spicy" sensation of burn moments after a finger comes into contact with an oven, or perhaps it's a dull pain over the forehead after a full day of tension and stress. Otherwise, the pain patient might recognize it as a sharp sting along the back after lifting something large. Chronic pain, in its more benign manifestation, warns people when something is not exactly right, when to take medication, or go to a doctor. At its worst, however, chronic pain robs individuals of efficiency, well-being—and for many struggling with extended sickness—life. In certain instances, chronic pain can be much worse than death itself. These days, chronic pain is among the most common medical problems and a critical and costly general public health issue.

HOW PAIN AFFECTS A PERSON'S LIFE

Psychological factors can also cause aches to a certain extent, which can be just as extreme as pain derived from bodily stimulus. Since pure physical pain is uncommon, it will be typically a mixture of physiological and psychological components. Treating emotional pain is as important as dealing with bodily pain. It is emotional anguish that accompanies or perhaps exacerbates physical pain. The victim may feel that he or she is missing his or her dignity, his or her sense of humor and therefore is "not himself or herself" as a result of bodily pain. Previous tragedies and losses, such as those involving divorce proceedings or deaths in the family can lead to the sufferer's overpowering anxiousness. There might be a feeling of helplessness as well. It's been found that previous psychiatric ailments sensitize people to their pain, which usually shows itself through major depression or perhaps frustration. Appreciation and concern on the side of the care team members could alleviate this very part of pain by encouraging the sufferer to talk about feelings of pain.

Spiritual Facets of Pain

In ways similar to psychological pain, spiritual factors can be involved with physical pain. Pain can make a spiritual person feel a new desolate meaninglessness regarding his or her existence. The sufferer's view of life continues to be broken. People are not destroyed by simply suffering; they might be struggling without purposefulness or meaning. This could be attributed to the breakup of a happy relationship or even the loss of someone close.[15]

Pain and Memories

Patients' past experiences associated with pain and its discomfort will also have an effect on how they judge that pain and what it implies. Therefore, the childhood recollection of one's palm on the scorching iron and the resulting pain experienced from the burn may give rise to learning to keep away from committing the same blunder again. The patient's view of his own existing pain can also be influenced by discomfort from earlier events, for instance, if a family member died from an identical procedure.[16]

Character

It turns out that introverts are more serious about pain, though they report it less often than their extroverted counterparts. People who fail to grumble of soreness tend to be a lot more emotional and less sociable.[17]

Age

Elderly individuals acquire much more rest from anesthetics compared to their younger counterparts. It is possible that younger sufferers have greater anticipation involving treatment, or perhaps they haven't experienced serious soreness before. This may be why dissatisfaction with treatment is more common among younger patients. The volume of pain tolerated by sufferers lessens with increase in age.[18]

PHYSICAL VS. PSYCHOLOGICAL

Choosing bodily over psychological pain is a concept that can't be approached without difficulty. With bodily pain, sufferers tend to acknowledge it for what it is and "deal with it." A person breaks a bone and sees a medical professional and gets healed. It's not a comfortable sensation, but people understand what causes the pain and so they can cope and get on with their life. Emotional or psychological pain, on the contrary, is generally caused by nonacceptance of what is happening as well as an inability to deny the facts. The focus is on the cause of the pain, and the more one thinks about it, the greater the discomfort.

Uncovering the Differences

Emotional pain can be a more agonizing experience than physical pain. As the sufferer screams in order to somehow "spell out" the pain sensation, the discomfort increasingly makes itself real, and therefore more valid. However, psychological pain might be dealt with more rapidly and easily by knowing the best way to target the mind. It is possible to relax and release the pain with thoughts, provided that they are understood. For example, people can use their imagination to be able to feel warm fingers placed on their heart, comforting them and piecing things back together again. They can visualize their inhalation and exhalation. They can focus on words and phrases that will soothe the pain, help them loosen up and heal. They will be able to heal their own mental pains using their mind. They do not have to go on a rampage and open up their current wounds. Simply put, it is extremely difficult to think clearly if you are going through mental chaos. When you take things easy, you might also manually program your mind to concentrate on another route, therefore gaining strength to handle your emotions in a beneficial way—essentially "rub salve" on your psychological wounds, cover up emotions, and move on with life.[19]

ANALYSIS

As a basic introduction to pain, this chapter showed how pain is an adverse feeling but may be regarded as a positive experience, since it serves as a warning that something is damaged within the body, or is going to be. In the absence of pain-sensing ability, a person might not seek required medical attention.[20] Pain encourages people to seek out medical help to get rid of, or at least lessen, the pain that they feel. Through this, they're able to prevent any health-threatening circumstances from taking place, thus saving themselves from potentially serious illnesses. Whether or not total eradication of the pain is possible, being familiar with the general concept of the pain may help with consideration of specific therapeutic alternatives.[21]

2

INTRODUCTION TO THE
NERVOUS SYSTEM

Pain is conducted by the nervous system, one of many body systems found in most multicellular animals such as human beings. The nervous system governs the actions of other body regions and coordinates these systems with each other. There are two main parts of the nervous system for most animals. These are the central nervous system and the peripheral nervous system, whose main role is to control the body.[1] This control is effected through information collected from the environment through signals sent from one cell to another. The central nervous system analyzes the gathered data and chooses the correct response. The intricacy of nervous systems varies from one organism to another.[2] Sponges, for example, lack the kind of intricate nervous system humans have, but parts of their genetic makeup have a similar function, enabling them to move about in a primitive manner. The study of the nervous system, called *neuroscience*, is important for the understanding of pain because without the collaboration between pain receptors and organs, pain would never have come to exist.

CENTRAL NERVOUS SYSTEM

The main parts of the nervous system, which transmit pain in most animals, are the central nervous system and the peripheral nervous system. The central nervous system of *bilaterian* (having bilateral symmetry) animals, or creatures with a back and a front end as well as a top and a bottom end, such as in humans—as opposed to radially symmetrical animals such as jellyfish—consists of the brain and the spinal cord. Some also classify the retina and the cranial nerves as part of the central nervous system. The bulk of the nervous system is found in the central nervous system, which is enclosed within the dorsal cavity and is protected by a system of membranes called meninges. The dorsal cavity contains the cranial cavity that houses the brain and the vertebral or spinal canal that holds the spinal cord. In conjunction with the peripheral nervous system, the central nervous system has an important role in the behavior of animals toward pain, among other sensations.[3]

Brain

The center of the nervous system of most animals is the brain. It is divided into four separate sections: (1) the brain stem, (2) diencephalon, (3) cerebellum, and (4) cerebrum. These four sections work together with the help of the spinal cord to control the animal's voluntary and involuntary behaviors. Because of the brain's complexity, there are also some parts that scientists have trouble categorizing. One of these parts is the limbic system, which influences emotion, behavior, motivation, long-term memory, and *olfaction* (smelling) among many other functions.

Brain Stem

The brain stem is located in the hindmost part of the brain. It connects the brain to the spinal cord. All signals sent from the cerebrum and cerebellum to the body and back travel via the brain stem through nerve connections of the motor and sensory systems, including (1) the *corticospinal tract*, responsible for motor functions; (2) the *posterior column-medial lemniscus pathway*, which has a sensory function; and (3) the *spinothalamic tract*, which governs the body's pain perception. These connections enable the brain stem to govern the body's basic and involuntary behaviors, such as reflexes, blood pressure, respiration, awareness, as well as the release of hormones during a painful "flight-or-fight" situation—namely *adrenaline, noradrenaline* or *norepinephrine,* and *cortisol.* These integral functions of the brain stem make it such that any damage to it can be fatal to an animal's survival. An important region of the brainstem is the medulla oblongata, or simply *medulla,* which controls the body's autonomic functions such as digestion, heart rate, and respiration.

Diencephalon

The diencephalon, or the interbrain, is located inside the cerebrum just on top of the brain stem. In unborn vertebrates, it is the region of the neural tube that develops into the central nervous system when an animal reaches adulthood. Part of its function includes regulating sleep patterns, appetite, and metabolism. The diencephalon is divided into four different sections. These sections are *thalamus*, the *subthalamus* or *prethalamus*, the *hypothalamus*, and the *epithalamus*.[4] The thalamus, also known as *dorsal thalamus*, found in the middle part of the brain in vertebrates, is a walnut-shaped and walnut-sized structure located between the cerebral cortex and the midbrain. It is likened to a relay station or an information switchboard, processing sensory and motor signals and sending them to the cerebral cortex. It also regulates consciousness, awareness and sleep.[5] Damage to the thalamus can send a person into a coma.

The *subthalamus*, also known as *prethalamus* or *ventral thalamus*, is wedged between the thalamus and the hypothalamus. It's found below the thalamus and is separated from it by the *zona limitans intrathalamica*, a compartment that serves as a border and a signaling center between the two sections. The subthalamus is responsible for regulating movements made by skeletal muscles. The bulk of the subthalamus is made up of the subthalamic nucleus, a small lens-shaped structure whose main function might be pain perception, but this has yet to be determined. Some theories state that the subthalamic nucleus is a functional part of the basal ganglia control system that performs action selections. An increase in impulsiveness when presented with two equal stimuli is a sign of dysfunction of the subthalamic nucleus in pain sufferers.[6]

The hypothalamus is a part of the brain that forms the lower end of the diencephalon. It contains several small multifunctional nuclei. It can be found between the thalamus and the brainstem. It monitors and controls appetite, thirst, fatigue, sleep, homeostasis, circadian rhythms, and other body urges. It links the nervous system to the endocrine system through the pituitary gland. Since the hypothalamus is so critical for a person's actions (whether harmful or safe), it thus indirectly determines whether an individual will experience pain or not. It creates and releases hypothalamic-releasing hormones that stimulate pituitary hormones such as the following:

- *Thyrotropin-releasing hormone*, which helps regulate metabolism;
- *Corticotropin-releasing hormone*, involved in stress and immune responses as well as the regulation of inflammation, carbohydrate metabolism, protein catabolism, blood electrolyte levels, and behavior;
- *Gonadotropin-releasing hormone*, which regulates normal growth, sexual development, and reproductive function;[7]
- *Growth hormone-releasing hormone*, a peptide hormone that stimulates growth, cell reproduction, and regeneration;
- *Pituitary inhibiting hormones*, such as somatostatin, which suppresses the release of the growth hormone and thyroid-stimulating hormone (TSH); and
- *Dopamine*, the "feel-good hormone," known to be crucial in reward-driven learning.

The epithalamus can be found in the rear part of the diencephalon. It connects the brain to the limbic system and controls the secretion of melatonin by the pineal gland and the regulation of motor pathways and emotions. It consists of (1) the *trigonum habenulae*, a small triangular structure that contains the *ganglion habenulae*, a group of nerve cells; (2) the pineal body, which produces *serotonin*, a neurotransmitter found in the gastrointestinal tract involved in pain perception, growth, reproduction, and aging as well as feelings of well-being and happiness; and (3) the posterior commissure, a rounded band of white fibers that contributes to the *bilateral pupillary light reflex* (when pupils increase or decrease in diameter due to light levels) because of its interconnection with the *pretectal nuclei* (nerves branches with the primary function of responding to light).[8]

Cerebellum

The cerebellum is the region of the brain found underneath the cerebrum, attached to the brain stem appearing as though a separate structure. It is classified by anatomists as a part of the *metencephalon*, which is the upper part of the *rhombencephalon*, or the hindbrain. It manages motor control, coordination, the body's ability to interpret painful stimuli, as well as cognitive functions that include attention, memory, language, problem-solving, and decision making, and in the regulation of fear and pleasure responses.[9] It doesn't initiate movement but has a fine-tuning functionality that contributes to equilibrium, posture, and motor learning.[10] The cerebellum is divided into three lobes: the *floccu-*

INTRODUCTION TO THE NERVOUS SYSTEM

lonodular lobe, anterior lobe, and posterior lobe. It has: (1) two types of neurons in its circuit, namely, the Purkinje cells and the granule cells; (2) three types of axons: mossy fibers, climbing fibers, and parallel fibers; and (3) three main layers: the thick granular layer found at the bottom of the cerebral cortex, the Purkinje layer that contains only Purkinje cells, and the molecular layer, which contains the dendritic trees of the Purkinje cells. They both originate from the mossy fibers and climbing fibers and go into the deep cerebellar nuclei. There, deep cerebellar nuclei come in a pair of each of the following nuclei: the dentate nucleus, the *emboliform nucleus*, the *globose nucleus*, and the *fastigial nucleus*. Two main pathways cross the cerebellar circuit that connects the axons to the deep nuclei. Clinical evidence proves that Purkenje cells have a modulatory function in pain reception.[11]

Three Lobes of the Cerebellum

The *flocculonodular lobe* influences head and eye movement with its connection to the vestibular nuclei. It can be found in the frontal and lower surface of the cerebellum. It consists of the nodule and *flocullus*, which are both connected to the *nodulus*, the midline structure, through thin *pedicles*. Infliction to this area can result in problems in visual tracking and movements related to eye control such as *nystagmus*, as well as trouble maintaining balance and equilibrium. The anterior lobe or the *paleocerebellum* is responsible for coordinating an individual's perception with the position of its body parts and employing strength of effort in movement. It is found in the front part of the cerebellum and receives data, including pain signals, from the spinal cord.[12] The anterior lobe can deteriorate with alcohol abuse.

The posterior lobe, or the *neocerebellum,* is found in the lower back side of the cerebellum. It is thought to be the youngest part of the cerebellum when evolution is considered. The neocerebellum controls fine motor coordination through the inhibition of involuntary movements with the help of involuntary neurotransmitters such as *gamma-aminobutyric acid*, more commonly known as GABA. The posterior lobe receives data from the brain stem, specifically from reticular information and the *inferior olivary nucleus*.[13]

Two Types of Pain-Related Neurons in the Cerebellum

The Purkinje cells or Purkinje neurons are a class of *gamma-aminobutyric neurons* found in the cerebellum and are its output neurons. They were discovered by Czech anatomist Jan Purkyně and are (1) one of the most unique neurons in the brain, and (2) among the earliest types to be identified. They are notable for their size, shape, and distinct activity patterns. Purkinje cells are some of the largest neurons in the brain. Like other neurons, they form a tree-like pattern that is aptly called a dendritic tree. Similar to an actual tree, dendritic spines branch out profusely. Each spine sends out synaptic data to another. A *synapse* is a structure that allows another neuron to transmit electrical or chemical signals (including that of pain) to another cell, and the Purkinje cells receive more synaptic pain data than any other cell in the brain. Purkinje cells dispatch inhibitory messages to the deep cerebellar nuclei, and they can send data for all motor coordination in the cerebellar cortex (the inner part of the cerebellum). Purkinje cells are found in the Purkinje and the molecular layers of the cerebellum.

The granule cells, unlike the Purkinje cells, are among the tiniest neurons in the brain, but they are also some of the most abundant. Granule cells get all of their data from mossy fibers, but they outnumber them. For example, in the human brain the ratio of granule cells to mossy fibers is 200 to 1. This enables the granule cells to expand the information gathered from the mossy fibers. Granule cells are densely packed and gather at the thick granular layer found at the bottom of the cerebellum. The number and structure of granule cells lets the cerebellum make much more accurate distinctions between input patterns than what the mossy fibers can allow.[14]

Two Types of Axons of the Cerebellum

An axon or nerve fiber is really a long slender projection of a neuron that normally sends electrical impulses from a neuron's cell body to another. There are two types of axons that will be discussed here. These are the mossy fibers and the "climbing" fibers.

Mossy fibers connect with granule cells inside the granular layer. Research demonstrates that these fibers are important for the nervous system's transmission of pain.[15] Their point of contact is called the glomeruli. They may arise from the *pontine nuclei*, the spinal cord, the vestibular nuclei or another point of origin, such as the cerebral cortex. The cerebral cortex has numerous pathways to the mossy fibers. They arrive at the cerebellum through *pontocerebellar fibers* that run through the middle cerebellar peduncles and the pons, a structure found in the brainstem. Within the granular layer, a mossy fiber creates an array of enlargements called the mossy fiber rosettes that can be found inside a glomerulus. Terminals from Golgi cells, inhibitory interneurons found within the granular layer, filter through the mossy fiber and make inhibitory synapses, which are crucial in the pain regulation process, onto the granule cell dendrites. The mossy fibers found in the cerebellum have very little similarity to those found in the hippocampus. Whereas the latter is more involved in different types of behavior such as spatial learning, the ones found in the cerebellum are merely pathways for pain-related information to reach the Purkinje for processing.

Climbing fibers send data to the Purkinje cells from the *inferior olivary nucleus*, the largest nucleus in the olivary bodies or "olives." They (the climbing fibers) carry information from various sources such as the spinal cord, vestibular system, red nucleus, *superior colliculus*, reticular formation, and sensory and motor cortices. There are two theories on the function of climbing fibers; one is that the climbing fiber input serves primarily as a training signal for other cells, while the other theory suggests that its function is to shape cerebellar output directly. For the majority of researchers, the climbing fibers signal errors in motor performance either in the usual manner of discharge frequency modulation, as a single announcement of an "unexpected event," or the degree of rhythmicity among a population of climbing fibers. This is how climbing fibers participate in the pain sensation process.[16]

Cerebrum

The cerebrum (often confused with *cerebellum*) is the topmost structure of the central nervous system in vertebrates. With the help of the cerebellum, it controls the pain patient's more conscious and voluntary behaviors, such as speech and emotional responses. The cerebrum also controls the memory and the senses. The cerebrum together with the diencephalon constitutes the forebrain. The cerebrum is divided into four different lobes. These lobes are the frontal, occipital, parietal, and temporal lobes.

There are two frontal lobes that make up the largest section of the cerebrum. They are associated with an individual's personality and logic. The lobes also control administrative functions such as thought patterns, planning, decision making, problem solving, and emotional control. The frontal lobe houses most of the dopamine-sensitive neurons in the cerebral cortex. Dopamine is a simple organic chemical responsible for reward-driven learning. Every type of "reward" increases the level of dopamine transmission in the brain, including the effects of a variety of highly addictive drugs such as cocaine and methamphetamine, both of which have pain-relieving properties. Too much dopamine in the system can be found in people with schizophrenia, whereas a lack of dopamine can be found in people suffering from depression, attention deficit hyperactivity disorder and restless legs syndrome.[17] Parkinson's disease is said to be caused by the loss of dopamine-secreting neurons in the *substantia nigra*.[18] The frontal lobes play an important part in keeping long-term memories that are not task based. These memories are regularly associated with emotions coming from data sent by the brain's limbic system. The frontal lobe analyzes those emotions and alters them to fit socially acceptable norms. Damage to the frontal lobe can lead to transient ischemic attacks or strokes, Alzheimer's disease, Parkinson's disease, and frontal lobe epilepsy.

The occipital lobes are the smallest set of lobes in the cerebrum and can be found in the back-most portion of the brain. An occipital lobe is a visual processing center of the mammalian brain and contains the visual cortex and controls an individual's sight, visual perception, and reaction to light. Recent studies show that certain epilepsies are triggered by a sensitivity of the occipital lobe, and that seizures in general can be painful.[19] Occipital seizures or photo-sensitivity seizures are brought about by flicker stimulation caused by flashes of images with multiple colors through television, video games or any other flicker stimulatory system, and they generally happen during daytime.

The parietal lobe, found above the occipital lobe and behind the frontal lobe, gathers sensory data from different locations to determine navigation and spatial sense. The somatosensory cortex enables the parietal lobe to map visually perceived objects and interpret them into body-coordinate positions. The temporal lobe, a region of the cerebral cortex, is located beneath the *Sylvian* or lateral fissure—a structure that divides the frontal lobe and the parietal lobe—and is found on both cerebral hemispheres of the mammalian brain.[20] The temporal lobe's main role is to influence auditory perception. It also helps in the process of understanding auditory and visual inputs and in the formation of long-term memory. There are three gyri, or ridges, found in the temporal lobe of the human brain. These are the *superior temporal gyrus*, the *fusiform gyrus*, and the *parahippocampal gyrus*. Another part of the temporal lobe is the medial temporal lobe, which contains the hippocampi.

The superior temporal gyrus contains parts of the Brodmann areas housing the primary auditory complex and the Wernicke's area. The primary auditory complex found within the Brodmann areas of the superior temporal gyrus is the first part of the cerebral complex to receive auditory signals that travel through several *subcortical* (below the cortex) nuclei. This primary complex is responsible for hearing and processing sounds. The Wernicke's area, on the other hand, is involved in processing of speech and comprehending languages. The superior temporal gyrus is found on the top, rear, and side parts of the temporal lobe. The *fusiform gyrus*, or the *discontinuous occipitotemporal gyrus*, is located between the *occipitotemporal gyrus* and the *parahippocam-pal gyrus*.[21]

Limbic System

Research suggests that the limbic system is highly involved in pain processing.[22] The limbic system, or the *"paleomammalian brain,"* is in fact a set of brain structures that includes the hippocampus, amygdalae, and the neocortex, as well as the hypothalamus and the thalamus. It's known to influence a variety of functions, such as emotion, behavior, motivation, long-term memory, and olfaction, or the sense of smell. It works through its influence on the endocrine and the autonomic nervous systems.

The hippocampus is a key component of the limbic system situated in the medial temporal lobe, underneath the cortex surface. The hippocampus creates forms, classifies and stores memory and plays an important role in spatial navigation and behavior. There are two hippocampi in mammals and they are both found in each side of the brain. Damages caused by stress, aging, oxygen starvation, encephalitis, or medial temporal lobe epilepsy may show up as posttraumatic stress disorder, severe depression, Alzheimer's disease, anterograde amnesia, or schizophrenia. Signals from the hippocampus to the hypothalamus and the septal nuclei are carried by a C-shaped axon called the *fornix*.

The amygdalae are small groups of nuclei found deep within the medial temporal lobes of the brains of complex vertebrates. They produce and process emotions, such as reward and fear as well as social interactions, sexual desires and aggression, and store emotionally charged memories. Emotional responses such as an increase in heartbeat, sweaty palms, and freezing are triggered through the amygdala. This region has an important role in mental states and is associated with many psychological disorders. Hyperactivity on the left amygdala can be found among people suffering from depression, whereas a lack of activity or size in this region contributes to anxiety, obsessive compulsive disorders, and posttraumatic stress.

Spinal Cord

The spinal cord is a long, thin, and tubular structure that begins from occipital bone and ends at the first and second lumbar vertebrae, which, in humans are found in the back region. It is made of nervous tissue that extends from the medulla oblongata, which transmits neural signals from the brain to the rest of the body and contains neutral circuits for independent control of several reflexes. It has three major roles, acting as a channel for motor information, as a channel for sensory information, and as a center for coordinating reflexes.[23] It is protected by the spinal column, a bony structure that starts at the base of the skull and extends to the pelvic region.

PERIPHERAL NERVOUS SYSTEM

The peripheral nervous system is made up of nerves and ganglia outside the brain and the spinal cord. It's not protected by any bone. Its main function is to connect the central nervous system to the limbs and organs. It is divided into two or three parts: the *somatic nervous system* and the *automatic nervous system*. Other sources consider the sensory systems to be part of the peripheral nervous system as well. The somatic nervous system is connected to the conscious and voluntary control of skeletal muscles through *efferent* (going toward muscles) nerves that stimulate muscle contraction. The automatic nervous system (otherwise known as the visceral or involuntary nervous system) is a control system that functions below the level of consciousness. It affects heart rate, digestion, respiratory rate, salivation, perspiration, pupillary dilation, urination, and sexual arousal. Sensory systems are responsible for processing sensory information such as vision, hearing, touch, taste and smell. They consist of sensory receptors and pathways that transmit data from the physical realm to be interpreted by the mind, thus, creating perception of the outside world.[24]

NERVOUS SYSTEM AND ITS RELATION TO OTHER BODY SYSTEMS

There are various body systems found in multicellular animals, and in a sense, the nervous system controls all the other body systems that can suffer from pain. The other body systems have distinct vital functions that can be dependent upon the other but they rely on the nervous system the most. It's important to know about this relation when studying how patients and caregivers address pain.

Circulatory System

This system includes the cardiovascular system, which distributes blood, and the lymphatic system, which brings lymphatic fluid to the heart and affects the immune system.[25] The nervous system and the circulatory system are mutually dependent. The circulatory system provides the nervous system with nutrients and oxygen, whereas the nervous system controls heart rate. It also changes the constriction or dilation rate of blood vessels (a great way to reduce certain pains), thereby altering blood flow and distribution of heat throughout the body. Parts of the nervous system that affect the circulatory system include the medulla oblongata and the autonomic nervous system.

Digestive System

The digestive system breaks down food that morphs into nutrients distributed in the body (which includes the nervous system) through the circulatory system. The nervous system through the diencephalon, hypothalamus, and epithalamus monitors and controls appetite, while the enteric nervous system, a subset of the autonomic nervous system, controls the movement of the digestive organs, especially the gastrointestinal tract.

Endocrine System

The endocrine system works closely with the nervous system to secrete different types of hormones into the bloodstream. These hormones are secreted through its glands and they regulate the body and affect behavior. Similar to the nervous system, the endocrine system is an information signal system, but unlike the former, where information travels rapidly, the endocrine system's effects on the body are slow but last longer. Hormones released by the endocrine system, including those involved in pain regulation, directly affect the nervous system. These hormones are as follows:

- Thyrotropin-releasing hormone;
- Gonadotropin-releasing hormone;
- Somatostatin;
- Vasopressin;
- Oxytocin;
- Dopamine;
- Growth hormone-releasing hormone; and
- Corticotropin-releasing hormone.

In response, the nervous system through the hypothalamus and the limbic system sends signals to the endocrine system to release the said hormones.

Excretory System

The excretory system is responsible for the elimination of the waste products from the body to maintain homeostasis or stability, and to prevent painful damage. The said waste products are a result of metabolism and may come in solid, liquid or gaseous forms. The excretory system includes the integumentary structures (skin, hair, nails, and other appendages), the digestive system, the respiratory system, and the urinary system. The excretory system maintains a healthy environment within the bloodstream to prevent any painful disorders of the nervous system.

Immune System

The immune system is the body's defense mechanism against disease. It affects all organs, including those of the nervous system. The nervous system in connection with the endocrine system release hormones for stress and relaxation. Too much stress hormones in the body in turn can negatively affect the immune system.

Musculoskeletal System

This system consists of the skeletal, smooth, and cardiac muscles. Through signals sent from the nervous system, these muscles are able to move. Skeletal muscles are voluntarily controlled by the nervous system through signals from the cerebellum to the somatic nervous system. They enable the body to do conscious physical actions such as dancing, running, and other such activities. The smooth and cardiac muscles, on the other hand, are involuntary muscles. Smooth muscles are found in

- lymphatic vessels;
- walls of blood vessels;
- uterus;
- urinary bladder;
- male and female reproductive tracts;
- gastrointestinal tract;
- respiratory tract;

- *arrector pili* of the skin; and
- ciliary muscle and the iris of the eye.

As the name suggests, cardiac muscles are the muscles of the heart. Both the smooth and the cardiac muscles are controlled by signals from the brainstem, through the autonomic nervous system.

Reproductive System

The organs of the reproductive system are controlled and regulated by hormones released by the pituitary gland through signals sent by the hypothalamus.[26] These hormones, because of their reproductive function, affect the organism's growth into sexual maturity—inadvertently affecting the organism's size and shape as well as the development of secondary sexual characteristics. They also affect pregnancy in females and the development of the fetus. Also, the amygdalae control sexual urges.

Respiratory System

The respiratory system allows the body to take in oxygen that is circulated throughout the bloodstream and to get rid of carbon dioxide. All body systems, including the nervous system, need oxygen. It is vital in the consumption and release of energy used for an organism's survival. As with other involuntary systems, the respiratory system is influenced by the brainstem and the autonomous nervous system.

Skeletal System

The skeletal system provides the structure supporting the body and protects vital nervous system components as well as organs such as the heart, the lungs, the brain, and the spinal cord. The growth of the skeletal muscles from infancy to childhood to maturity is affected by hormones released by the brain through the pituitary gland.[27] Aside from sensory pain receptors within the bone structure, the skeletal system's movement isn't directly affected by the nervous system. It could be *indirectly* affected, however, through the movements of the skeletal muscles, which are controlled by the cerebellum through the somatic nervous system.

ARGUABLE PARTS OF THE NERVOUS SYSTEM

Some scientists consider the retina and the cranial nerves to be distinct structures of the central nervous system because these parts actually originate and emerge from the brain. The retina is a light-sensitive structure that lines the inner surfaces of the eyes.[28] It receives information from the visual world through light that is interpreted as chemical and electrical events that eventually trigger nerve impulses. These impulses then travel through fibers of the optic nerve to several visual centers of the brain. Cranial nerves are also considered part of the peripheral nervous system (with the exception of the optic nerve, which is a tract of the diencephalon) and have various functions. There are twelve pairs of cranial nerves in humans, the first two of which emerge from the cerebrum while the rest come from the brainstem. These nerves have either motor or sensory functions or both. The cranial nerves are as follows:

- Olfactory
- Optic
- Oculomotor
- Trochlear
- Trigeminal
- Abducens

- Facial
- Vestibulocochlear
- Glosopharyngeal
- Vagus
- Accessory
- Hypoglossal nerves

Three of these nerves, the oculomotor, trochlear, and the abducens nerves, transmit signals for eye movement. The rest of the cranial nerves channel signals for smell, vision, facial sensations and control, sound, taste, respiratory and digestive sensations and control, neck and shoulder control, and tongue control.

ANALYSIS

Pain patients and caregivers must understand that the nervous system, which plays a crucial role in pain, is a vital component of vertebrates, as it controls all bodily functions, from conscious thought to memory to involuntary movements such as a heartbeat. The nervous system contains an intricate network of information delivering neurons more complex than any computer system in existence. However, it can be susceptible to painful damage through substance abuse and physical injuries to the head and spine.

3

PHYSIOLOGY OF THE NERVOUS SYSTEM

The nervous system is a network of specialized cells that can send, transmit, receive, or keep messages associated with the organism and its environment. By processing those messages, the nervous system stimulates reactions in other body parts. Nervous tissue consists of nervous (nerve) cells and glial cells, and nervous cells are the functional units of the nervous system. Different glial cells usually perform many auxiliary functions, such as fixing damaged nervous tissue and nutrition of nervous cells. While the basic structures of various parts of the nervous system have been covered in the preceding chapters, this chapter explains the specific *physiology* (functioning) of these parts as they relate to pain perception.

STRUCTURE AND FUNCTION OF THE NERVOUS SYSTEM

The nervous system can be divided into two categories—central and peripheral. The central nervous system is located inside of the spine and skull bones. It consists of the spinal cord and brain. As far as parts of the brain are concerned, one can recognize three major areas: brainstem, cerebellum (based on the Latin term for "little brain"). and cerebrum (based on the Latin term for "large brain"). The peripheral nervous system includes (1) some small clusters of nervous cells located outside the central parts, and (2) "shoots" of nerve cells, which connect the central nervous system with various structures on the periphery, such as sensory organs, muscles, and glands. These shoots are arranged in bundles referred to as nerve bundles, which are essential for properly sensing pain. A total of twelve pairs of nerves originate from the brain and are called cerebral or cranial nerves, and thirty-one pairs attached to the spinal cord are called *spinal nerves*. Nerve fibers that connect the sensory organs with the central nervous system are called sensory fibers. Fibers connecting the central nervous system with muscles are called motor fibers.

The part of the peripheral nervous system associated with the sensory organs and the striated or skeletal muscles is called the somatic nervous system. Through it the information about changes in the environment (such as painful injury) of living creatures is transmitted from the sensory organs to certain parts of the central nervous system. Furthermore, through the fibers of the somatic nervous system the commands from the central nervous system are transmitted to the skeletal muscles, which allow for responses to painful environmental stimuli. The second part of the peripheral nervous system is connected to internal organs such as the stomach and lungs. That part of the peripheral nervous system is called the *vegetative* or *autonomic* nervous system. It allows regulation of processes in the organism that serve to sustain life. The autonomic nervous system also has an important role in the development of various physiological changes, such as pain, that accompany emotions.

Spinal Cord

The central part of the spinal cord consists of nerve cell bodies—visually seen as a gray mass. Around the central part of the spinal cord is the *white matter*, which consists of a bundled series of nerve fibers that connect the sensory organs and the executive organs on the periphery with the structures in the central nervous system. Sensory fibers enter the spinal cord through the posterior roots of spinal nerves and motor fibers exit the spinal cord through the *anterior* (front) roots. The spinal cord has two physiological roles. The first is a so called *conductive function*. From sensory organs located in the trunk and extremities, impulses are sent through the spinal cord to higher parts of the central nervous system. Likewise, nerve impulses are carried from different parts of the central nervous system through the spinal cord to the muscles. Second, centers of various reflexes are located in the spinal cord. Muscle reflexes are the reactions of a gland that occur when nerve impulses are transmitted from sensory organs to the executive branch of the nerve through the designated heritage.[1] Therefore, these are reactions that don't require any prior learning. For example, when a finger touches a candle flame, it causes a reflexive movement of the finger. When the heat of the flame stimulates receptors for warmth that are found in the skin, it generates painful nerve impulses in sensory nerve fibers. These fibers transmit impulses to the spinal cord gray matter, and, there, they're submitted to the motor fibers. When nerve impulses through motor fibers reach the muscle, the muscle shortens and the finger moves away from the flames. In order to cause such a reaction to pain, it's not always necessary for nerve impulses to reach the brain. The spinal cord contains a series of reflex centers. Part of the reflex center provides protection of the organism from harmful stimuli. The second part of the reflex center regulates reflex reactions necessary for the normal performance of a series of motor actions, such as standing and walking. It should be mentioned that the reflex centers are under the influence of some of the following structures of the central nervous system.

Brainstem

The brainstem is composed of three parts: the medulla oblongata, *mesencephalon* (midbrain), and *pons*. Bundles of fibers pass through the brainstem, connecting the spinal cord to the brain. Through the middle of the brainstem stretches a nerve structure called the *reticular formation*, which is linked with many other parts of the nervous system and is necessary to keep the organism awake. In other words, the general physiology of the nervous system depends on the number of active cells in the reticular formation. In this way, the part of the nerve impulse that is evoked by stimuli to sensory organs leads to the reticular formation. These impulses increase the activity of cells in the *reticular formation* (in this case, specific nerve fibers in the brain) and thus contribute to the maintenance of nervous system vigilance (when nerve cells are alert). This is the reason why it's easier to fall asleep in a room that is dark and silent than in one that is noisy and well lit. In the medulla oblongata are nerve centers for breathing, heartbeat, and blood pressure control. Thus, there are some reflexes involved here that are necessary to sustain life for the pain patient. Furthermore, fibers pass through the pons, connecting the cerebellum with some parts of the central nervous system, primarily with the cerebral cortex. Through these fibers, the cerebellum can control voluntary movements. This is how the physiology of the cerebellum can indirectly determine whether a person will experience pain from injury.

In the midbrain, one can find a larger number of clusters of nerve cells. Some of these clusters are related to the sensory organs of sight and hearing. Due to their function, for example, a person can avoid collisions with objects. Ten pairs of cerebral nerves come out of the brainstem and they primarily connect different sensory organs and muscles in the head with the central nervous system.

Cerebellum

The cerebellum is located in the rear of the brainstem. It (1) allows the pain patient to maintain body balance, (2) regulates muscle tone, and (3) conducts movement.[2] Some nerve cells in the cerebellum are sensitive to the increased amount of alcohol in the blood. That's why, after consuming large amounts of alcohol, one can become groggy. Diseases of the cerebellum, some of which are painful, are evident in a series of disorders in motor skills. Thus, pain patients with problems of cerebellar physiology may have difficulty in coordinating movements. One of the ways to check whether there is a disorder is, like a sobriety test, to have the subject extend his arms, close his eyes, and then touch his nose with the tip of the forefinger.

Thalamus

The thalamus consists of a large number of small clusters of nerve cells or ganglia. Toward the thalamus, are nerve impulses transmitted from specific sensory organs. Impulses from the thalamus go to different areas in the cerebral cortex of the cerebrum where sensations arise. Some parts of the thalamus are directly connected with reticular formations. These areas of the thalamus (in conjunction with the cerebral cortex) process information that comes from the different sensory organs. Therefore, these areas of the thalamus are important for the processes of so-called *selective attention*. Some parts of the thalamus are connected to the front part of the cerebral cortex and regions of the limbic system. These connections are important for the physiology of emotion—something that can, at times, cause mental and physical pain in the long run. The thalamus is connected to the main endocrine gland: the pituitary gland. Some parts of the hypothalamus secrete specific chemical substances that affect the secretion of certain hormones from the pituitary gland. In this way, the nervous system (by way of the hypothalamus) influences the performance of the endocrine glands. The hypothalamus, through the vegetative nervous system, coordinates the work of various systems in the organism that are necessary to sustain a pain-free life. For example, it regulates body temperature and blood pressure.[3] In it are the main centers for thirst and hunger, as well as centers for the physiology of sexual behavior of both healthy individuals and pain patients. Along with parts of the limbic system, the hypothalamus plays an important role in the regulation of emotion.

The limbic system includes a series of structures located on the inner side of each hemisphere. It's connected with nearly all parts of the nervous system, particularly with the reticular formation and the front parts of the cerebral cortex. Electrical stimulation of the front parts of the limbic system in animal experiments has shown that animals can quickly learn to handle the device that irritates these parts of the limbic system.[4] The hippocampus is a structure that's part of the limbic system. It is involved in memory processes. Individuals who have a damaged hippocampus can't memorize any new information, but they can remember what they've learned or experienced before the injury.

Cerebrum

The cerebrum consists of two hemispheres. The hemispheres are interconnected by transverse nerve fibers that enable physiological collaboration between the hemispheres. On the surface of the cerebrum is a thin layer of nerve cell bodies that form the cerebral cortex. The human cerebral cortex is wrinkled, and below the cerebral cortex is a multitude of nerve fiber bundles that are home to several clusters of nerve cell bodies.[5] The cerebrum has four sections called lobes. The frontal lobe is located in the front of the cerebrum. Damage to the frontal lobe can result in social difficulties and mood changes. On the upper back side of the cerebrum is the parietal lobe, which has a great role in visual perception. The temporal lobe is located on the side of the cerebrum involved in the processing of complex stimuli such as faces and scenes. In the back of the cerebrum is the occipital lobe, which is responsible for sight.[6]

Cerebral Cortex

The cerebral cortex is part of the nervous system that developed last in the course of evolution. In the cerebral cortex, nerve activity may switch to *psychonervous* (mind and nervous system) activity. The cerebral cortex can be divided physiologically into sensory, motor, and associative areas. The nervous impulses arrive from certain sensory organs to the sensory areas. In these areas sensations are stacked into the complex, structured experiences known as perceptions. Therefore, these parts of the cerebral cortex allow cognition of what's happening in the environment. The areas responsible for processing information received from the receptors for vision are located in the occipital lobe; for hearing in the temporal lobe; and for touch, cold, warmth, and pain in the parietal lobe. While the majority of fibers that transmit nerve impulses from the sensory organs intersect each other, the neuronal stimulation that arises from the sensory organs in the left half of the body ends up in the right hemisphere, and vice versa. Motor areas are located in the frontal lobe. From these areas, nerve impulses are transmitted to the muscles, allowing the physiological development of movements of varying complexity. Unlike the various reflex and automatic movements whose occurrence is controlled by the lower parts of the nervous system, the cerebral cortex controls voluntary movements. Pathways that transmit the stimuli to the muscles intersect, so that the nerve impulses from motor areas in the left hemisphere are transmitted to the muscles in the right half of the body and vice versa. Major associative areas are located in the frontal lobe and on the border between the parietal, occipital, and temporal lobe. Associative areas of the frontal lobe are also called the *areas of general integration*. The associative areas of the frontal lobe are responsible for the physiological programming and control of the overall behavior of the pain patient.

Associative areas in the frontal lobe allow for the management of activities toward certain goals. People with injuries in this area of the brain can experience changes due to the action of some random stimuli from the environment, and hence they can forget their original intentions. In the overlapping zone, the information units processed in different sensory areas are linked. These areas allow for memorization of newly received information. In essence, the function of the overlapping zone is related to the ability to orient oneself in space. Patients with injuries in this area confuse "left," "right," "up," and "down" positions. The functions of associative areas include a series of complex physiological processes, such as learning, memory, and thinking. The performance of these processes isn't limited to a narrowly localized center in the cerebral cortex, for their execution requires cooperation between different brain areas.

It is necessary for pain patients and caregivers to understand the physiology of speech since words alone can often instill pain in the form of slander. Important areas of the cerebral cortex are involved in the understanding and production of speech. Most people have these centers located in the left hemisphere of the brain. The center for speech understanding is located in the back of the temporal lobe, but the center for the production of speech—that is—for uttering words, is located at the bottom rear of the frontal lobe. Words are registered in the "visual" sensory area. In one region of the *gyrus angularis* (overlapping zone), visual information is encoded properly so that it can be "understood" by the center for speech understanding (Wernicke's area).[7] From that area, information is relayed for the production of speech (Broca's area), where, through the motor areas, are located muscles whose activation is necessary for uttering words. A simple way to describe how the cerebral cortex functions in receiving information from the environment and responding to it is as follows: Information received through the sensory organs is initially processed in certain sensory areas and then integrated into the overlapping zone. In accordance with this physiological process, signals are generated in the motor areas and then through motor nerve pathways nerve impulses are transmitted to specific muscles. It should be noted that the cerebral cortex doesn't perform its complex functions independently, but in close cooperation with a number of other parts of the central nervous system.

The vegetative (autonomic) nervous system relates to the various internal organs, blood vessels, and glands. Processes that the vegetative nervous system influences, including pain reception, are achieved through reflex. There are two parts of the vegetative nervous system: the sympathetic and parasympathetic. Increased activity of the sympathetic nervous system causes rapid heartbeat, elevated blood pressure, rapid breathing, and pupil expansion and enhances the secretion of certain hormones, particularly adrenaline. It also hampers digestion.[8] All these changes allow increased motor activity: a physiological event necessary for pain moderation. Most emotions are accompanied by an intensified response of the sympathetic nervous system. Emotions of fear, anger, and the increased activity of the sympathetic nervous system are especially important when an individual is in a life-threatening situation. Fear accompanied by increased performance of the sympathetic nervous system may provide for a temporary physiological escape from the source of a pain stimulus, but not for permanent relief. As opposed to the response of the sympathetic nervous system, the parasympathetic nervous system has an inverse effect, as its increased activity slows down heart rate, blood pressure, and breathing and "encourages" the digestive system to begin digestion. The central structure that coordinates the work of the vegetative nervous system is the hypothalamus.

Looking into Nerve Cells

A nerve cell or neuron consists of a "body" and a "shoot." The body is wrapped in a semipermeable membrane and contains cytoplasm and the cell *nucleus*. In the cytoplasm, one can find a series of structures called organelles. The nerve cell bodies form the so-called *gray matter* of the nervous system. The nerve cell contains two kinds of shoots:

dendrite and *axon*. A typical neuron has two or more branches of dendrites and only one axon. Bundles of nerve cell shoots form a white mass of the nervous tissue. A neuron usually has several dendrites. In reality, dendrites are extracted parts of the protoplasm of the body cell and have the same structural form and physiology as the body cells. They are usually shorter than axons. Their function is to receive information from the sensory organs or other nerve cells, and to transmit this information to the axon via the nerve cell body. An axon originates in a body cell in a place called *the axon hillock*. Some cells have axons that are only a few micrometers long. There are also cells whose axons are longer than one meter. Inside the toe muscles, for example, are axons whose body cells are located in the spinal cord. The main physiological function of axons is transmission of information from one nerve cell to another nerve cell or to muscles and glands. An axon can be wrapped with a myelin sheath, or *myelinated*. When axons lose this protective cover, conditions such as multiple sclerosis can ensue. The axon branches into a number of thin *terminal branches*. At the end of each terminal branch is a thickening that is called a *terminal button*, which allows for chemical communication with other cells. In the terminal buttons are stored special chemical substances called neurotransmitters. When in their basic element, neurotransmitters allow the transmission of nervous system information, including pain from one nerve cell to another.

A place where the terminal button (end) of one nerve cell touches the membrane of another cell is called *a synapse*. Most commonly, synapses are between the axons of one cell and dendrites or cell body of another cell.[9] Nerve impulses from one nerve cell are transmitted through the synapse to the other cell mostly via neurotransmitters. When the nerve impulse arrives at the end of a nerve cell, the neurotransmitter is released. Neurotransmitters on one nerve cell (the postsynaptic neuron) bind to specially built molecules called receptors. Moreover, there are several various neurotransmitters. A single neurotransmitter can only bind to certain receptors. Depending on the type of neurotransmitter and the type of receptors, that binding causes either the increase of electrical potential on the membrane of the postsynaptic neuron or its decrease. In case of increased potential, there is breakage or inhibition. In case of decreased potential, there is excitation. Each neural cell contains a large number of synapses. There can be several thousand. Some inhibition occurs in these synapses, along with some excitation. If at a given moment excitation dominates, the nerve impulses go through the postsynaptic neuron. In most nerve cells, there are constant spontaneous outbreaks of the nerve impulses. This means that the *excitation* of the postsynaptic neuron enhances outbreaks of nerve impulses and *inhibition* completely halts the out-breaks.[10]

Here's one example that shows that the processes of synaptic excitation and inhibition are important for the function of the nervous system and therefore the overall process of pain: The arm muscles allow the pain patient to extend and retract his forearm. Contraction of the biceps allows retraction of the forearm and contraction of *the triceps* facilitates its extension. If the patient wants to stretch his forearm, the excitation of those nerve cells that cause nerve impulses in the triceps is necessary. When the nerve impulses arrive at the triceps, the muscle fibers that build the muscle will shorten, while the tendon attached to the bone of the forearm extends the forearm. To extend the forearm properly, it's necessary to relax the biceps. That means that the nerve cells that transmit nerve impulses to the biceps have to be inhibited. The nature of nerve impulses in all of the nerve cells is the same. In other words, there's no difference in the nature of signals (including pain signals) to which the nerve cells mutually agree. Thus, all the variations of stimuli that can affect sensory organs turn into a series of impulses that are transmitted to different parts of the nervous system. This can be explained in the following way: Whether someone is reading a book or listening to someone saying something, the way in which the information from the environment is transmitted to his brain is the same—by means of nerve impulses that are transmitted through nerve cells and their shoots from the sensory organs of vision and hearing to certain areas of the brain.

Nerve impulses that have reached the center for vision will cause physiological sensations that differ from those taking place when nerve impulses reach the center for hearing. If equal nerve impulses are the only language that the nerve cells understand, the question is more about how the nervous system can accomplish incredibly complex functions. One of the physiological characteristics of the nervous system is the virtually limitless possibilities of connections between the nerve cells themselves. Certain groups of these cells may command extremely complex physiological functions, such as pain regulation. The connections between cells can be modified under the influence of experience. Another factor that is the base of the complex function of the nervous system is the multitude of neurotransmitters that the system has. There are neuronal circuits in the brain (clusters of the nerve cells and nerve cell shoots linking these clusters) that are using a specific neurotransmitter. The type of neurotransmitter determines the function of each neuronal circuit. Well-known neurotransmitters are acetylcholine, norepinephrine, dopamine, serotonin, and *gamma-aminobutyric acid.*

A special group of neurotransmitters consists of *neuroactive pep-tides*. It is interesting that neuroactive peptides aren't only secreted from nerve cells, but also from other tissues in the organism. From these tissues, they're carried by the blood and subsequently transmitted to the nerve cells in the brain and affect the latter's ability to recognize pain. Among various neuroactive peptides, a particular interest among scientists is *endogenous opiates* or *endorphins*. These are substances that are secreted from nerve cells in different brain areas and from some cells in the spinal cord. One of the physiological functions of endogenous opiates is that they regulate pain sensitivity. For example, some nerve cells that secrete endogenous opiates in the spinal cord are related to the nerve cells that transmit nerve impulses from receptors for pain. It is considered that these cells, through specific endogenous opiates, can, more or less, inhibit the further conduction of nerve impulses from pain receptors and thus affect the intensity of the pain stimulus.

When death from painful injury occurs, chemical and physiological changes affecting the neurons take place. Neuronal loss can happen after each serious injury that affects these cells. Cell death and the elimination of cellular remains is an important phenomenon that can be seen in normal and pathological conditions of the nervous system. There are two main types of processes that lead to cell death: necrosis and programmed cell death. Necrosis is the process of death that occurs under the influence of external pathological factors, usually due to an acute process that damages the membrane and allows entry of calcium ions, sodium and water. Thus, swelling of the cell is the first change, which results in the dissolution of the cell. *Apoptosis* (programmed cell death) is essential for normal development and processes for cell proliferation with limitations that prevent an excessive amount of cells. Research has shown that apoptosis is actively involved in pain regulation.[11]

ANALYSIS

The ability to respond physiologically to painful stimuli is a fundamental property of all living organisms. The nervous system is a vast "coordinator" that uses chemical agents called neurotransmitters for inter-neuronal communication via synapses. The function of the nervous system—transmission, processing, and retention of information—is governed by the synthesis and emission of chemical mediators.

4

OCCURRENCE OF PAIN

Pain and suffering are an integral part of life. Man has been trying to understand the "wherefores" and "whys" of pain and suffering for a long time; there have been many studies devoted to this theme, examining it from all imaginable angles. Today's medical science explains the occurrence of pain as the manner in which the central nervous system interprets any, but mostly harmful, stimulations, or to simplify: the way unpleasant sensations are perceived with the associated feeling of discomfort. Pain is an experience that is both physical and emotional. This chapter investigates what actually happens inside the body while pain takes place.

GENERAL CHANGES IN THE BODY WHILE EXPERIENCING PAIN

Difference between Acute Pain and Chronic Pain

There has to be a distinction made between acute (short-term/temporary) pain, and chronic (persistent/long-term) pain. Acute pain passes relatively quickly. By general considerations, it should not last longer than three to six months from the time of the onset. At times, it lasts for a shorter period—just a few seconds.

The sensation of pain serves as a signal that something isn't right, but as soon as the cause of the pain is taken care of, such as when an injury is healed, the hurting sensation ceases and the body suffers no lasting damage. Chronic pain, however, exists much longer or beyond the expected time of healing. As such, it places its mark on the rest of the body in much more definite terms. While in general it is considered to be a symptom of a sickness of sorts, on many occasions, chronic pain is a condition in itself and distinct from any other disorder.

Real Effect of Pain on the Nervous System

When experiencing a painful injury or when some abnormal processes happening in the body are causing pain, the nervous system will certainly go through changes. These changes can differ depending on the type of the pain. Acute pain won't cause any lasting changes or damage to the body. In the case of chronic pain, however, the processing of pain seems to become abnormal. One of the functions of the central nervous system is to automatically inhibit any unpleasant sensations, yet with chronic pain patients this function gets altered and becomes much more sensitive to pain than usual. In such cases the nerve cells may become so sensitive that even a gentle touch can feel painful to the patient.

How the Occurrence of Pain Influences the Brain

There have been several studies on the effect of pain on the brain. It's a known fact that the pain people feel is the result of the signal from the site of the injury in the body. However, it is even more so the result of the signal being processed in the brain. There's evidence that chronic pain actually can cause physical changes in the brain. A situation known as *brain morphology* (in this case, the altering of brain tissue) in areas related to pain processing was found in patients suffering from the following disorders: chronic back pain, fibromyalgia, complex regional brain syndrome, irritable bowel syndrome, tension-type headache, and migraine.[1]

What causes the change in the brain? Is it the source of the hurting sensation and inflammation, or is it the pain itself? The results of studies at the University of California greatly help in answering this question. [2] Researchers studied patients with "phantom limb" pain. These patients lost a limb, yet continued to have painful sensations in their missing limb. How is this possible? Well, if anything, their brain is giving mistaken signals, as it remembers the chronic pain the patient experienced before losing the limb. They don't have the aching limb anymore, but the pain continues because of the wrong brain signal.

Other studies shed more light on how the structure of the brain itself can change due to long-term pain.[3] These structural changes include cell atrophy, synaptic loss, cell size, blood volume, and even gray matter destruction. It becomes evident that while short-term pain has the function of "setting the alarm off" that something is amiss the usefulness of pain is arguably lost when it becomes chronic. It actually gets to be quite problematic for the patient. Naturally, when chronic pain is occurring along with negative changes in the brain, the patient will experience other consequences in life: his brain will start underperforming, which will have an influence on his work and quality of life in general. Thankfully, the process can be reversed by making the changes necessary to turn the tide. As the brain can suffer due to long-term pain, it can also go through a healing process. Even simple advancements, including (1) better exercise, (2) more wholesome and nutritious food, and (3) a positive, can-be-done attitude, could be a start to set the individual suffering from pain on to the path to recovery.

HOW AND WHY PAIN OCCURS

Actual Process

When the body gets injured, it responds in an automatic manner by stimulating pain receptors. These pain receptors continue the process by releasing chemicals and sending them to the spinal cord. The chemicals carry the message of "hurting" with them, and from the receptors of the spinal cord the message goes all the way up to the brain, where the thalamus receives it and passes it on to the cerebral cortex—the part of the brain where the message gets processed and registered as "pain"—after which the pain message is sent back to the site of the injury. It all happens very quickly. When an individual bumps his head, he feels the pain right away; not five minutes later.

Pain perception actually starts from a stimulus that's sensed by the receptors (*nociceptors*) and is transmitted to the brain by signals passing through neurons after the brain processes the signal. It then "orders" the body to perform different evasive measures to stop further damage. Some neurons with nociceptors have little *myelin*—a substance first introduced in the preceding chapter, that enables fast transmission of signals—thus slowing the signal of pain. The pain is probably a feeling that a person doesn't want to feel, yet feeling pain can sometimes turn out to be a positive feeling to be grateful for after the painful occurrence. When a person is going to experience an injury, for example, a burn due to touching a hot pan, the body quickly reacts to the immediate pain by pulling the hand away. This would cause a sharp pain in the hand, yet when inspected carefully, the pain that the person felt is minimal compared to what the person would've experienced had the hand been in contact with the pan for a long time, which would have resulted in extensive burns.[4] In this example, pain acts as an "emergency alarm," preventing further injury to the body. Pain can cause a particular region of the body to be immobilized, to prevent further complication or damage to that specific part. Pain perception mostly acts as a reflex action to prevent an injury, before substantial injury occurs in the body.

Nociception

There is, in fact, more to the process of pain, scientifically called *nociception*, taking place than written in the above paragraph. Nociceptors in mammals are sensory neurons. These neurons are cells that serve as the basic building blocks of the nervous system, with the function of transmitting information throughout the body. They are found in body regions capable of sensing pain. These locations can be internal or external. Some external examples of body regions with nociceptors are in the tissues (skin, cornea of the eye, and mucous membranes). Internal samples are in different organs (bladder, gut, muscle, joint, and continuing along the digestive tract).

Types of Nociceptors

Several types of nociceptors can be noted with their separate functions: thermal, mechanical, chemical, sleeping, and *polymodal*. Thermal nociceptors respond to excess heat or cold. Mechanical ones are activated when excess pressure or mechanical deformation is present. Chemical nociceptors can respond to a range of things: from a variety of spices used in cooking, to different environmental irritants (such as *acrolein*, a cigarette smoke component as well as a chemical weapon used during World War I); and to internal irritants such as some fatty acids formed when changes take place in internal tissues. Sleeping nociceptors only respond to stimuli—whether thermal, mechanical, or chemical—if the surrounding tissue gets inflamed. Polymodal nociceptors don't perform a single function, but many in combination.

NATURE OF PAIN

Categorizing Pain According to Its Source in the Body

Pain (acute or chronic) can also be categorized according to its source of origin in the body. Neuropathic pain or nerve-injury pain happens when the nervous system is injured in some way. The injury can be caused by some sort of nerve damage, or perhaps a compression of a nerve. The problem could also originate in the brain or in the spinal cord. It's a burning kind of pain, which can feel like a dagger piercing through and can surface along with tingling and numbness.

Radicular pain is also a type of neuropathic pain. However, in the case of radicular pain, there's pressure on the nerve roots, and the pain travels directly down the path of the nerve. The patient with such pain most likely has compressed or irritated nerves in the neck or spine while experiencing the pain shooting down the arm or the leg. Somatic pain (occasionally called *musculoskeletal pain*) occurs when the pain receptors are stimulated either in the musculoskeletal tissues inside or on the surface of the body. Here the source is the skin, bones, muscles, tendons or ligaments. A common but often-overlooked type of somatic pain is *myofascial* pain, which includes either a single muscle or a group of them. The (1) muscles, (2) *fascia* (connective tissue covering the muscles), and (3) soft tissues, all play a part in causing such pain. The source of visceral pain is in the main body organs such as the heart, lungs, kidney, and others. A vague kind of pain is felt, and at times it's even difficult to know where it actually originates from.

Things May Not Be So Obvious

When it comes to the occurrence of pain, there are cases that are quite difficult to judge. Recovery can take a long time and it can be a frustrating process for both patient and caregiver to find the causes (see chapter 10) of chronic pain. After all, the pain can originate from a large variety of ailments. In order to determine the right specialist, it is important to take a close look at the patient's history concerning the pain. Perhaps the sufferer will have to undergo a CAT scan or other examination as part of a broad diagnostic process, such as magnetic resonance interferometry or electromyography. Still, there are cases where a definite description of the occurrence of pain cannot be found.

Such a situation can be debilitating for the patient: not only do they have to deal with the pain, but also, there seems to be no "proper" explanation as to what is wrong with them. This can lead to their being judged and misunderstood by associates and in the workplace; unfortunately they can even end up losing their jobs. It's evident that behind these difficult-to-detect-and-treat cases there might be psychological and emotional reasons, perhaps stress or some childhood trauma. This issue will be dealt with in more detail later in this chapter, but for now, the susceptibility of pain in individuals will be explored.

Pain Proneness

Two patients could suffer from the same type of injury and one might end up with chronic pain while the other might not. Among survivors of traffic accidents, cancer, or AIDS, why do certain individuals end up with an unusual amount of pain? Some experts believe that it takes tissue damage to initiate and maintain chronic pain (i.e., neuropathic pain after surgery). Recently, researchers from Northwestern University came to an intriguing conclusion regarding this matter.[5] They reportedly found evidence of the involvement of the sections of the brain related to emotional and motivational behavior: the more communication these two regions have with each other, the more likely the development of chronic pain in the patient.

With 85 percent accuracy, the researchers predicted which patients would develop long-term pain. They made their prediction based on the level of neurological interaction taking place between the frontal cortex and the *nucleus accumbens*, a small region of the brain believed to be involved in addiction and impulsivity. It seems that the more emotional the brain's reaction is to the initial injury, the more likely that the pain will continue even after the injury has healed. Perhaps this section of the brain tends to get more excited with some individuals. Also, there might be environmental or genetic influences that condition the brain so that the nucleus accumbens interacts at an excitable level. The ongoing pain, then, is the result of the injury combined with the state of the brain. Actually, a major function of the nucleus accumbens is to train the rest of the brain on how to react to the external environment; it also has an evaluative role. It's possible that this brain section may react to the pain signal by somehow "training" the rest of the brain to develop chronic pain.

Risk Factors Leading to Long-Term Pain

While specific *causes* of pain are discussed later in this book, it's very helpful to be aware of the *general risk factors* that can contribute to the occurrence of chronic pain, especially for the purposes of easier prevention, recognition, and treatment. Risk factors for pain can be divided into three major categories: biological, psychological, and lifestyle factors. Biological risk factors stem from the pain patient's physical characteristics. Psychological risk factors are connected to the pain sufferer's personality and mood, while lifestyle risk factors are, of course, connected to the person's lifestyle.

Biological Risk Factors

Some of the leading biological risk factors are as follows:

- *Old age*: Elderly people, who have stood the wear and tear of time longer, are many times afflicted by pain.
- *Genetics*: Chronic pain conditions such as migraine headaches are connected to genetics. Some individuals have genetic conditions that can make them more sensitive to pain.
- *Race*: Certain races such as Hispanics or African-Americans seem to be at greater risk for experiencing chronic pain in their lives (see chapter 10).
- *Obesity*: Carrying a lot of extra weight is definitely a risk factor in more ways than one.
- *Previous injury*: The main neurotransmitter is released in significantly greater quantities in individuals with previous pain problems. For this reason, people who've recovered from a previous injury are at a greater risk of chronic pain.

Psychological Risk Factors

- *Childhood trauma*: Individuals who experienced physical or sexual abuse or parental neglect as children are at a higher risk to develop long-term pain.
- *Mood disorders, such as depression or anxiety problems*: Quite a few brain areas and neurotransmitters that have the function of handling pain signals also act as mood "managers."

Lifestyle Risk Factors

- *Stress*: Chronic pain is connected to chronic stress and posttraumatic stress disorder.
- *Smoking*: Smokers are more at risk of chronic pain. They also seem to respond less to pain-management therapies.

- *High-risk jobs*: Work that requires strenuous physical activity or heavy lifting often has adverse effects on individuals; chronic pain can be one of these.

Gender Differences in Relation to Pain

Strong clinical evidence suggests that women are more prone to long-term pain and seem to experience pain more intensely than their male counterparts.[6] First, women suffer more from chronic pain in general, including that from headaches, neck, shoulder, knee, or back pains; oral pains; or facial pains. What causes these differences? There are several possible explanations, with the first one pointing to some differences between male and female brain structure and chemistry. Even when a man and a woman experience similar levels of pain, the woman's central pain processors show greater activity. A possible reason why men and women have different reactions to opioid painkillers is that the painkillers work on different sections of the brain. Other theories point to the differences in sex hormones. Female hormones such as progesterone and estrogen appear to have a strong connection with pain reception because neurochemical changes caused by these female hormones can intensify pain sensations. The menstrual cycle in women also plays a major role. Several pain conditions (i.e., migraines) tend to fluctuate along with the cycle.

The next explanation leads the reader to the biological differences between genders. Quite a bit of pain that women experience is part of the process of menstruation, pregnancy, and childbirth. There are genetic differences between men and women, and it's known that long-term pain conditions are linked to genetics. Some people believe that women are also more expressive about pain than men; therefore they report pain more frequently.

Age and the Occurrence of Pain

It is observed that the variations of age and gender—in relation to chronic pain—are amazingly consistent across the globe. Furthermore, it's safe to say that there's an increase with age when addressing pain that interferes with life, on a global level. Chronic pain being more prevalent in women than men is also true worldwide. Another significant observation is that musculoskeletal pain, especially that of the back and the joints, is the single dominant type of chronic pain in the world.[7] At the same time, most chronic pain patients have multiple sites of pain, including patients suffering from chronic, disabling back pains. Headaches comprise another type of pain that's prevalent worldwide.

The abovementioned facts explain why results of studies of individual sites in the body—especially of musculoskeletal sites, such as the back, or the head—can be relied on and considered on a large scale when studying the occurrence of chronic pain at any age.

Pain Prevalence by Age-Groups

Chronic pain is common in children, adolescents and adults. Children do have less chronic pain in general, while the prevalence increases as they grow into adolescence. As an example: only 1–6 percent of children, but 18–51 percent of adolescents, suffer from back pains. The latter group's statistics are closer to the percentage that is prevalent in adults, which is 45–80 percent in communities as well as in institutional settings.[8]

Adult Chronic Pain Often Originates during Childhood

Early studies of chronic pain epidemiology focused mainly on adults, and there was a large concern for the short- and medium-term risk factors of causing long-term pain. Researchers were investigating the onset of the type of pain (such as back pain) happening for the first time in individuals in order to possibly modify potential risk factors for future episodes of pain. However, there was a difficulty: few adults experienced such regional pains for the first time. Most individuals reported having suffered the first onset of pain many years earlier; many of them had the first onset in their teenage years. Subsequent studies confirmed that previously experiencing pain (i.e., in childhood) is a common risk factor for the occurrence of pain.[9]

Dominant Type of Pain in Elders

The topic of pain occurrence in older adults is under-investigated, and there have been relatively few studies that specifically aim at research of chronic pain in the age group of the elderly. The main reasons for pain occurrence in older people are musculoskeletal conditions, especially osteoarthritis in multiple joints (pain in the knee, hip, hands, and feet). Much pain is associated with sleep problems, limitations in activities, and increased uses of health care resources.

RESEARCH OF CHRONIC PAIN ACROSS THE LIFE-COURSE

In comparison to other areas of medicine, the study of chronic pain across the life-course (considering possible risk factors in the patients' lives) is still in its infancy. The studies taking these factors into account were published in 1995 in an issue of *Arthritis and Rheumatism*.[10] The experiments were concerning fibromyalgia, a condition where patients experience muscle pain, extreme tiredness, and "tender points" on the neck, shoulders, back, hips, arms, or legs that hurt when touched.

While conducting these researches, a group of women with fibromyalgia and a control group of female subjects were tested. Both groups reported quite high levels of physical and sexual abuse—events where pain almost always occurs. While the group with the women who had fibromyalgia had a higher percentage of abuse reported, the differences in the percentage of abuse cases between them and the control group weren't significant. Frequent, severe cases of abuse were associated with fibromyalgia, as well as the number and severity of the symptoms. Another finding was that the majority of significant abuses reported had taken place during the patients' childhood.

A study conducted in 1998 implied that among patients with fibromyalgia, the ones that had reported abuse suffered higher levels of fatigue, pain, stress, and disability.[11] They also had higher health care usage. Subsequent studies used alternative methods to find connections of chronic pain with trauma in childhood or adolescence; the results were varied in how past events were recalled among persons with or without current chronic pain. Nevertheless, there has been a definite association found between the events taking place early on in life, and chronic pain in adulthood. In cases where a parent reports common chronic symptoms of pain in his child, the probability of chronic pain occurring in a youngster is greater once adulthood is reached.

ANALYSIS

Pain occurrence is an integral part of life that experts have studied for many centuries. Medically speaking, pain is the way the central nervous system interprets any—but mostly harmful—stimulations, and it serves as an alarm signal that something is not up to par. Pain patients and their caregivers should also note that the occurrence of pain can be divided into two categories according to the length of its duration: acute (short-term), and chronic (long-term).

5

HISTORY OF PAIN

Pain has existed since living creatures (animals, to be more scientifically specific) have been around. Ancient civilizations recorded their own experiences of pain through stone tablets.[1] Historically, pain was closely related to "the dark side of the world," which is comprised of demons, evil beings, magic, and sorcery. The expulsion of pain was to be the sole responsibility of the tribal shamans, priests, and sorcerers, who used different tactics, such as herbs, incantations, and ceremonial rites to cure painful ailments. The Greeks and Romans were the first to consolidate the idea of how pain is actually felt. They thought that the brain and nervous system were causing the sensation of pain. During the Middle Ages, evidence supporting that idea began to come to light. In the Renaissance, Leonardo da Vinci was one of the contributors to the idea that the spinal cord is responsible for transmitting the pain sensation to the brain and then to the parts of the body.[2] Research on the mechanisms of pain has continued to the present day.

ETYMOLOGY OF THE WORD

In English the word *pain* is derived from the Old French *peine*, Latin *poena*, (penalty, hardship, torment, punishment, suffering), and in turn from Greek ποινή (*poinē*), generally meaning "price paid," "penalty," or "punishment."[3] The word *pain* is also present in the Frisian language as *pine*, which in turn is connected to the English verb phrase "to pine," meaning "to long for." Historically the word was first used as a sign of penalty for sins, wherein the pain is due to wrongdoing or as punishment that can only be appeased by atonement. By experiencing pain, the sufferer would atone for the sins committed. Another more modern term for pain, *nociception*, meaning "injury perception," was coined by Charles Scott Sherrington (1857–1952) from the original Latin word *nocere*, which means to injure.[4]

EVOLUTION OF BELIEFS ABOUT PAIN

The attempt to understand the origins of pain may have begun with a belief that pain was a form of punishment for the folly of human beings, believing that the solution is to perform penance or other rites and rituals, which include sacrificial offerings and ceremonies. Ancient civilizations had their own concepts of pain, as well as their own processes for treating it. As time passed, pain evolved into a theory that painful sensation is caused by different stimuli, an idea that led to the conclusion that pain is a feeling connected to the brain. The Greeks and Romans were pioneers of the description of pain in these terms, contributing to the foundation of pain's history. Further along the timeline lay the knowledge that pain is felt by a person through a series of receptors that pass the signals to fibers, which then deliver the message to the brain. Scientists have proven this concept of pain, and they have asserted further that pain is felt through *completely different* receptors, independent to that of the other senses.

Part of the variation in theories about pain stems from the fact that pain is very subjective, since there are different ways of feeling it, as well as different ways of explaining what it really is. Pain can be perceived as minor by one individual, but severe by another. Different kinds of pain perception exist in different cultures and for different historical periods. Indeed, research has shown that pain can be felt differently than the usual negative effect.[5] For instance Native Americans during their rituals do not experience pain. They perform ceremonial acts for hours, subjecting a person to tremendous amounts of what would normally be painful experiences, yet the person doesn't feel the actual, physical nature of the pain. Instead, the individual somehow negates pain and its effects.[6] The following sections explain some of the thinking about pain in throughout the progression of civilization.

Beginnings

It was said that the Greek goddess of revenge, Poina, in the form of pain, punished mortals who angered gods.[7] Ancient cultures have long thought that pain was divine punishment for human foolishness; they thought that appeasing the gods would also appease the pain. During this period, many thought of pain as a disorder that must be treated and appeased, while others believed pain to be a necessary feeling, that it's only right that a person experiences pain, and that one should welcome the pain as a blessing rather than a disorder. Dating back to ancient times around 5000 BCE, records about pain were etched on stone tablets indicating that pain was partially relieved by using opium, referred to as the "joy plant." By 800 BCE, we find Homer mentions in *The Odyssey* that a man forgets his worries and soothes his pain by using opium.[8] It was believed that opium was a form of analgesic, and gaining this knowledge initiated the research of different kinds of analgesics by different cultures in the past. Another such analgesic was willow tree bark, of which research was essentially spearheaded by Hippocrates. Aristotle first interpreted pain as emotion rather than sensation. He thought that pain was unrelated to the brain and was an emotion caused by spirits entering the body when a person experiences an injury.[9] Hippocrates (460–370 BCE), on the other hand, believed that pain was due to an imbalance in vital fluids. He used willow tree leaves and barks to provide relief from pain. The Greek physician Pedanius Dioscorides (40–90 CE) also recommended willow bark as a cure for pain and shared his knowledge about such cures during his time, as compiled in his five-volume pharmacopeia.

Middle Ages Theories

Religious groups of the Middle Ages had their own versions of pain theories. Some even thought that pain existed outside of the human body and that deities created pain to remind their subjects to do penance and practice their faith in God, as prayer was believed to be their only treatment. These religious theories were supported by the other religious groups, resulting in a rise in the number of religious theories regarding pain and its origins. They also compared pain with the suffering of Christ, thinking that the suffering that they endure is the same as Christ's sacrifice on the cross for the sake of humanity. But even among the religious there were contending beliefs. The Franciscans believed that pain and suffering led the way to knowledge, while the Dominicans, on the other hand, believed that learning is the pathway to divinity and that pain is a distraction from the acquisition of knowledge. During the thirteenth century, academics agreed that pain is caused by an imbalance of the bodily fluids, the Hippocratic "humors" (blood, phlegm, bile, and black bile). They believed that pain would occur when the mixture of humors was altered. Use of narcotics to balance out the humors was also believed to be an effective remedy during that time.[10]

Renaissance and Early Modern Theories

It was during the Renaissance that the idea of sensations' connection to the brain resurfaced. Leonardo da Vinci believed that pain is from the sensation being delivered by the spinal cord to the central organ, the brain, which is mainly responsible for all sensations in a human being. René Descartes (1596–1650) in his *Treatise of Man* theorized that the body feels pain as a disturbance of the brain's functions, explaining that the human body was similar to a machine. This theory implied that pain is not religious punishment, but is a mechanical sensation found in the brain. Essentially, Descartes eliminated the religious belief in experiencing pain. Descartes explained this through his example of a man being struck by a hammer that has a hollow tube with a cord (symbolizing an arm) and a bell at the end (symbolizing the brain). The mechanism works when the hand is struck by the hammer and the cord is pulled and the bell is rung, indicating that the brain finished receiving the painful "message" from the hand. From this example, researchers started to focus on treating pain starting with the initial culprit in the occurrence of pain: by cutting the pain fibers (the cords in the arm), the pain signal doesn't reach the brain (the bell), eliminating the feeling of pain itself even though the body experienced injury.

Thomas Sydenham (1624–1689), also known as the English Hippocrates, popularized an effective medicine called *laudanum*, formed by mixture of opium and alcohol.[11] A theory known as the *specificity theory* states that a sensation can only be felt by its own sensory components, independent to that of the other senses.[12] This theory was the foundation of Charles Bell's proposal of specific sets of sensory receptors, responding to only their respective stimuli.[13] Further research of the historical theories of pain led to Johannes Müller's (1801–1858) single-stimulus type theory, stating that some energy types are perceived by a specific set of receptors mainly broken down to Aristotle's five senses. He characterized itching, pain, heat, and other varieties of sensation to be "feeling and touch."[14] He concluded that pain can be sensed by touch only, and not by the other four senses. After his discovery, the era of sensory psychology began, primarily aiming to secure knowledge about variations of stimuli. Later, Wilhelm Erb (1840–1921) argued that pain is a sensation actually *generated* if the source of pain is intense enough, thus giving birth to the *intensive theory* of pain.[15]

MODERN-DAY PAIN THEORIES

Overview

In 1953, an observation by Willem Noordenbros explained how the signal carried by smaller pain receptors is dispersed or alleviated by larger "touch, pressure or vibration" sensors. Simply put, Noordenbros maintained that when a person experiences an injury, such as that from a direct physical hit, the person rubs the assaulted part in order to neutralize the pain by the hand's touch receptors.[16] Touching the painful part can relieve part of its pain. A later theory regarding the reasons for pain soon surfaced. The *gate control theory* was introduced by Patrick Wall and Ronald Melzack in 1965. Their article, titled "Pain Mechanisms: A New Theory," explained that nerve fibers carry information from the injured part, sending the information to the spinal cord, and later the signals are received by the brain.[17] This theory has given the world a physiological explanation for pain perception. Roughly ten years after the gate control theory was proposed, the International Association for the Study of Pain proposed a clear-cut definition of pain, combining their knowledge of the past. The organization has described pain as a sensory or emotional phenomenon that can lead to actual or potential tissue impairment.[18] Based on historical definitions, pain is a physical phenomenon that, when linked with trauma, can induce not only physical trauma, but also, emotional and mental trauma if the painful event resurfaces. A simple example can further elaborate this pain phenomenon: Assuming there are two persons with the same painful injury and one of them experienced a greater amount of emotional stress than the other, the former would feel a more intense sensation of pain *physically* than the other when the event happens again.

Religion vs. Science

William James states that the *full* understanding of pain has been an enigma throughout history.[19] Treating pain with anesthetics by means of surgery puzzled physiologists for ages. Further contemplation with regard to treating pain led to the understanding that pain originated from other sources and not from God. Yet an English novelist, Harriet Martineau, wrote a book in the mid-1800s that claimed that pain is the chastisement of a priestly being.[20] She believed without doubt that pain is the work of a deity, believing that pain was meant to be desirable in some way or another. After much further research, the religious belief of pain began to decline and the scientific explanations began to flourish. Gradual knowledge of the field of medicine throughout history began to unveil the real reason behind pain, and it became clear that pain is an uncomfortable feeling that should be alleviated by chemical or surgical means rather than by strict religious ritual.[21] Essentially, science has proven that pain can be identified and its relief can be sought. The religious beliefs regarding the reason for pain faded out by the end of the nineteenth century.

An example in modern pain perception theories is an experiment that tested the visual perception of pain by humans, where investigators subjected the hand of a person to heat.[22] When the person is visualizing the hand directly, a stronger resistance against pain is reported; when looking away, the person feels a greater amount of pain. This research has demonstrated how the person perceives pain in accordance with visual input, that there is greater pain threshold when the part subjected to pain is viewed as opposed to it not being seen. Another perception proven by experiment is that pain can be felt differently depending on the belief of the sufferer. The experiment consisted of people with varying religious beliefs (Roman Catholics, atheists, and agnostics) who were subjected to electrical shocks after being shown a painting of the Virgin Mary and the *Lady with an Ermine*. The subjects' brain scan results had the same rating of pain when they were presented with *The Lady with an Ermine* painting before they were shocked, but the results for the other painting were strikingly different. The Roman Catholics reported experiencing lesser pain when they were presented with the Virgin Mary before they were shocked as compared to the others. A review of this experiment leads one to the placebo effect, wherein the pain is simply *thought* to be less threatening or not dangerous at all. This is possible due to the activation of the part of the brain that is regulating the perception of pain signals. The Catholics felt that they were somehow safe under the eyes of the Virgin Mary, and though their belief in the latter may have helped them reduce the pain, the experiment did not prove that religion really appeases pain. The placebo effect however does reduce pain, and it can be achieved by anyone as long as they can channel the pain into something that is less threatening, by means of meditation or mental strategies.[23]

ANALYSIS

Pain—whether considered an undesirable sensation, a sign of underlying sickness, or a supernatural punishment—has always been part of human life. Pain continues to be perceived and defined differently by people up until this day, both a negative experience, such as from an injury, and a positive experience, as it prevents further injury because of reflex action. But one thing is for sure: members of modern society will be born with it, live with it, and die with it, since people will inevitably experience pain in different forms throughout life.

6

DIFFERENT INTERPRETATIONS OF PAIN

A discourse on the different interpretations of pain requires a review of the diverse factors that contribute to how an individual measures the painfulness of any given experience. Such factors include, but are not limited to: age, socioeconomic status, culture, past experiences (especially during childhood development), and gender. Consideration of these factors brings forth one of the most peculiar and problematic aspects that one confronts when dealing with pain and its diagnosis, which is its subjective nature. Certain experiences that might be painful or unpleasant to some people might not cause the same feelings of discomfort in another individual. What one person might consider as painful might not be interpreted by another individual as such, since the latter doesn't feel the usual sensory qualities associated with what he or she commonly identifies as "pain." Taking these points into account, this chapter provides a better understanding of (1) why pain is perceived differently from one person to another, and (2) how interpretation ultimately affects patients' and caregivers' management of pain.

REASON FOR DIFFERENCES IN INTERPRETATION

Age and Socioeconomic Status

The idea that pain is a vague phenomenon instead of an objectifiable experience seems to be an axiom. Indeed, what one person might consider as a painful experience might be considered by another as just one more mundane, trifling sensation. The difference between people's interpretations of pain has constantly been a source of interest and concern in a wide variety of scientific fields. Some individuals have been found to bear stimuli that normally cause severe pain with mere indifference, while others react to relatively moderate pain with extreme reactions and emotional turmoil.

One factor contributing to this perceived difference in pain interpretation is age. Studies conducted on pain tolerance capabilities between different age groups yielded clear-cut, evident differences when it comes to pain interpretation. One such study, performed jointly by the Stanford University Medical Center and The Permanente Medical Group in the 1970s showed that pain tolerance generally decreases with age.[1] It's worth noting, however, that when the results of this study were compared to earlier work, it seemed that along with increasing age, tolerance to cutaneous pain increases while tolerance to deep pain decreases. Another more recent study indicates that not only do the differences in pain interpretation among people from different age groups exist, but that people's reactions to different kinds of pain stimuli also vary depending on this same factor.[2] These details may be critical when understanding the root or nature of pain that a particular person experiences, therefore paving the way for a well-suited form of treatment.

A person's current socioeconomic status is yet another factor that might contribute to the topic of pain interpretation. While an individual's socioeconomic disposition can lead to a wide variety of effects on his health and well-being at several different levels, it's also highly relevant when trying to deal with how any particular person responds to pain. An individual's socioeconomic status is comprised of several different attributes, such as place of residency, financial capability, occupation, education, and degree of access to basic health care services. It is well known that socioeconomic inequality has a fundamental effect on all aspects of human existence. Therefore, it is unsurprising that socioeconomic position should also have a tremendous impact on how a certain person interprets pain. A study conducted in 2008 indicates that people who come from households with an average annual income of $30,000 and below have higher instances of feeling pain and feel a higher degree of pain severity.[3] This is twice the number of pain occurrences and severity compared to people who come from households with an average annual income ranging above $100,000. The same study indicates that blue-collar employees have a higher average pain rating compared to white-collar workers. Test participants who have less than a high school degree also displayed double the average pain ratings as did the participants who graduated from college. The investigators even noted in an interview from 2008 that the people who have higher incomes seem to welcome pain and that the pain usually results from exercising, while people who have lower incomes report that their pain usually comes from doing their work.[4] Furthermore, a recent study published in *The European Journal of Pain* showed that people from the lower end of the socioeconomic ladder feel that they suffer from a greater degree of disability through pain compared to those who come from the higher end of the socioeconomic rankings, even though the pain intensity and the number of painful body areas were the same for all survey participants.[5] Clearly, a person's income, degree of education, and occupation imparts a very significant contribution on how he or she interprets any form of pain in their lives, since pain itself has a direct impact on a person's daily productivity and role effectiveness in society.

Cross-Cultural Differences

In spite of the ubiquitous nature of pain in human lives, the interpretations, definitions, and perceptions of it seem to be culturally specific. The several ways that people express and control pain, manifests itself as a learned behavioral attitude that is distinct from one culture to another.[6] Some individuals might display stoicism in the face of experiencing pain and consider it as the norm. They tend to withdraw socially and just turn to themselves, bearing the discomfort with a grin and a "stiff upper lip." Others are extremely expressive both verbally and physically wherein some scream, cry, or sometimes even succumb to episodes of *hysteria* (uncontrolled emotion). It's been suggested that people who come from an Eastern cultural background have a more stoic approach or response to pain compared to people who were raised in a Western culture upbringing.[7] During case studies made by The University of California, the researchers observed that people from Hispanic, Mediterranean, and Middle Eastern cultures are mostly very expressive with their pain, while most people of Asian and Northern European cultural backgrounds tend to exhibit stoicism.[8] Some cultures tend to view pain as a punishment from a higher being brought about by spiritual failings and thus, believe that it must simply be borne with fortitude. Pain might be a result of failure to heed traditional rituals designed to please deities, thereby apparently invoking divine punishment.

Others still, interpret the pain that they're experiencing as a result of negative karma and must therefore endure pain willingly as a necessary evil to maintain the proper balance and harmony of the environment. Notably, in most of these cultures where pain and illnesses are usually seen as the work of a divine hand, people tend to interpret painful experiences as a test of religious faith. In the same study by the University of California, the primary investigator studied a patient who underwent a shoulder surgery telling his nurse that he was experiencing severe pain, but refused to take pain medication, because it was supposedly the will of a god that he go through this painful experience and that a god will give him the strength to bear it for the exact same reason. The main researcher also noted a Nigerian farmer who had to undergo arthroscopic knee surgery due to injuries sustained from a charging bull. He never asked for pain medication afterward because, being a Muslim, his pain was apparently an "offering to Allah" in return for the good fortune of getting such a surgery.[9] People from cultures that value stoicism when it comes to dealing with pain are also mostly unvocal about what exactly they are feeling. They may feel that admitting to pain or showing signs of pain is a sign of weakness. Thus, they hide it and make a conscious effort of not letting it show on their faces. They might even deny feeling pain when asked. On the flip side, some people from other cultural groups tend to be very descriptive of the pain that they're feeling. This may be correlated to experiences or behaviors learned and acquired during childhood. Certain cultural groups believe that expressing their pain through groaning, grimacing, screaming, and howling actually help to relieve and ease the pain.[10] They don't subscribe to the idea that pain is something to be endured, but instead, they interpret it as something that must be alleviated as soon as possible.

The manner by which a pain patient interprets the pain that he experiences is highly affected by culture and belief systems, therefore leaving pain subject to a wide and diverse variety of interpretations differing from one cultural group to another. Currently, existing studies on the correlation between pain interpretation and culture are at the most, mere "benchmarks" and do not provide a set of solid qualitative data from which a concrete culture-specific treatment for pain may be administered. It is of absolute importance to note that the usage of current study results regarding the relation between culture and pain interpretation is restricted to just guidelines, since culture provides only a basic outline of any particular person's behavior.

Not everyone in every culture strictly conforms to a specifically expected set of behaviors and beliefs. The current, existing descriptions about any particular culture may even be considered as merely wide generalizations. A strict observance of cultural generalizations in dealing with pain leads to stereotyping. Stereotyping can lead to grave inaccuracies in diagnosis and potentially harmful or inappropriate prescriptions of pain-treatment methods. Even though pain is a universal human condition, the fact remains that it is culture-specific as well, further reinforcing the significance of pain's subjectivity and susceptibility to individual-specific interpretations, as a crucial aspect to be considered—when dealing with its treatment and medication.

In relation to different cultural upbringings, an individual's past experiences with pain also contribute largely to how he'll respond to succeeding pain episodes that may be encountered throughout his lifetime. It has been recognized that the differing degrees of pain tolerance capabilities from one person to another are directly affected by how a certain person learns to cope or respond to past encounters with pain while growing up. Parenting style is of great importance, as the parents serve as models for their children on how to respond to a painful experience.[11] This still has a direct relation to a person's cultural background, since a person's development of his own pain threshold parameters are directly acquired as a result of learned experience, mostly from the formative years and in reaction to the environment. The development of this set of behaviors and attitudes will directly affect how the person interprets and responds to pain later on in life.

Sexual Differences in Pain Interpretation

Experiments referenced throughout this writing indicate that there's consistent, supporting data to suggest that sex or gender has an effect on the way that a person interprets pain. However, current studies on the relationship between sex differences and pain interpretation have varying results and seem to raise even more questions than answers. Nonetheless, sex differences in pain interpretation appear to be existent even though it's not always explicable. In one of her studies regarding the relationship between childhood pain and gender, an expert observed that in general, boys and girls have a different conceptualization of what's considered to be painful.[12] She noted that the pain reactions between boys and girls differ. Generally, girls tend to feel fear and anxiousness when encountering pain. Boys tend to feel anger. Boys interpreted the tightening of braces as severely painful while girls on the other hand, reported having a broken arm as being more painful in comparison. These observations however, may be more related to the way that boys, in virtually all cultures, are raised to be more stoic when it comes to dealing with pain as compared to girls. This may affect the males as they grow older for they may possibly underreport feelings of painful discomfort. Girls on the other hand aren't necessarily encouraged but neither are they admonished when they get emotive or expressive of their feelings and emotions. In the elderly, sex hormones and anatomical differences might contribute to the differing pain interpretations. Evidence indicates that pain thresholds and pain tolerance for human females vary along with the different stages of the menstrual cycle.[13] It's also now well-known that there are ailments that are more common among women than men such as fibromyalgia, migraine, irritable bowel syndrome, and abdominal pains. The sexual differences regarding some painful experiences, such as those in relation to migraine, even diminish gradually after menopause.[14] The *American Pain Society* published an extensive study in 2009 affirming the existence of sexually-influenced interpretations of pain. However, a completely realized method of its application in handling different responses to pain perception based on sex remains beyond reach. The bottom line: pain will always be subjective from one person to another, and interpreting it also requires certain sensitivity to anatomical and psychosocial differences between males and females.

ADVANCEMENTS IN PAIN INTERPRETATION

Currently, there are several modern technological advancements that are capable of interpreting pain. Medical image processing can reveal areas of the body that have sustained tissue or nerve damage. Several less-technological methods are also already in place for quite some time now, capable of interpreting the nature of any particular pain sensation. These methods are anchored mainly on language and the prerequisite that both the patient and the person trying to administer treatment understand each other. However, due to pain's subjective nature, its severity may not always be interpreted by the degree of tissue or nerve damage shown through imaging studies. As such, a more thorough and accurate diagnosis of pain relies heavily on the person's own self-reports and descriptions. This is where the efficiency of treatment and accurate prescription of medication starts to depend on the particular individual's interpretations and beliefs. In light of this, a mere understanding of each other (patient and caregiver) through the ability to speak in the same language doesn't provide a fully satisfactory way of dealing with pain, for it's still subject to personal biases: both from the pain patient and the caregiver's point of view. It is therefore of great importance that individual interpretations of patients as based on age, culture, sex, and socioeconomic status be taken into consideration in order to provide the most effective and most applicable form of pain relief method available.

DOCTORS' PERCEPTION OF PATIENTS' PAIN

Since pain's subjective nature requires that the experiencing individual's circumstances be taken into account, a closer look must also be directed toward the other end of the spectrum to consider the manner in which the health worker interprets a patient's pain. Patients and doctors often seem to have differing ideas or perceptions when it comes to interpreting pain. This shouldn't really be a surprise since it has been well established that even though objective assessment of a source of pain may show little or no difference between individuals with a certain kind of injury, the perception of the severity and intensity of pain being felt still rests upon the specific patient's own interpretation. Doctors and nurses often seem to incorrectly assess pain intensity and severity, or at least disagree with a patient's own interpretation. One study asked a group of patients to rate pain intensity from zero to ten, where zero represents painlessness and ten is unbearable pain.[15] As part of the study, a group of doctors were asked to do the same using a similar pain rating scale. Findings show that the doctors underestimated the pain that their patients self-reported about 40 percent of the time, even though the former group had full access to patient records. Forty-six percent of participating physicians gave the same pain intensity ratings that the patients did, while 15 percent overestimated the pain intensity that their patients felt by a slight margin. Clearly, the different factors influencing how a person interprets pain not only affects the person experiencing it but must also be taken into account by whoever is providing the treatment. While overestimation of a patient's pain might not necessarily be detrimental toward proper diagnosis, underestimating a patient's pain can definitely lead to under-treatment. For many years now, health care organizations have been lobbying for a proposal that health care providers should simply accept the patients' self-reports of pain as the basis for providing pain treatments. Furthermore, a patient's own interpretation of the pain being experienced plays a very significant role in the processes of pain management (see chapter 14).

Self-reports shouldn't, however, be regarded as the only basis for determining the most efficient methods required to alleviate a patient's pain. A doctor's knowledge and expertise of the conditions of the human body, brought about by years of education and training, is also instrumental in ensuring that the most appropriate form of treatment is received by the patient. Nonetheless, just as is the case with patients, health care professionals are also potentially subject to their own personal biases based on the different factors that affect an individual's interpretation of pain. In order to achieve the most effective pain management, caregivers must consistently take all the factors that affect a person's pain interpretation into consideration. Effective communication with a patient is needed in every clinical encounter to reduce misunderstandings and differences regarding the intensity of pain being experienced. This will ensure that there are no discrepancies between the pain treatment method being provided and the actual pain severity the patient is experiencing, thereby resulting in better management of pain.

COMMUNICATION AND ITS ROLE IN THE INTERPRETATION OF PAIN

Linguistic Challenges

A huge part of dealing with the different subjective ways that a person interprets pain involves having a firm grasp on the terms that people normally use to describe such experiences. The words people use for describing pain are as varied as the factors that affect a person's interpretation of it. Terms such as "waxing and waning," "throbbing," "tingling," "shooting," "intermittent," "numbing," and "gnawing" are just some of the words that people use to ascribe some form of measurement to the intensity of any particular pain sensation. This puts the interpretation of pain under an even more idiosyncratic light.

Within the medical and scientific community, the different interpretations of painful sensations usually fall under the two broad categories of either acute or chronic pain, and then into several subcategories. This categorization still doesn't resolve the basic need to describe the nature or intensity of a painful experience, which varies from one person to another even though the root cause might be the same. In everyday instances, people may use a broad expanse of terms to describe the degree or intensity of a painful experience. A "dull" kind of pain is that which may normally be used by patients to describe a pain that doesn't prevent the performance of daily activities. It's usually the type of pain that is just barely noticeable and negligible. This type of pain is generally classified as just a slight, vague, or trifling sensation that doesn't provide so much discomfort that an individual cannot perform daily tasks. A "mild" pain generally describes the same kind of pain as a dull one, except for the aspect that the latter is usually consistent and nagging. Dull pain is something that is more spread out and not focused on one specific area of the body. A mild pain might usually be referred to in the context of describing the intensity of a particular pain, while a dull pain may refer more to the persistence of any particular painful experience over a period of time. A sharp pain is generally something that is the opposite of these two descriptions. It's most often used by patients to describe the kind of pain that has a definite and clear location on the body. It is the "stabbing" kind of pain that is keenly and suddenly felt. "Severe" pain, on the other hand, is most often used by people to describe a kind of pain that is extreme in nature. It is the form of pain that rating systems place in the highest and most intense categories. Physicians seem to agree that a severe pain is the kind of pain that awakens the patient in the middle of the night, and, if experienced, is usually interpreted as a more serious bodily ailment that needs to be addressed immediately through clinical intervention.

ANALYSIS

Scientists appear to have been constantly struggling to devise a way to objectively interpret pain. In spite of several extensive studies and educated attempts, its realization still remains elusive. Health care workers have already accepted patients' self-reports as the most valid measure of the pain experience. Pain caregivers should strive to be sensitive regarding differences in age, sex, socioeconomic status, culture, and medical history when trying to address pain-related issues. Pain *patients* should be encouraged to describe their pain as accurately as possible. That is how the individual differences and interpretations of pain that people naturally have will be less of a hindrance in providing efficient medical services.

7

THE CHANGING CULTURE OF PAIN

The preceding chapter discussed *some* cultural interpretations of pain; now this chapter explores in much more detail how people of distinct cultures perceive and deal with pain in everyday life. Pain can be defined with respect to (1) time, (2) the body portion or tissue type involved, or (3) the way that it was generated. The perception of pain differs for every individual because it is influenced by both the present situation and past experience.[1] Even though pain is universally treated with some kind of painkiller, more often than not, people tend to prefer to deal with their pain first using home remedies and over-the-counter remedies rather than immediately consulting with a physician. Throughout the years, various studies have been conducted regarding the phenomenon of pain and the possible treatments to alleviate it, but its complexity still leaves researchers with a lot of things to consider. In research done in 2000, it was discovered that 80 percent of Americans viewed pain as an inevitable part of getting older and something they have to live with.[2]

Pain exists in spite of the continuous advancements in science because it requires a multidisciplinary viewpoint. While there are many culturally distinct therapies available, including acupuncture, pharmaceuticals, nutrition, supplementation, yoga, and psychology among others, pain reduction still relies heavily on the patient, and a chosen healing therapy must complement the sufferer's cultural needs and beliefs.[3]

A CULTURE OF PAIN

By definition, culture is an integrated and patterned idea through domi-nant economic forces, social patterns, symbols, and values.[4] Culture is said to be present only in humans. Although animals can learn certain methods and practices and develop attitudes based on the natural in-stinct for survival, only humans have what is called cultural learning, which depends on symbols attached to certain phenomena, allowing people to give meaning to events.[5]

Culture can be best defined by highlighting its core characteristics. The first is that culture can be learned consciously or unconsciously through the process known as *enculturation*, which is defined to be a conditioning process (both conscious and unconscious) wherein hu-mans achieve competence and internalize their culture.[6] Culture is also shared; it is a feature of individuals as members of groups and not something of one's own making. In addition, culture depends on the human ability to assign meaning to events, which allows people to eval-uate phenomena.[7] Culture can be adaptive or maladaptive in the sense that it may offer short-term benefits as well as threaten a group's long-term existence.[8]

Why Cultural Perceptions of Pain Change

Pain patients and caregivers must also realize that culture is also known to be all encompassing, which basically means that a certain culture may include otherwise painful things that may sometimes be regarded as trivial. Eventually, changes are bound to influence cultures, and three distinct forces are determined to be responsible for these changes: the various influences within a society, the interaction be-tween societies, and changes in the natural environment.[9] Within a society, changes can be attributed to technological or ideological inno-vation and to cultural loss, which is essentially the replacement of old cultural patterns with new ones. Diffusion, acculturation, and transcul-turation are identified as the leading factors for changes that happen through interaction between societies. Diffusion allows for the spread-ing of certain cultural traits (e.g., how pain is to be defined) to different areas, and allows these traits to be shared in different territories.[10] Acculturation is the process of change that results from the interplay of cultures, while *transculturation* describes an individual's experience when moving to a new place with a different culture that is then adopted.[11]

Introduction to the Changing Culture of Pain

Pain depends upon the meaning that one gives it, and this constantly changes across time, culture, and social contexts.[12] Over the years, the notion of pain has transformed from a cultural and personal phenomenon to being an entirely medical problem.[13] The current cultural perception in the West is based largely on the research and breakthroughs presented by science. In America alone, this huge dependence on science to treat pain is evident in Americans' expenditure of more than $4 billion annually for painkillers.[14]

As early as 428 BCE, the classical Greek philosopher Plato presented his ideas on pleasure and pain through *Timaeus*, one of Plato's published dialogues that explore the nature of the physical world and of human beings.[15] In this dialogue, Plato states that pain largely depends on the senses. All pain has some meaning associated with it, and within cultural limitations, pain is viewed by a person as a form of suffering when it is rendered useless otherwise.[16] Pain stems from many cultural experiences, and is usually interrelated with various occurrences in a person's life. Throughout the years, pain was seen in relation to other factors, including religion, sex, and even comedy. Through an analysis of literature and other works of art, there's been a link seen between the perception of pain and brilliance.[17] David B. Morris in *The Culture of Pain* states that a majority of patients are suffering from pain because of physicians' refusal to acknowledge pain as a phenomenon that should include cultural and social factors.[18]

In the present day, some researchers and professional caregivers essentially depend on the medical viewpoint in understanding pain and in treating it. Aspirin, the popular name for *acetylsalicylic acid*, has been used largely to treat mild to moderate pain, as well as to reduce fever and inflammation. This drug, manufactured and patented by a major Germany-based corporation, became prominent during World War I and since then has established a huge presence in the market worldwide.[19] Over the years, more and more medicines and drugs have been manufactured, claiming to be a solution for pain, but recent experiences present contradictions that prove that pain cannot be seen only from a purely medicinal viewpoint and as a brain problem.

The cultural resources that were available in the past have been generally forgotten because of the world's complete trust in medical "cures." Today, however, those in the field of medicine and even those who are not, have already begun to explore new methods of pain relief.[20] These changing (cultural) viewpoints play a large part in the world's understanding of pain, and also hold the future of pain medications.

Regulatory Barriers and Culture

Regulatory organizations can indirectly shape the way pain is dealt with in a specific culture. The basic food and drug law present in the United States, which is considered to be the most extensive law of its kind in the world, is the Federal Food, Drug, and Cosmetic Act, while the Secure and Responsible Drug Disposal Act of 2010 acknowledges that the nonmedical use of prescription pain drugs is a continuously growing issue in the country, and that the number of deaths related to this has significantly increased.[21] There has also been a recorded increase in violent crime and property crime due to the abuse of controlled prescription drugs (CPDs) in the past years, and for this reason, there's greater concern and necessity for the government and related agencies to impose strict restrictions and guidelines related to prescription pain medications and their public sales to consumers.

In the United States, the Food and Drug Administration (FDA) aims to promote and protect consumers' health by monitoring and providing regulatory guidelines for food, drugs, medical devices, vaccines, cosmetics, radiation-emitting products, and tobacco products. In relation to pain medications, the FDA is responsible for providing consumers and health professionals with information on new drug warnings and safety information. At present, as many as three billion prescriptions are written annually in the United States alone, but many people die as a result of errors given in preventable medications.[22] The Food and Drug Administration created the *Safe Use Initiative* in order to facilitate public and private collaborations within the health care community. By identifying risks linked with various pain medications, preventable harm can be drastically reduced for any particular culture— not just the American one. The potential partners of this project could include federal agencies, health care professionals and professional societies, pharmacies, hospitals, and the consumers.

The U.S. Food and Drug Administration's Center for Drug Evaluation and Research (CDER) is tasked with evaluating pain drugs before they can be allowed to be sold publicly, therefore allowing the consumers to have a guaranteed safe medication. Companies who wish to sell drugs in the United States have to send CDER certain test results to prove that the drugs are safe and that they work for their intended purpose. This is then reviewed by the CDER to ensure that the company is to sell drugs that are true to their labels, and when it's already made certain that the health benefits of the drugs outweigh its known risks, the drug is approved for public sale. The drug company first performs routine laboratory and animal tests to show how the drug works, before it's tested on pain patients.[23]

In the United Kingdom, the Medicines and Healthcare products Regulatory Agency (MHRA) examines the safety and quality of health care products. While there may be cultural differences between the United States and UK, the MHRA makes sure that companies comply with European and local (UK) laws, which are somewhat similar to those in the States. In December of 2009, the (MHRA) had a press release that launched a set of new guidelines for the sale of pain killers in the UK, which is yet another expanding culture. This is in line with the MHRA's partnership with stakeholders, including large and small retailers, pharmacists, trading standards offices, and the pharmaceutical industry. The British Retail Consortium (BRC) and the Association of Convenience Stores (ACS) are also part of the stakeholders. The guidelines stated the following restrictions on the sales of pain killers:[24]

- No more than two packs of painkillers should be sold per transaction.
- Retailers are discouraged from encouraging the sale of more than one packet at a time.
- "Buy one get one free" or price promotions that hint a discount for buying more than one pack would merely encourage customers to purchase a lot more than necessary.
- In a general sales outlet, the maximum pack-size for pain relief medicines is sixteen tablets or capsules. Pharmacies under the supervision of a pharmacist may sell larger packs of up to thirty tablets or capsules.
- Sales of more than 100 tablets or capsules of *paracetamol* or aspirin in one retail transaction is illegal as per legislation.

The above points help to minimize stockpiling and overdosing (whether it is accidental or impulsive) within a specific culture of society. Moreover, the medications would be effective and safer if the instructions for the use and dosage of the medicines are followed. The laws can be implemented through the use of regular training of staff on the imposition of restrictions, and notices for customers so as to raise awareness. In the UK, all medicines that go to the market are first scrutinized by the MHRA before they are approved to be sold publicly. The MHRA also issues a so-called marketing authorization or license, and manufacturers and distributors are also directly licensed by the agency. Apart from the MHRA, there are other organizations concerned with ensuring the quality and safety of publicly sold drugs, including (1) a Notified Body, (2) member states of the European Union, and (3) ethics committees.[25] In Europe, Notified Bodies are organizations who carry out compliance assessments. Member States of the

European Union (EU) aid in sharing problems that they encounter with certain drugs, thus improving the regulation. Lastly, ethics committees are the ones responsible for clinical trials of the products, whereas the MHRA is responsible for scientific evidence.

The MHRA and the FDA are both significant agencies when it comes to medications, particularly in ensuring their safety for public consumption, as well as in setting standards and performing tests before drugs are sold in the market. This way, the consumers can be more confident that the medications they are using are medically tested to be safe and that consumption will result in improvement rather than risk.

FEAR AND THE CULTURE OF PAIN

There are cases in which patients are said to suffer from pain because the doctors are afraid to prescribe medicines to alleviate pain. This is in line with the fact that there is a significant number of people who abuse prescription drugs by using them way above their dosage limits, or by selling them to other people. This is a growing issue in the United States, and as more doctors hold this fear, more and more patients become agitated and bothered by pain that doctors refuse to manage. Patients are thus going to the pharmacies without prescriptions from their physicians in an attempt to get drugs that might reduce or numb the pain that they are feeling. This has further caused growing concern with regard to drug use. Patients affected by inadequate treatments include both types: those who are suffering from chronic pain and those experiencing severe acute pain.

A renowned pain management professional stated that fears of pain medications being abused are irrational and are often caused by inade- quate medical training.[26] He further argued that there are other ways to manage pain, including massage, opioids, and behavioral therapy, and that any medication could easily be misused or abused. In truth, Kath- ryn Hahn, an expert and practicing pharmacist notes that abuse of pain medications has indeed been worsening throughout the years, given that federal treatment programs for drug abuse have more than tripled within the past decade. Additionally, she states that there are alternative pain management techniques available but doctors are not yet fully informed about these new options. Doctors need to have full knowl- edge of their patients' pain and be well informed about other pain relieving options. Patients also need to take the prescriptions seriously and acknowledge their seriousness so as to make doctors more confident in prescribing them, including opioids, over-the-counter pain relievers, and antidepressants.[27]

In light of these rising problems, organizations and agencies (who undoubtedly contribute to the culture) feel more compelled to impose guidelines regarding pain management. Most importantly, the direction for pain management experts in dealing with these problems is to educate professionals with the best drug- and non-drug methods to reduce and control pain.[28]

PRODUCTIVITY AND SCIENTIFIC ADVANCEMENTS IN THE CULTURE OF PAIN

Emergence of Electronic Medical Records

An electronic medical record is a computerized medical record created by an organization that delivers medical care, and includes a *clinical data repository* (CDR), a *clinical decision support system* (CDSS), a *controlled medical vocabulary* (CMV), a *computerized provider order entry* (CPOE), and other pharmacy and clinical documentation applications.[29] Ideally, electronic medical records (EMRs) should serve to save all of the patient's information such that all records are secure and easily accessible not only to physicians, but to the patients as well. This method, which is increasing in certain cultures, also allows a patient to see several specialists without worrying about the specialist not knowing the patient's medical history, which is crucial to treatment and recovery in most cases.

The downside to such an information system is that it may be costly, with an estimated cost (for hardware and software) of up to $20,000 for every physician.[30] Furthermore, doctors will need to dedicate many hours of their time to properly learn how to handle and use the system, which is undeniably a great deal of time, and this may even take longer for doctors who are not acquainted with the new technology. Despite its downsides, hopes for the EMRs' benefits are continuously increasing. Solid research studies show how electronic medical records can lead to a higher quality of care because of interactive features that include regular e-mail reminders to patients for their checkups and other services.[31] This allows professional caregivers to serve their patients more fully with a reduction of risks associated with the much older paper-based system. Eight core capabilities possessed by electronic medical records are[32]

- health information and data;
- electronic communication and connectivity;
- decision support—the use of reminders and alerts to ensure regular screenings and preventive practices for the patient;
- patient support;
- result management—increases patient safety by allowing providers and other professions to new and past test results of a patient;
- order management;
- administrative processes; and
- reporting.

With continuous improvements in technology, the cultural changes presented by EMRs are expected to be solved sooner rather than later, and eventually, the benefits presented by the system will be fully utilized by the professional world to better serve the patients and aid in their treatments, especially when it comes to sensitive issues such as pain.

Research and Products

With the changing culture of pain, the world has been adapting along with the way that people understand it. At present, pain is seen as a disease that alters the nervous system, thus increasing the need to improve research and methods on how to deal with it. Seeing pain in this light lends more hope for resolving the patient's problem, particularly with the belief that pain as a disease means that the patient can alter it with his emotional, professional, and family settings. Ongoing research about pain and the medications for controlling it within a given culture are said to be more promising, allowing for optimism that pain and its associated risks will be less of a problem in the future.

The goal of current research is to educate patients on how to deal with the pain they are feeling, which is mostly an interaction between the mind and the body. The president of the American Pain Foundation stated that several long-acting products are now being developed, and there are new drugs that are set to appear to deal with nerve damage pain.[33] Researchers have acknowledged that better treatments are needed to alleviate pain, which is a growing problem in the United States and worldwide.

ANALYSIS

Pain research has indeed taken on different cultural approaches. By recognizing pain in its medicinal aspect *and* in its cultural terms, researchers are better off in providing people with treatment modalities to alleviate their pain. The future of pain research largely depends on: (1) the acknowledgement of the interplay between the mind and body and the results of it, and (2) the further education of caregivers across various cultures.

II

Clinical Picture

8

PATHOLOGY OF PAIN

In order to understand and treat pain effectively, it is vital for patients and caregivers to know the pathology of pain. Pain is an unpleasant feeling that might be alleviated by different remedies. It is also a bodily alarm that serves as a warning sign when something is wrong. In this chapter, *pathology* will be defined and explored to provide a further understanding of the structure of pain. The four factors involved in pathology are also identified, since recognizing the different disciplines of pathology is essential to alleviate pain that may be associated with different diseases.

DEFINITION OF PATHOLOGY

Pathology is a study that deals with the transformation of structures and functions in the human body that is a result of an illness or disease.[1] Pathology: (1) focuses more on the alterations that the cells, tissues, and body organs undergo due to the nature of the disease, and (2) is a medical specialty that touches virtually all of medicine. It is relevant for the development of a permanent cure for pain and treatment for illnesses that affect humanity.[2]

Four Pathological Bases of Painful Disorders

Because pain is so interrelated with the concept of disease, we should explore the latter in depth. Pathology addresses four facets of disease: *etiology* (cause), mechanisms of development (pathogenesis), change of cell structure (morphological changes), and the result of these of changes (clinical manifestations).[3]

Etiology is the first component of pathology and refers to the origin of the disease, which could be from (1) biological agents, (2) physical forces, or (3) nutritional excess or deficit. These agents may affect one or more organs or body structures. A disease, including one that is responsible for pain, could have several predisposing factors as the cause. For example, diseases can be the consequence of a genetic predisposition along with events that trigger disease development.[4]

Pathogenesis focuses on the development of the disease process. After determining the cause, it is vital to be aware of the progression of the illness. Before the effects of the illness are evident, the body undergoes changes that are caused by risk factors or predisposing conditions. The primary structure of cells and tissues is referred to as *morphology*. This primary structure is altered with the onset of a disease, which is known as morphological change. To study the changes, several laboratory tests are done, including blood testing and internal imaging. The changes that take place are known as *clinical manifestation*. Manifestations such as fever, dizziness, difficulty in breathing, and pain are all possible by-products of a disease. A particular symptom may be a manifestation of one or more diseases.[5]

Disciplines of Pathology

It is essential to trace the pain's progression, which is sometimes misinterpreted as the pathology of pain itself. To some, pathology *is* medicine since it plays a vital role in treating illnesses from conception to *post mortem* (following death).[6] Pathology has many disciplines, namely: anatomical, chemical, clinical, forensic, genetic, hematological, immunopathological, and microbiological. It is important for pain patients and caregivers to understand these categories fully, in case professional referral is necessitated.

Anatomical Pathology

Anatomical pathology deals with the study of diseased organs. To determine the cause of the disease, specialists obtain a tissue sample from the patient during operation or post mortem. Pathologists examine these tissues to examine the cause of the disease or the death of a patient. Separated cells from different body organs can also be examined by pathologists.[7]

Chemical Pathology

Chemical pathology is another branch of pathology that focuses on the complete scope of the pain. It identifies painful disorders through examination of body fluids or components of the blood during an illness to determine the electrolytes and enzymes. It also aims to detect signs of cancer as well as chemical origins of pain. Chemical pathology is very important in detecting chemical changes, as well as ensuring accurate medical intervention and treatment.[8]

Clinical Pathology

Clinical pathologists are well trained in chemical pathology, microbiology, hematology, and blood banking, though not as specialists in each of these fields. They are familiar with clinical branches of laboratory medicine. For concerns that require a more detailed evaluation of a painful disease, they usually consult experts in a specific field. They work closely with medical technologists.[9]

Forensic Pathology

Forensic pathology involves the investigation of unexpected deaths for *medico-legal* purposes. This mainly involves an autopsy or examining external and internal body parts to identify the cause of death.[10]

Genetic Pathology

Genetic pathology is the latest field of pathology to emerge, and it focuses more on the genetic makeup of the patient to identify the underlying cause of an illness, especially those that are congenital. Genetic pathologists provide families with advice on hereditary diseases from different specialists.[11]

Haematology

Hematology is a discipline closely related to pathology that is developing fast. It specializes in studying diseases that affect the blood, such as anemia, leukemia, and bleeding or clotting disorders. Hematologists are also involved in the management of blood transfusion services.[12]

Immunopathology

Immunopathology involves laboratory evaluation of the patient's immune system. An example is testing for allergy *antibodies* (specialized protective proteins) to determine if the individual is allergic to a particular substance. The immune system is the body's defense against foreign particles that may arise in the form of bacteria and viruses. Immunopathologists manage disorders that result from malfunction of the immune system, such as lupus erythematosus and rheumatoid arthritis, and AIDS, as well as transplantation medicine. [13]

Microbiologists

While microbiologists aren't formally considered pathologists, the scope of microbiology can involve the evaluation of painful disorders caused by infectious agents such as bacteria, viruses, fungi, and parasites. This field of pathology is very critical to society since it deals with outbreaks. New organisms and infectious diseases have been discovered by microbiologists through history. [14]

GENERAL PATHOLOGY OF PAIN

From a general standpoint, physical malfunction of the body occurs when something fails to operate normally. [15] The nervous system is an intricate "machine" comprised of structures already explained in the preceding chapters. These structures in humans are relatively advanced, but once illness takes over or when these organs sustain sudden or violent injury, the welfare of the entire pain patient is at risk. When the nervous system malfunctions (i.e., it becomes pathological), there are many varied effects that the body experiences, and these effects will mainly depend on the area that is malfunctioning. General effects range from altered levels of consciousness to problems in motor function. [16]

Developmental Defects as Pathology

Some nervous system disorders are caused by developmental defects. These defects can be congenital, such as *hydrocephalus* (swelling and fluid build-up in the brain). Painful infections and inflammation are also a common cause of nervous system problems. Toxic, metabolic, and nutritional disorders such as *phenylketonuria* are also responsible for some disorders. Vascular disorder wherein blood vessels become diseased and with interrupted, blood flow to the brain and other organs is also a cause of a painful developmental disorder. In addition, tumors are also life-threatening problems of the nervous system that often require surgery. [17]

Brain Malfunction

Since the brain and spinal cord are the two main parts of the nervous system, there are major effects when these parts malfunction. Injuries to these parts may result to impaired consciousness. This may range from confusion to coma. The ability to think clearly or alertness is easily disturbed in this instance, once the nervous system malfunctions. These effects may be accompanied by unresponsive pupils, inability to respond to stimuli, and impaired motor and verbal response. A seizure can also be an effect for any brain malfunction. All of these are evident in pain patients experiencing problems with the nervous system in general, but more specifically, the brain.[18]

Spinal Cord Malfunction

Malfunctions in the spinal cord also have devastating effects on body functions. An injury in the white matter of the spinal cord leads to problems in the function of the upper extremities. Spinal cord problems in the anterior part may result in an inability to feel pain and temperature. Sacral and lumbar cord injuries will impair bowel, bladder, and sexual functions. Complete spinal cord injuries may result in paralysis. Furthermore, the resultant paralysis impairs circulatory function. *Bradycardia* (slow heart rate), *hypotension* (poor blood pressure in comparison to normal perfusion), and oxygenation are experienced.[19]

Disorders in Motor Function

Nervous system pathology has detrimental effects such as involuntary reflexes. Spasms or involuntary muscle contractions may cause delays and disturbances in simple activities such as eating, dressing, or walking. This can also be dangerous for a person experiencing pain since the reflexes cannot be controlled and spasms may occur at any time. Tremors and tics are also involuntary movements that may be experienced by the individual suffering from pain. Movements of the face such as grimacing, rolling of the eyes, and raising the eyebrows occur unintentionally. Limbs may move also. These involuntary movements may range from brief and rapid, to slow and irregular.[20]

Disorders in Bladder, Bowel, and Sexual Function

Pain is also a common effect of any malfunction, and it can be quite devastating depending on the severity. Impaired bladder and bowel function is one of the substantial problems in nervous system malfunction. Sexual function may also get impaired. Men may experience erectile dysfunction and women may have fertility problems. There could also be problems with responding to sexual stimuli.[21]

Peripheral Nerve Pathology

There are also long-term effects for any nervous system malfunction that is not treated promptly. Paralysis can last a lifetime due to cerebrovascular diseases such as stroke. Disorders of the peripheral nerves can cause weakness that leads to difficulty in chewing, climbing stairs, or lifting objects.[22] Carpal tunnel syndrome is another effect of malfunction of the peripheral nerves, but it can also be associated with different pathological disorders such as diabetes mellitus, which comes with pain in the wrist and hands, along with numbness of the thumb. There is also *paresthesia* or a feeling of "pins and needles" and a weak grip.[23]

Nervous System Pathology in the Elderly

Some disorders of brain function can lead to memory loss and personality change in a senior, and therefore these disorders indirectly contribute to the general pathology of pain. Such problems often occur in the elderly but may also affect much younger individuals. As people get older, there is a greater chance that the brain may malfunction and hence may, by extension, affect the level of pain in the patient. Older people may exhibit unusual behavior such as restlessness, abstract thinking, agitation, and wandering. This may prevent them from carrying out activities of daily living normally. Inability to communicate along with urinary and fecal incontinence is also evident. These effects do not only concern the patient but the patient's family as well. Elderly people experiencing dementia and other malfunctions of the brain require thorough assistance and quality caregiving.[24]

Sleep Disorders

Sleep disorders are also the result of nervous system pathology. The most common sleep disorder is insomnia. *Chronic insomnia* usually results in mood changes such as depression and irritability. *Dyssomnia* is a disorder wherein the person has excessive sleepiness or impaired wakefulness. *Narcolepsy* is also known as "sleep attack" where the patient may fall asleep while doing daily routines such as driving and eating. This disorder can be harmful and is also difficult to treat. Some also experience motor disorders of sleep, characterized by an irresistible urge to move the limbs. *Sleep apnea* is the cessation of airflow through the nose and mouth, which usually lasts for at least ten seconds. Changes in behavior may be the only treatment for patients with mild sleep apnea. These changes include weight loss and eliminating alcohol and sedatives. Proper bed positioning during sleep can also help.[25]

PATHOLOGY OF PAIN AT THE MOLECULAR LEVEL

For pain patients and health care professionals to develop accurate and effective approaches, the pathology of pain can be studied extensively in molecular detail.[26] A molecule is actually "the smallest identifiable unit into which a pure substance can be divided and still retain the composition and chemical properties of that substance."[27] Common examples would be oxygen (O_2) which has one element and water (H_2O) which has multiple elements.

N-methyl-D-aspartate Activation

Activation of *N-methyl-D-aspartate* (NMDA) receptors would allow calcium ions (Ca^{2+}) entry, which in turn activates calcium-sensitive intracellular signal cascades that lead to the combination of the NMDA receptor and other receptor-ion channels with *phosphoric acid*, instigating extended increases in the excitability of spinal cord neurons.[28]

Since the cell properties of the magnesium ion (Mg^{2+}) are unique, generally NMDA receptors are inactive under normal conditions. As a result, synapses containing only NMDA receptors are called silent synapses. Research showed the presence of silent synapses among sensory fibers in dorsal horn neurons.[29] Moreover, *5-hydroxytryptamine* (5-HT), a neurotransmitter with a crucial role in pain pathology, transforms inactive *glutamatergic* (pertaining to the behavior of glutamate, a salt molecule) synapses into useful ones. The basic way this conversion occurs is (1) 5-HT induced *protein kinase-C* activation, (2) *a-amino-3-hydroxy-5-methyl-4-isoxazolepropionic acid receptor* (AMPA) activation, (3) PDZ interactions, and (4) the addition of AMPA receptors. PDZ stands for *post synaptic density protein, drosophila tumor suppressor*, and *zonula occludens protein*. [30]

Opioid Receptors

Mu, *delta*, and *kappa* are different types of opioid receptors. The endorphinergic pain modulatory pathways are represented by multiple *endogenous ligands* (binding molecules) and the opioid receptors. Endorphins are visible in the periphery, on nerve endings, immune-related cells and other tissues, and generally circulate in the central nervous system (CNS). They are involved in many neuroregulatory processes apart from pain control, including the stress and motor responses.

Depolarization

Depolarization involves an intricate neurochemistry where molecules produced by tissues, inflammatory cells, and the neuron itself, influence transduction. As depolarization takes place, the transmission of information continues nearest to the axon and spinal cord and then on to upper centers. Complex systems that modulate this input exist on all levels of the neuraxis and are greatly characterized in the spinal cord. Transmission across the first central synapse may be influenced by activity in the *afferent* (toward the brain and spinal cord) pathway and modulatory neural pathways that originate segmentally or *supraspinally* (above the spine). Further modulation results from processes initiated by *glial cells* ("glue" cells that protect the nervous system).[31] The molecular chemistry of these processes involves an amazing array of compounds, including endorphins, neurokinins, prostaglandins, biogenic amines, GABA, neurotensin, cannabinoids, purines, and others.

Anterior Cingulated Cortex

The *anterior cingulated cortex* (ACC) neurons react to nociceptive stimuli (chapter 4), and movement within the ACC is related to the discomfort of somatosensory stimuli.[32] Electrical and chemical activation of the ACC leads to sensitization to heat or shock in animals, whereas blocking *cyclic adenosine monophosphate* (CAMP) inhibits pain.[33]

Neural activity activated by injury boosts the release of glutamate at the ACC synapse. This leads to an increase in postsynaptic calcium in the spine. Calcium attaches to *calcium/calmodulin-dependent protein kinase* (CaMK), leading to the activation of calcium-stimulated pain pathways. Activation of CaMK, a molecule which is mainly produced in the nucleus of the neuron, generates *CaMK-dependent CREB*. Together with other premature genes, *CAMP response element binding proteins* (CREBs) set off targets known to cause long-term changes in synaptic make-up and hence, pain function. Upcoming studies are required to map pathological pain pathways that enhance the maintenance of long term potentiation (LTP), plus late-phase LTP, in the ACC.[34]

Activated *microgliae* also increase the synthesis and emission of the following during pain:

- A range of cytokines and chemokines;
- Interleukin-1β (IL-1β);
- Interleukin-6 (IL-6);
- Prostaglandin E2;
- Tumor necrosis factor (TNF) alpha; and
- Nitric oxide.

PATHOLOGY OF PAIN AT THE CELL AND TISSUE LEVELS

The cell is the fundamental structural and functional unit of the pain patient's body. The body is composed of billions of cells. The brain and spinal cord cells include neurons and glial cells. Neurons are cells that send and receive electro-chemical signals to and from the brain and nervous system. Glial cells, or glia, are supportive cells that provide protection for the neurons (see below). Neurons vary in structure but they all carry *electro-chemical* nerve signals. Most cells are replaced with new ones after painful damage, but neurons are not.[35]

Nociceptive Neurons

Pain can be branded as "nociceptive" when it is due to the ongoing activation of the nociceptive system by tissue injury. The nociceptors are responsible for the detection of painful stimuli such as temperature, mechanical force, acidity, and tissue inflammation. When a pathological disorder ensues, nociceptors conduct electrical signals to the spinal cord via the sodium channels, which will trigger neurotransmitters to activate nerve cells in the brain where the sensation of pain is realized. Although *neuroplastic* (brain versatility) alterations such as underlying tissue sensitization are involved, nociceptive pain is presumed to transpire as an effect of the activation of the nociceptive system by irritating stimuli, a process that involves transduction, transmission, modulation, and perception of pain at the cell and tissue level.[36]

Tissue injury triggers afferent neurons—namely nociceptors, which are small-diameter afferent neurons—that react to pain and are found in skin, muscles, joints, and some visceral tissues. These fibers have specific receptors that may be responsible for irritating mechanical, chemical, or thermal stimuli that often cause pain.[37] Nociceptive afferent neurons are wide ranging. Most neurons are "silent." They're only active when stimuli of sufficient strength or quantity invade. Some neurons only respond to one type of stimulus, such as heat, but most respond to several different forms of sensory stimulation. Research regarding various types of nociceptors to disease states, or to possible therapeutic targets, is still at a nascent stage.[38]

Somatic and Visceral Pain

Nociceptive pain may be chronic or acute. It may mainly entail damage to somatic or visceral tissues. Somatic pain is caused by constant activation of nociceptors stimulating nerves in the bones, joints, muscles, and connective tissues. Somatic pain is often described as an aching, squeezing, throbbing, and stabbing pain experience and is often associated with a lesion. The pain coming from stimulation of afferent receptors in the viscera is called *visceral pain* and is usually described as constricting and gnawing with varying intensity. Nociceptive pain of any kind can be "referred" (i.e., the pain is felt somewhere other than the site of injury), and some referral patterns are medically significant. For example, an injury to the hip joint may pertain to the knee, while bile duct clotting may create pain closer to the right shoulder blade. Nociceptive pain may pertain to acute or chronic inflammation. The functioning of inflammation is often difficult to understand. Moreover, the prostaglandins (hormonelike compounds that have regulating properties) produced by injured tissues may increase the nociceptive response to irritation by lowering the threshold to noxious stimuli.[39]

Astrocytes

The knowledge about pathological pain has developed from *neuronal* mechanisms to *neuroglial* interactions. Mainly, *astrocytes* (star-shaped nerve cells) and microglia serve as potential modulators of pain by discharging cytokines and chemokines. Astrocytes and microglia have dissimilar roles in relation to pain pathology but they do have some overlapping functions in mediating CNS natural immune response. Astrocytes and microglia are stimulated in neuropathic pain, and their activation leads to pro-inflammatory responses with pathological effects, such as nerve hyperexcitability, neurotoxicity, and chronic inflammation.[40]

Glial Cells

Glial cells provide support functions for nerve cells involved in pain. Ninety percent of brain cells are composed of glial cells. The different glial cells carry out several important functions, including: (1) digestion of components of dead neurons, (2) manufacturing myelin for neurons, and (3) physical and nutritional maintenance of neurons. These cells play important roles in transmitting pain reception.[41]

Microgliae

Microgliae act as primary immune defense barriers of the central nervous system. These cells are (1) scattered throughout the brain and spinal cord, and (2) are highly sensitive to any changes in the environment. Due to evidence that microglia play an important part in pain modulation, specialists are now aiming to study them and their related signaling molecules in hopes of better pain control. This will be beneficial to pain patients due the fewer number of side effects involved. Some *immunosuppressive* (inhibiting over-responsiveness of the immune system) compounds are being generated to ease microglial activation and inflammation and have been confirmed to be effective in lab animals.[42]

Microgliae are the existing macrophages and major immune-responsive cells in the central nervous system.[43] They are equally scattered in the brain. Presently, there isn't much information about the function of inactive microglia under regular conditions, but it was discovered that inactive microglia have vastly active processes and survey the microenvironment in the brain.[44] In pathological conditions, these cells are stimulated and produce movements related to chemical agents and defend the body by destructing foreign matter.[45] An inactive microglia quickly transforms into an activated state in the following:

- Host defense against infectious organisms;
- Trauma;
- Autoimmune inflammation;
- Neurodegeneration;
- Ischemia; and
- Neuropathic pain.[46]

Changes in morphology, up-regulation of immune surface antigens, and the creation of cytotoxic or neurotrophic molecules is accompanied by activation of microglia.[47] In neuropathic pain conditions, microglial creation in the spinal dorsal horn has been established by at least three different methods. Initially, the structure of microglia transforms from "dormant" states, which have thin and branched processes, to "activated" states, which is pathologically manifested with *hypertrophy*. The morphological change is also associated with proliferation or microgliosis.[48]

Nerve Axons

Painful injury to a peripheral nerve axon can result in an abnormal nerve structure. The damaged axon may develop multiple nerve sprouts, which may form *neuromas* (nerve cell tumors). The nerve sprouts, including these growing neuromas, can generate spontaneous activity that intensifies several weeks after injury. The heightened sensitivity: (1) is associated with a change in sodium receptor concentration and other cell and tissue processes, and (2) can take place at spots of *demyelination* (when the protective cover is removed) or nerve fiber injury. These damaged areas are more insightful to physical stimuli, which is clinically associated with tenderness and the manifestation of Tinel's sign (i.e., pain or tingling when the area over a nerve is tapped). Atypical connections may develop between nerve sprouts or demyelinated axons in the area of the nerve injury, allowing "crosstalk" between somatic or sympathetic efferent nerves and nociceptors in the long run. Dorsal root fibers may also grow following injury to peripheral nerves.

Peripheral Nerve Pain

Other pathological changes occur in peripheral nerves that are related to pain and yet are poorly characterized. *Anterograde* (forward) and *retrograde* (backward) transport of compounds may shift, and chemical messages received in neurons may turn on specific genes. Some of these changes in structure and function produce peripheral sensitization, which may be connected to a lower pain threshold or a development in receptive fields. In contrast to the still underdeveloped understanding of the mechanisms of peripheral-generated pain, there is almost no information about the processes that induce or sustain centrally-generated pain syndromes. Functional neuroimaging has demonstrated the extraordinary neuroplasticity of the brain in the setting of a neuropathic pain, such as phantom pain, but the mechanism responsible is still largely unknown.[49]

ANALYSIS

The pathology of pain has been studied, researched, and experimented for centuries. Even now, specialists are finding new ways to understand pain pathology in its entirety. Furthermore: molecules, cells, and tissues at the pathological level are explored by pain experts in hopes of finding more avenues for treatment.

9

DIAGNOSTICS OF PAIN

When it comes to diagnosis, it is important to understand that pain is a natural, organic occurrence without which a person could not survive. However, with pain that is acute or severe or becomes chronic, there is no advantage involved. Pain should therefore be transitory, lasting only until the harmful stimuli are completely removed or the original damage or pathology has recovered.[1] As such, pain is a symptom of a medical problem, and thus it is crucial to diagnose. Knowing the time of onset, location, and intensity of the pain, as well as the pattern of occurrences, such as continuous or intermittent and exacerbating, will assist the examining doctor to precisely diagnose the pain.[2] Even though pain is a part of life, doctors and other professional caregivers have many methods for reducing the harshness of the pain.[3]

Pain is diagnostically useful for a number of reasons. These reasons include alerting pain patients that something isn't physiologically correct with their body. From a diagnostic standpoint, pain is a "good thing" because it warns patients of impending damage. For instance, pain may alert someone about structural damage in the spine.[4] Pain itself can also be diagnostically—to a certain extent—a sign of infection, such as an abscess. In addition, pain can warn a person who has had previous surgeries; the reoccurring pain then become a warning sign signaling that something may have changed or slipped. It may also indicate that a new fracture has occurred.[5]

INTRODUCTION TO DIAGNOSING PAIN

This section pertains to the diagnosis of painful disorders and the proper recognition of painful signs by professional caregivers. Pain is a part of everyone's life and therefore care must often be taken to not make it go away completely in the diagnosis and treatment of both chronic *and* acute pain.[6] The major objective of diagnosing generalized pain is to examine the patient over the course of a given period of time to see if the pain is getting worse or if it goes away on its own, which therefore informs the diagnosis and indicates how to proceed.[7]

Chronic pain originates in social and personal norms. Since the source of pain is frequently elusive in many ways, techniques for diagnosis tend to look at the purpose of the pain.[8] Diagnostics also tend to get separated into those that depend on mechanical, chemical, and nerve-related reactions.[9]

It is important to be able to diagnose pain properly in order to treat it the right way. The question as to why a patient's pain care is not working cannot be addressed if the diagnosis of pain is erroneous. This is made more challenging because pain doesn't have any objective biological markers—groans, moaning, and such cannot necessarily be taken as definitive signs of pain. Thus the subjectivity of pain presents barriers to communicating the pain felt by the sufferer.

Surveying the ways to diagnose the type of pain felt by the patient and its intensity, one comes to a single conclusion: it is the patient who knows what he or she is feeling and experiencing, and the caregiver needs to take the patient's word for it. The one suffering is the most reliable source of information regarding the intensity, duration, onset, and aggravating factors of the discomfort experienced, and what relieves it. Therefore, trust between the sufferer and the health care provider is essential to properly diagnose pain.

THREE PRIMARY AGENTS OF DIAGNOSIS

First Agent: The Doctor

To the general public, a "doctor" is a person with clinical expertise and medical knowledge. However, doctors in the field of medicine specialize in different medical subfields, such as pain diagnosis, pediatric diseases, and surgery, among many other fields. When people experience sickness, physicians investigate to discover possible causes as well as the treatment required. They examine patients, ask them to describe their health problems, and carry out tests to diagnose the problem.[10] They also administer medicine to patients as well as provide advice on diet, exercise, and sleep schedules.[11]

Family physicians and general medical practitioners are usually the first doctors visited by patients who have a painful condition. These doctors attend to common problems of illness and refer the patient to other doctors who specialize in specific types of health issues. For instance, internists pay attention to internal organs. *Pediatricians* focus on care for young children as well as babies

Second Agent: The Pain Patient

A patient is any individual who seeks medical care services from the physician or other professional caregiver. These patients seek medical attention for diagnosis as well as treatment. Pain patients can be treated in two different settings: *outpatient* or *inpatient*. An outpatient is a pain patient who is hospitalized for less than twenty-four hours after a medical issue is diagnosed. The treatment provided in this mode of medical attention is known as *ambulatory care*. An inpatient is a patient admitted to the hospital and stays overnight or for an indefinite time. The hospital stay can run for several days or weeks. The treatment administered in this fashion is known as *inpatient care*.[12]

Ideally, when a person experiences pain or any other type of illness and it remains unresolved, he or she considers visiting a doctor. However, some may feel stigmatized when asking for diagnostic help. Stigmatization may cause pain patients to shy away from seeking medical attention, hindering the diagnostic process as well as worsening the overall level of pain, since most pain or illness exists because of weakened tissue (chapter 8). If the patient has shoulder pain, for example, then some painful tissues in the body need to be strengthened. Therefore, medical attention is essential to stimulate healing as well as strengthening of the affected tissues. But the treatment for pain is not universal. Some patients depend on pain killers, while others seek the assistance of doctors simply to certify that they are well and have only a minor temporary problem.[13]

Third Agent: Imaging Technology

Imaging technology is used to produce, preserve, or reproduce images as part of the diagnostic process of painful medical conditions. There are several different kinds of diagnostic imaging technologies and techniques available to assist doctors in diagnosing the injury that is responsible for the pain.[14] The technology involves the use of X-rays, which are electromagnetic radiations that create shadows of the structure of an object upon passing through it. X-rays penetrate the skin tissue as well as other soft tissues and form a shadow-gram of the bones within the body of the patient, which assists doctors as a diagnostic tool. The X-ray imaging test allows doctors to look at bony structures inside the body of the patient without surgery. The results of the X-ray films are used by doctors to spot the cause as well as the degree of the injury causing pain and to develop a treatment program. In addition, imaging technology also uses infrared imaging, ultra-sound detection, *electro-optical* sensors, as well as electron microscope and imagery analysis.[15] Functional magnetic resource imaging (MRI) allows the diagnosing specialist to look at brain activity and indicates whether a patient is in pain.

Three Agents in Unison

Before diagnosing generalized pain in its totality, it is significant to know different facts about pain. The key factor to always keep in mind is that the pain might be exactly what the individual going through states it is, occurring where and when the patient describes it.[16] If an individual can communicate his pain, it will most likely be simple to relay it to a pain physician. When the individual cannot communicate what he or she is experiencing, it may be tougher to evaluate the discomfort, but it is still possible. To do this, the assessor must be aware of the physical signs and symptoms that convey what the individual is feeling. Physical diagnosis for pain involves identifying the nature of the pain. Pain is subjective, but a quick overall assessment can illuminate relevant factors. Vital signs may suggest the presence of pain, usually with regard to breathing, heartbeat, and blood pressure.[17]

When the patient decides to visit the doctor because of the severity of the pain, the doctor performs a physical examination to develop a medical history of the patient. Information such as the location as well as the intensity of the pain, pain pattern, what relieves it as well as what makes it worse are given to the doctor by the patient. The doctor also asks how the pain affects the proper functioning of the individual and seeks information about the past medical conditions of the patient.[18]

For diagnostic purposes, it is important for the pain patient to be honest when discussing the present and past medical history with the doctor. This information helps physicians plan the treatment program as well as select any appropriate drugs. If the pain is originating from an internal source and seems to be severe, the doctor will order the patient to be examined with imaging techniques such as X-ray, ultrasound, magnetic resonance imaging (MRI), computed tomography (CT) scans, or bone scans.[19] In some instances, imaging as well as lab tests are carried on to help interrelate the conditions of pain with the symptoms given by the patient. The imaging tests that the doctor may order depend on the location of the pain. For example, X-rays are used for imaging bones and teeth, MRIs are used for imaging soft tissue.[20]

While the tests can be revealing, doctors do not rely on them exclusively as diagnostic tools. Sometimes the examination results (as well as medical history) signal the need for advanced testing.[21] It is essential to note that physical examination as well as lab tests are meant to indicate the normal as well as abnormal manifestations of pain. The doctor will then compare signs as well as symptoms with the result of the examination and lab tests to come up with an accurate diagnosis. However, caregivers sometimes do not find a clear anatomical cause of the pain in the examined region of the body, and, conversely, imaging studies may disclose an internal stress for which the patient might not experience any pain.[22]

MISDIAGNOSIS

Misdiagnosis is prevalent enough for pain sufferers to be concerned that possible treatments they require will not be applied. Most empirical studies on diagnosis indicate that 30 percent of cases are misdiagnosed.[23] If a patient continues to experience symptoms despite medication, then the diagnosis could be incorrect.

Several factors can lead to misdiagnosis of patients' conditions. For example, misdiagnosis may occur if the symptoms as well as other medical information of the patient or results of checkup tests are misinterpreted or wrongly dismissed. Also, a pain patient might supply incomplete or misleading information. Moreover, laboratory tests are not always foolproof and can be misleading without any fault of the doctor. Medical personnel are human beings and everyone makes mistakes. A misdiagnosis could be one that is missed, delayed, or inaccurate.

Missed Diagnosis

Diagnosis is said to be "missed" when particular signs or symptoms do not come to light or are ignored, leading to inaccurate or no treatment. For instance, a patient might be told that a small lump in his elbow is benign, only to discover later that it is in fact malignant. In some instances, a missed diagnosis is no different from incorrect diagnosis. Unfortunately, any pain patient can experience a missed diagnosis on occasion.[24]

Physicians use a sequence of questions designed to capture the relevant diagnostic information from the pain sufferer to obtain the possible cause as well as the extent of the pain. Possible diagnostic results range from neurologic conditions such as sciatica to *foraminal stenosis* (narrowing of the holes in the skull). If the symptoms are acute, the cause may be determined to be more life-threatening such as meningitis. Unfortunately, it is often more difficult to get an accurate "pain diagnosis" than a diagnosis for other medical problems.

Delayed Diagnosis

Delayed diagnosis is diagnosis of a medical situation that comes later than the ideal. The delay in diagnosing health issues is likely to result in more serious health complications or possibly even death because of the delay in proper treatment. Delayed or incorrect diagnosis of any painful medical condition can result in

- an incorrect form of medical therapy for the patient;
- failure to order indicated as well as essential diagnostic tests;
- misinterpretation of the results of medical tests; and
- incorrect tests being ordered.

Delayed diagnosis may preclude the possibility of necessary surgery or reduce treatment options, especially during critical health situations. problematic complications or even eventual incapacitation or death may result.[25]

Inaccurate Diagnosis

Inaccurate pain diagnosis occurs when the professional caregiver fails to correctly diagnose the medical condition of a patient, possibly because of inaccurate laboratory results. These lab results can include imaging as well as other types of test results. Inaccurate diagnosis also arises due to (1) instances of human error, such as contaminating or mixing samples or incorrectly reading imaging or other test results, (2) the use of improper procedures by the technician, as well as (3) use of faulty diagnostic equipment.[26]

Effects of Misdiagnosis on the Pain Patient

When misdiagnosis occurs, pain sufferers can be left with heavy medical expenses as well as the inescapable pain. Diagnosis is an essential stage of the pain treatment process, and if it is to be accurate the doctor has to have sufficient knowledge about the pain sufferer.

If a patient's pain is diagnosed as severe when it is in fact very minor, the error may result in the patient undergoing unnecessary medical procedures. As a consequence, the health of the pain patient is adversely affected and this may lead to a medical malpractice claim. Conversely, when a false negative diagnosis is given to a patient, it results in the disease or condition going undetected. This can cause deterioration of the patient's painful condition to the point that the pain will require advanced medical care. The condition may deteriorate to the point that even extensive intervention may not yield good results.[27]

In conjunction with persisting symptoms of the pain, misdiagnosed patients unfortunately also suffer increased stress and anxiety. It is worrisome when pain symptoms are not improving despite medical attention or when the illness has progressively worsened. Patients and family members may also be concerned because of lost income and increased costs in the prolonged treatment process.[28]

Consequences of receiving a misdiagnosis of pain can vary because different people have different immune responses. Sometimes no real harm is experienced, despite a condition being repeatedly misdiagnosed. On the other hand, missing or misdiagnosing pain from serious conditions such as meningitis can have devastating effects on the patient's quality of life or even cause death. Patients with misdiagnosed pain and those who eventually receive incorrect medical attention may also be forced to hire pain specialists, adding to medical costs.[29]

DIAGNOSING THE PSYCHOLOGICAL ASPECTS OF PAIN

The personal handling of the psychological aspects of pain will be covered in detail in chapter 26, but it is important to look at the *diagnostics* of the psychological ramifications of pain here. Since pain causes both mental and physical problems, it can be diagnostically considered both a psychological and physical issue.[30] Recently, there has been a growing recognition that acute pain and chronic pain need very different diagnostic approaches from a psychological standpoint. Acute pain is the warning sign to stop something that is likely to be harmful. Conversely, chronic pain is referred to as the alarm signal that keeps on "ringing" long after the original source of the pain has been addressed. This sort of pain can affect the attention as well as the emotional center of a person's brain. This is because chronic pain is a multidimensional health problem with both sensory as well as affective components. It is viewed by medical professionals as a *biopsychological* phenomenon in which biological, psychological, and social factors dynamically interact with each other. Therefore, it is essential for doctors to comprehend ("diagnose") the psychological factors in the case of chronic and disabling pain.

Approximately 60 percent of all patients diagnosed with chronic pain exhibit various levels of psychological distress.[31] A considerable proportion of patients with chronic pain are diagnosed with reactive disorders such as depression, anxiety and somatization, personality disorders, as well as various nonspecific issues. These nonspecific issues include intense emotion, anger, and loss of self-esteem. The high rate of reactive disorders diagnosed in patients with chronic pain, even though well acknowledged, is poorly understood. Therefore, psychological abnormalities, their diagnosis, and management are an essential part of interventional pain management. Psychological issues may significantly influence the diagnosis and prognosis as well as the outcome of treatment.[32]

Effective chronic pain diagnosis is more likely when doctors and other formal caregivers undergo additional training. Pain has long been recognized as a major symptom that is suitable to diagnose acute injury or illness. However, an injury may heal or a disease may subside and leave patients with undiagnosed chronic pain.

ANALYSIS

Pain patients and caregivers have a lot to do so as to come up with proper and accurate diagnostic procedures. Pain can sometimes present a diagnostic challenge for doctors since it involves a physical examination as well as diagnostic tests used for a myriad of other ailments. Lasting pain affects social behaviors as well as daily norms of the affected individuals. In this and in many other ways, pain presents accurate symptoms which are appropriate for diagnosing acute injuries or health problems. Pain diagnosis therefore requires a detailed history of previous painful disorders, if any, to be taken from the patient.

10

CAUSES OF PAIN

The English word *pain* originated from the Latin *poene*, which means "to punish." Yet pain does not always come from punishment; it comes from the perception of different stimuli leading to the feeling of pain. René Descartes proposed that the mind and body are separate parts of the human being and are connected by the *pineal gland*, which is the "seat of the soul." Even though Descartes's conception has been discredited, it has led to the study of different genres of pain. Thus, the cause of pain has either a physical or a mental basis, depending on the person, thanks to Descartes's theory.[1]

LIFESTYLE IN CONNECTION TO PAIN

The perception of pain is affected by various factors, including thoughts, emotions, and stress. A large part of pain can be exacerbated by stress, since stress is linked to the mind, while the mind in turn is linked to pain reception. It is all dependent on the way that a person classifies *what pain is*. Pain can be differentiated as two types: hyperactivity and immobility. Both these kinds of pain can greatly affect the lifestyle of a person, and with that in mind, the following sections present a deeper look into each, to further understand the overall causes of pain.

Hyperactivity

Hyperactivity-related pain usually occurs due to tissue injury. In fact, scientific reports suggest that hyperactivity-related pain occurs often in the muscles.[2] Even though just "being a really active person" does not itself lead to pain, the injuries resulting from hyperactivity can result in pain. Moreover, pain can originate from anxiety, stress, and other sources. This may then lead to different reactions in the body that, though not deadly, can be worrisome, since these might be underlying manifestations of pain that may be even worse than the pain currently being experienced. These manifestations include[3]

- increased respiratory rate;
- increased blood pressure;
- dilation of the pupils; and
- hyperventilation.

How can the above affect the lifestyle of a person? A person might experience *attention deficit hyperactivity disorder* (ADHD) disorder that leads to mental pain in the form of irritability, a feeling of restlessness, and depression in worse cases.

Immobility

With regard to the causes of pain, immobility is specifically a condition wherein the person is unable to move a part of the body due to accident or sickness. There are many sources of immobility; such sources include sports-related mishaps, vehicle accidents, stroke, and severe injury of a part of the body. This kind of pain usually affects the older generation, since they have less resilience against these conditions. Immobility is not a lethal condition, yet the person experiencing immobility can feel depressed due to inability to accomplish simple tasks such as walking about the house, going to the bathroom, or making meals. Some of the difficulties that the body may experience with immobility-related pain are[4]

- problems with using crutches or wheelchairs;
- severe pain whenever the injured part touches anything (e.g., an injured foot touching the ground);
- dependency due to inability to perform simple tasks; and
- side effects due to taking medications.

OPIOID-INDUCED HYPERALGESIA

Medications can be effective in treating the sickness they are prescribed for, but they often come with harmful side effects. Some medications cause pain for certain people. Some examples of these pain-inducing substances include prescription drugs and medications prescribed in the wrong dosages. Caution must be exercised in taking these kinds of medications, since they can be harmful to the pain patient's body. Ironically, sometimes pain medications themselves are the cause of pain. This is especially true for a class of drug called opioids, and while these prescription drugs come in various forms, they all have relatively the same mechanism of treating pain. Negligence on the part of the medical practitioner or abuse on the part of the patient may lead to undesirable situations. *Opioid-induced hyperalgesia* (OIH) is the paradoxical condition of opioid medications causing pain, a side effect of long-term taking of opioids for treatment of chronic pain. Opioids can be administered to a patient without the risk of addiction or dependency, yet they can eventually be a cause of pain that may complicate the treatment of the chronic pain that the patient is experiencing.

Tolerance versus Sensitization

Tolerance is a condition wherein a person taking medication grows familiar with the drug, resulting in a decrease in the desired effect of the drug, which may lead to increase in dosage. This increase then leads to overdose or other harm to the person. Sensitization to pain comes from increased dosage of opioids, which may lead to faulty operation of the nervous system—specifically, its transmission of pain.[5] Two types of sensitization can occur; the first is primary hyperalgesia wherein the peripheral nerves are the ones injured. The other is secondary hyperalgesia, which originates from the reception of the stimuli itself.

Sensitization is often synonymous with OIH, since the excessive intake of opioids for treatment of chronic pain may lead to pain from stimuli that were not previously painful to the person. Simply put, tolerance can be treated with increased dosage of the opioid, whereas sensitization can be treated with reduced dosage or eliminating the opioid.

Approaches to Opioid-Induced Hyperalgesia

There are three areas studied by medical experts involving body systems activated by OIH:

1. *Central glutaminergic system*: This system, when inhibited, activates NMDA (N methyl-D-aspartate) receptors in order to prevent the further development of OIH and tolerance in a person.[6]
2. *Spinal dynorphin*: The spinal dynorphin, in increased levels, releases spinal excitatory neuropeptides that in turn develop into OIH.
3. *Descending facilitation*: This prevents the increase in excitatory neuropeptides, thus preventing the development of OIH.[7]

There are two research approaches to OIH:

1. *Basic science*: Tests are conducted using rodents responsive to opioids, indicating that their pain thresholds are reduced when administered these drugs.[8]
2. *Clinical evidence*: Pain reduction tests conducted with patients that were detoxified from high-dose opioids.[9]

Treatment of chronic pain when opioids are involved can be rather difficult since both and tolerance can result. The question is how do we identify the main condition that the pain patient is facing? Different solutions for lack of success with the opioids may involve opioid rotation, reduction of dosage, or detoxification. Identification of the condition before further treatment is important, since tolerance and OIH have different treatment procedures. The clinician also faces the problem of distinguishing whether the pain that the patient is experiencing is due to OIH or the chronic pain the opioids are being used for.

Tolerance may be another cause for an increase in pain. OIH can be identified clinically by the changes in the pain threshold of the patient, as well as by the tolerance to the opioid. If the patient's tolerance to opioids is still high, an increase in dosage may relieve the patient's pain, but the patient could still be developing or facing a worsening OIH.[10]

When faced with a patient with chronic pain, the practitioner may include non-opioid medication in the patient's treatment. This helps to reduce the amount of opioid used, thereby reducing the possibility of contracting the side effects of the opioid and ultimately OIH, which could be a cause for the pain in the first place. Another strategy would be to rotate the type of opioid used in order to reduce the tendency to be dependent on a single form of opioid, which is more immediate when only a single type of opioid is administered. Other strategies include interventional pain management and behavioral management, both aiming to reduce the need for pharmacotherapy, thereby eliminating the use of opioids altogether. If the above options are unavailable or ill advised, the physician can then look to the following options for diagnosis and treatment of OIH:

- Increase dosage of the opioid and take note of changes in efficacy or tolerance.
- Reduce or eliminate opioid medication and take note of whether there is a change in pain threshold.
- Consider NMDA receptor antagonists (with limitation) for the pain patient.
- Use opioids that may mitigate OIH: This can be done with either *methadone* or *buprenorphine*, which both have the ability to prevent or reduce OIH, but buprenorphine can treat chronic pain and may even treat OIH.

As with all therapies, there are side effects that can't be prevented, no matter what. When treating a pain patient with opioids, there must be a backup plan in case complications such as tolerance, opioid dependence, addiction, and even OIH occur. The caregiver should also consider the possibility of OIH when the therapy fails. Most of all, the treatment of a patient with opioids should be initiated in a mutual agreement between the patient and the pain caregiver.

STRESS AS A CAUSE OF PAIN

While everyone will likely experience stress at times, some people are so used to living with stress that they don't feel pain from it or even identify stress at all. There are two different kinds of indicators of stress: physical and mental. A discussion of each of these kinds of stress reactions and their role as a cause of pain follows.

Physical Signs of Stress

Physical signs of stress show up in body organs and tissues in reaction to stressful conditions, and these reactions may lead to pain. Typically, there are two types of physical signs of stress: short term and a long term. Here are some physical reactions that occur with stress:[11]

- increased heart rate;
- increased sweating;
- cold extremities and cold skin;
- malaise (a "sickening" feeling);

- tense muscles;
- dry mouth;
- frequent urges to use the bathroom;
- fatigue, headaches, shortness of breath;
- changes in appetite;
- changes in sleeping habits;
- nervous responses such as nail biting, twitching, or other repetitive actions; and
- reduced immunity to sickness.

An example of chronic pain induced by stress is a headache. Severe cases of headache may lead to nausea, vomiting, and irritability. This kind of pain can originate from stressors such as an abusive conversation with a boss or a recollection of a traumatic event from the past. Severe physical conditions can also result from recurrent stress; some examples are cardiac arrest, stroke, and even death. Prevention of pain from stress is not possible since stress is part of everyone's life. Here are some ways to cope with physical stressors known to cause pain:[12]

- stress management therapy;
- taking medication prescribed by a doctor to relieve stress, such as painkillers and steroids; or
- as a last resort, the pain patient can undergo surgical procedures to block the nerves that cause the pain during highly stressful situations.

Mental Signs of Stress

Mental signs of stress appear when the mind and its capabilities of functioning properly are affected as a product of stress. Some of the short-term mental signs of stress that appear in patients are:[13]

- panic;
- interference with judgment resulting in bad decisions;
- feeling threatened by difficult situations;
- loss of enjoyment in an activity;
- difficulty in concentration;
- anxious or frustrated feelings;
- feelings of rejection.

Some long-term mental stress indicators are:

- successive anxiety/panic attacks;
- dependency on food, tobacco, alcohol, and/or drugs;
- confusion resulting in inability to make decisions;
- sudden mood swings;
- negligence in school, work, or personal hygiene; and
- phobias.

As well as severe psychological issues such as behavioral disorders, these reactions of the mind may lead to some mild physical pain problems such as toothache.[14] Other evidence has been found supporting pain caused specifically by mental stress.[15] One research project focused on how stress can affect the effectiveness of *cortisol* to regulate inflammatory response. Immune cells are activated by cortisol (a stress hormone) when there is inflammation. The inflammatory response to a virus may lead to a common cold, as it is the sign of the body fighting off the infection. The scientists found out that a prolonged stressful event can hinder the response of the immune cells to the signal of cortisol, and people affected by stress have the likelihood of developing a common cold or other sickness. Another experiment within the same study involved about eighty participants who were tested for their capabilities to regulate inflammatory responses before exposure to the virus. They were also monitored for the production of chemicals that aid the inflammation process. The tests showed that people with lesser capabilities of regulating inflammatory responses produced more chemicals when exposed to the virus.[16] These tests have proven that stress can be a source of physical diseases; thus, stress can also be an indirect source of pain.

CULTURAL, ENVIRONMENTAL, AND GENETIC FACTORS OF PAIN

There are several factors that can cause pain, including cultural, environmental and genetic elements. Definitions and other important details of each factor will be discussed in the following paragraphs.

Cultural Factors

Culture can affect a person's way of assessing pain. For example, a person who has a belief that walking on coal is a sacred ritual, may not feel any pain, whereas an individual who has a different belief may get hurt, not because the method of walking on coal is different for each person, but because the mind interprets what is and what is not "painful." In this case, walking on coal is not painful for the believer because that person's cultural beliefs are able to block the sensation, whereas the nonbeliever tends to focus on it. Medical practitioners also face cultural factors in determining how pain patients classify their pain and how they respond to painful situations. Cultural factors involved in assessing the etiology of pain are portrayed in the following five examples:[17]

- Stoic persons are the type that mask the pain and hide it from others, thereby giving the impression that they're strong enough to withstand the pain on their own.
- Expressivity would be the opposite case. Cultural subtypes with this characteristic tend to seek attention when in pain. Moaning or even crying, are also demonstrative of this group.
- Language barriers can pose a cultural factor since the patient and the caregiver may not fully understand each other, even while an interpreter is present.
- Cultural beliefs also have control on a person's reluctance to take certain medications. Some people do not believe in medication at all, and thus difficulty arises in finding the cause of the pain.
- Racism is a subcultural factor that can lead to improper treatment and pain management.

Different cultural factors can make finding the actual cause of a pain difficult. Therefore, the professional caregiver should always consider the above factors in the treatment for every pain patient.

Patients from different cultures use different cognitive frameworks to conceptualize and describe the pain they experience, making it difficult for a professional caregiver to unearth the true cause of the pain. Gaps in proper understanding of the patient's experience of pain may result from the failure to understand particular descriptive content. For example, a Native American patient may reference their "sacred number" to describe the level of pain being experienced, in contrast to the usual understanding of numbers in pain assessment, wherein the intensity of pain coincides with the progression of the numbers in a scale.[18] Patients from some cultures may reference or avoid lucky and unlucky numbers when rating their pain. A culture may have many different words for pain, each describing a particular type. For example, in the Tagalog language, words with different nuances differentiate (1) pain from general sickness (*sakit*), (2) burning or searing pain (*hapdi*), and (3) regular muscle or cramp-like pains (*kirot*).

Hispanic patients frequently describe pain as "suffering," while African American patients usually use the word "hurt" to describe pain.[19] They also employ different methods to cope with their pain once they have determined its cause: while Hispanic patients usually ignore their pain, African American patients tend to turn to distractions, prayers, and hope. Patients from cultures that value stoicism are less likely to complain of pain, or show signs of discomfort, for fear of being perceived as "weak" or of losing control. On the other hand, some patients will groan and scream with pain, as their cultural background has taught them to be expressive. Some cultures emphasize collective decision making, and people from these cultures tend not to seek treatment for their pain without first consulting family, friends, and spiritual or traditional leaders. Clearly, then, there are cultural gaps that must be bridged in order to assess the actual cause of pain in patients.[20]

However, language and cultural barriers are not enough to explain the glaring disparities between pain assessments received by the white majority population and minorities. It seems that in a clinical setting where the minority patient has not established a relationship with the medical practitioner, ethnic bias and stereotypes may influence or shift clinical decisions. These biases and stereotypes may influence the physician's perception of the true cause of the minority patient's pain. Also, nurses, physicians, and other health care providers may have certain convictions about how to properly react to the patient's pain that may cause misunderstandings that hinder the process of finding out the cause of the pain.[21]

Most physicians are advocates of equal medical opportunities for people of all cultural and ethnic groups. However, recent studies suggest that disparities are caused by implicitly held biases and preferences.[22] It is possible that an individual who strongly denies racist and prejudicial sentiments harbors biases that take the form of unacknowledged acceptance of negative characteristics and stereotypes associated with a particular group. Thus, a person may hold a certain conviction to pain in a "rule-based" (gauging pain based on logic or language) cognitive fashion, but will also hold beliefs associatively (gauging pain based on other constituents in the environment). In the clinical setting, medical practitioners are particularly prone to *cognitive overload*. Busy schedules, numerous patients, fatigue, and other factors may make the associative cognitive function dominate the rule-based cognitive function. The physician, due to cognitive overload and the need to process information quickly, may tend to think in terms of associative cognitive models.[23]

In the expanding world of medicine, it is important for pain patients and their caregivers to be sensitive to the specific needs of patients who belong to other ethnicities and cultural groups, and realize that race, language, and culture play a noteworthy role in medical care, especially the treatment of pain. When considering these needs, finding an accurate cause of pain is not a one-dimensional experience. As a subjective experience, pain is multidimensional, and its perception and interpretation is significantly influenced by the cultural and societal makeup of the one suffering from it, as well as the experts trying to figure out the underlying cause of it. Steps need to be taken by the current health care system to ensure that medical practitioners are made aware that racial and ethnic disparities do exist so that further steps can be taken to significantly reduce—if not eliminate—the broad gap between the pain assessments received by majority patients versus those received by patients belonging to minority groups.

Environmental Factors

Environment can exacerbate pain depending on how a person reacts to a certain event. Inadequate sleep, for example, because of too much light or noise in the room can intensify a person's chronic pain. Personal habits for coping with environmentally induced lack of sleep can include:[24]

- Keeping the body temperature cool or warm, depending on the weather;
- Self-distraction methods such as watching TV, reading books; and
- Avoiding daytime naps that disturb sleep patterns.

Some can experience muscle pain due to a sudden change in the environmental temperature. Strenuous daily routines and poor nutrition are also among the factors that cause muscle pain. Since nutrition is a general factor in experiencing pain, it is considered an environmental influence: the diet is dependent on the environment where food is produced, prepared, and consumed.[25] In addition, daily stress is normally a result of environmental factors around a person.

Genetic Factors

Genetic factors may affect pain tolerance. Research shows that hand dominancy can be an important feature affecting one's tolerance of pain. According to a 2009 Israeli study from the University of Haifa, right-handed people are more tolerant of pain than left-handed individuals.[26] Moreover, studies have been presented at a meeting of the

American Society of Anesthesiologists that surprisingly revealed that redheads have less pain tolerance as compared to people with other hair color.[27] This is due to the fact that a mutated gene causing their hair to become red, known as the *melanocortin-1 receptor*, also belongs to pain receptors in the brain, thus making redheads more sensitive to pain. Due to the complexity of pain, one can never accurately quantify whether part of the pain is caused by genetics psychological elements, or environmental factors. That said, genetic factors that "cause" pain are typically related to multiple genes. Here are some of the genetic factors that contribute to the pain experience of a person:[28]

- Gender difference is an example of a genetic cause of pain since females experience different kinds of pain that are not experienced by a male. Moreover, males have higher pain thresholds and thus can tolerate pain longer than their female counterparts.[29]
- Heredity of illness varies depending on the genes of a person. For example: siblings may have the same illness as their parents, or it may be that only one of them is genetically affected by the disease.
- Genetic factors also apply to two different persons undergoing the same medical procedure who report different *postoperative* (after surgery) pain levels.
- Inherited characteristics such as race, ethnicity, and personality type affect pain perception.
- Other factors influenced by genetic makeup include stress threshold, overall mood, and cognitive processes of the brain.

Genetic factors play an important role in differentiating pain perception of every individual. Knowledge of these factors may prove vital in the process of assessing the true cause of a person's pain. Though noted as different kinds of factors causing pain, genetic factors are also relevant for determining methods of pain relief.

ANALYSIS

The perception of pain can be traced to different sources beyond physical problems, including medications, beliefs, environment, psychological stress, and the genes of a person. Since each individual perceives pain differently, one of the duties of formal caregivers is to pinpoint the cause of it. Furthermore, it's of great importance that the cause of pain is known in order to prevent the development of pain into worse situations. Knowledge about the causes of pain may prevent pain itself, and experience in identifying the cause of pain will definitely increase the chances of successful pain care.

I I

DAMAGING EFFECTS

Many illnesses are accompanied by pain. As such, pain has an important preventative function in the human organism. Technically, pain is
an essential helper in understanding problems and averting further det-
riment of the organism.[1] As soon as pain becomes severe, intense, or,
nagging and chronic, it might pose considerable threat to one's existence, lead to depression, and affect quality of life in a damaging way.[2]
For instance, a severe headache might have damaging effects, utterly
disrupt one's everyday existence, inflict serious suffering upon the pain
patient, and have far-reaching implications for personal and social lifestyle.[3] There is no clear blueprint for studying *every single* damaging
effect of pain. Yet, to form a departure point and create a structure, this
chapter has been divided into three sections that in themselves represent general areas for identifying the damaging effects of pain: personal,
social, and economic.

PERSONAL IMPACTS OF PAIN

Pain is highly romanticized in popular culture. It is thought to be a great
source of inspiration for artists. In movies, heroic crime victims derive
their strength from it. And the motto "no pain, no gain" promises greater power through it. In many respects, the ideas people have about pain
share common features. Pain is in fact really a very damaging, but also a
very personal experience. There are scores of studies that prove this
argument.[4] Two different people may experience pain differently,
though suffering from the same type of injury. When it comes to personal experience of pain in real life, there is not much "romanticism" in

it. Pain may transform one's personal life in many unexpected, mostly negative ways; it may turn an individual from an effective and hard-working person into a disabled one, or from a person with a healthy desire for sex into a sexually unresponsive individual.[5] The social and economic damages of pain are explained later, but for now, one of the most personal segments of life, sexuality, will be investigated.

Pain and Sexuality

Psychological problems may be a substrate for physical pain during sex. In many instances, physical pain during sex might be a serious issue. It is indicative of gynecological disorders of the female reproductive system. Irrespective of the cause, the pain makes women sexually unresponsive. Sigmund Freud pioneered in studying the primacy of sex and the sexual drive.[6] Today it is taken for granted that sexual intercourse has one of the central roles in life; it is not only essential for reproduction, but also for keeping partners together as a functioning pair.[7] It is possible to say with a high degree of confidence that an irregular sex life will inevitably lead to strife in a marriage and, in the extreme, to its dissolution. A person in pain often has little desire for sexual contact. During illnesses or recovery periods, doctors sometimes warn: "No Sex!"[8] If a physician prohibits intercourse, the first thing the pain patient must do is discuss it with his or her partner to avoid damaging complications of the relationship.

A well-qualified caregiver is aware of the fact that it is always difficult, especially for a man, to stop to having intercourse. After a prolonged period of abstinence from sex, a man might find it difficult to react to sexual stimulation, or his reaction to sexual stimulation might change. Secondly, abstinence from sex can create stress and aggression, hamper functioning, and engender psychological damages. Thus, it is very important to consider alternatives to absolutely abstaining from sex. "Soft" sex—or intercourse that is not very intense and does not generate too much physical strain—is a reasonable practice in many instances. Research has shown that healthy intercourse can [9]

- reduce blood pressure;
- improve immunity;
- burn calories;
- improve heart health;
- develop self-esteem;
- lower chances of incontinence;
- gives a person better sleep; and

- cut pain threshold.

It is important that the pain patient discuss his or her sexual life with a doctor. In some instances the doctor might prohibit the patient from having sex "just in case," but there should be objective reasons for such a recommendation. In some cases, an individual seeking help from a pain doctor might be reluctant to discuss his or her sexual life with a doctor, but health should not be compromised for the sake of protecting privacy in this matter. Consulting with a doctor might help an individual to maintain sexual activity without compromising health or aggravating pain during sex. A caregiver has to advise and assist his patients in finding a healthy sexual lifestyle, since sex has a vital role in maintaining the psychological well-being of an individual.

The topics of pain and sexual effects have many inherent controversies. On one hand, there is sexual desire, which is rooted in human nature. On the other, there are religious and moral mores, as well as sociocultural dictums.[10] In essence, a sexual life may have a positive impact, on the pain patient, such as increased stamina or personal power.[11] In some cultures it also might not conform to an individual's sense of honor and purity.[12] All in all, the effects of a sex life for pain patients boils down to individual preferences and priorities.

SOCIAL DAMAGE FROM PAIN

Chronic pain is one of the underlying causes and contributors to psychological illnesses such as depression and anxiety.[13] Pain and depression in tandem create a vicious circle. In an attempt to understand better the social bearing of pain, a number of studies present the following correlation: pain causes depression and anxiety while depression and anxiety reinforce the pain.[14] As a result, the social life of an individual starts decaying in varying degrees. A deeper look into the social impacts of pain inevitably leads to discussion about painful, damaging effects of depression and anxiety.

Depression and Anxiety

From a social perspective, depressed persons often attempt to isolate themselves from the larger social milieu and develop social phobia. This entails much more than isolation of an individual from society, be it actively or passively. Research findings suggest it is important to medically and scientifically validate the damaging effects of pain to make it socially acceptable.[15] Absence of medical validation of pain leads to antipathy and caution by society. Since pain is not understood in entirety, its psychological factors may be misunderstood, and ultimately, people may ostracize and stigmatize the pain patient. Two important lessons follow from this observation: First, it is essential to clearly define pain and increase social awareness of it in order to have it socially accepted. Otherwise, the individual might be personally held accountable for the pain and suffering as well as considered weak, further excluding the patient from society. Second, misjudgment of pain by society re-creates the vicious circle of pain and depression, which means more and more pain for the individual and for society as a whole. Based on research data, the World Health Organization (WHO) argues that depression is one of the greatest sources of disability in the world.[16] The burden of depression (1) puts strain on an individual by limiting quality of life or imposing difficulties in carrying out everyday activities, and (2) entails enormous costs on the social and employment sectors.

Many visionaries and artists were labeled as mad people, yet in their cases, their individuality and uniqueness was ultimately valued, especially in hindsight as the benefits to society of the person's accomplishments came to be recognized. An ordinary member of society, however, is more likely to have no reprieve from being isolated from the larger social world, and their contributions at work and other social sectors never given a chance to be appreciated. A study conducted by WHO suggests that average person suffering from depression is likely to end up laid off from work and with a financial disaster.[17]

Suicidal Tendencies

Every year, about one million people commit suicide, which is yet another damaging effect of depression that may be caused by pain.[18] Failure to treat depression or inadequate treatment of it leads to complications such as development of suicidal tendencies. Surveys suggest that depression is one of the leading causes of death among teens.[19] Clinical research also shows that suicidal behavior is very common during the adolescence period, again due to the painful, damaging effects of depression.[20]

A number of factors are usually invoked in analyzing risk factors and explaining suicidal drive. Studies conducted by U.S. scientists maintain that pain damages the brain tissues of a child.[21] The longer a child is exposed to pain, the more damage it inflicts upon the youngster's brain. As a general rule, the younger the age, the more the child is vulnerable to the damage. Pain is a huge enough challenge for an adult, but for a child the suffering is manifold. It is vital to stop the pathological process from further progress in children, since long exposure of the brain to pain damages nerve cells and deters physical and psychological development. Thus, to prevent further deterioration of a child's health, it is imperative to use the appropriate pain medication. The problem is that it can be difficult to predict the effects of psychoactive medications. A number of studies have documented that the medications in themselves may lead to suicide, thus contributing to the already-damaging effects of pain.[22]

Differences in gender (females are more likely to commit suicide) and social standing are yet additional factors affecting rates and methods of self-inflicted death.[23] A case in point is the social upheaval in China in the 1980s, which led to changes in social roles. Clashes between the popular representation of freedom, right to choose one's personal life, and traditional mores led to gossip about improper sexual behavior of certain women. Inability to cope with the social pressure drove young women from rural areas to commit suicide.[24] The women were caught between the new and the traditional Chinese values.

Works of research also suggest that depression, known to be a damaging effect of pain, leads to lowering of self-esteem.[25] Therefore, a discussion of depression and suicide in relation to pain would be incomplete without inclusion of the situation in Japan. Depression and suicide are one of the most pressing social issues in Japanese society. Every year, more than 30,000 people commit suicide there.[26] Research from the University of Hiroshima has found a way to objectively diagnose the state of depression by blood analysis.[27] Until now, the only way to diagnose depression in treating patients was to study subjective experience. The investigators managed to detect a gene that is accountable for *brain-derived neurotropic factor* (BDNF). The research results were based on a blood sample analysis taken from two groups of people: healthy, and depressed. The analysis revealed that chemical reactions taking place in genes have strongly pronounced features. For the first time in the history of medical science, scientists managed to discover the protein that could highlight depression.[28]

Pain Affecting Culture

While the preceding chapter explored how cultural elements can cause pain, this section briefly discusses how pain in turn affects culture in a damaging way. Changing cultural perception of pain is oftentimes vital. In many cultures, stoicism is a commonly accepted norm of conduct, and to endure hardship without complaint is important for one's social standing.[29] Many people around the globe suffer from various forms of psychological illnesses and depression, yet some are reluctant to seek help because of certain cultural imperatives and painful social stigma.[30]

ECONOMIC DAMAGE FROM PAIN

The prevalence of pain makes it one of the most important problems in world economies. The financial burden of pain and depression in the U.S. alone is tens of billions of dollars.[31] Much of the burden is associated with loss of work productivity and reduced work performance. That said, it is important to discuss the damaging economic impacts of pain.

Fiscal damages associated with pain can be divided into two categories: direct and indirect costs. Direct costs are primarily the medical ones associated with the cost of treatment. Indirect costs include lost productivity and absenteeism from work due to sick leaves. There are also a number of other intangible costs, such as hampered concentration, low efficiency, and diminished ability to work in a productive way. It is estimated that with millions of people suffering from various forms of pain, the economic burden is worth at least $560 to $625 billion each year.[32]

Example

Due to the vast number of physically and mentally painful disorders existing today, the economic burden of all these conditions would be impossible to address here. Therefore, depression will be used as an example here. In the 1990s, the economic burden associated with depression was roughly $40 billion. Nowadays, it's estimated to be around $50 billion.[33] A study that observed individuals for forty years to examine the effects of psychological issues and their consequences on personal, social, and economic realms has determined that people suffering from depression have: (1) lower income as opposed to healthier counterparts, (2) do not have high educational achievements, and (3) often take sick days. The study also found lifetime economic loss for an individual with psychological problems is estimated at $300,000, and that people who suffer from depression are reluctant to get married and, on average, have a loss of $10,400 income by the age of fifty, which is a 35 percent decrease in lifetime income.[34]

Depression is a global issue. The situation in the United States in many respects is similar to the one in the UK. Pain and depression puts enormous strain on the British economy. Research suggests that indirect financial damage associated with the issue is far greater than the direct ones. A recent economic survey estimated that the cost is over £9 billion. Of the total, £370 million is associated with direct costs, while the rest comes from roughly one hundred million lost working days and around two thousand six hundred suicides due to depression.[35] It's no surprise that the National Health Service of UK (NHS-UK) has developed a similar program to that of the Japanese—with goals of effective treatment of depression to reverse social and economic costs.[36]

The Japanese government says that the economic burden of pain, depression and suicide of a Japanese national is $1 million per individual.[37] The suicides of 32,000 Japanese last year inflicted a fiscal damage of $32 billion to the Japanese economy due to the lost income and the cost of treatment of the people in pain. To counter the problem, the government of Japan might organize a special group of experts to develop a mental health intervention program. Such a program might give people access to effective ways of treating depression and other damaging psychological problems connected to pain. Some might consider this a cynical and a rather commercial proposal, but the main argument behind such an initiative is economic. Japan is also a good example of a culture where it is common for an individual not to complain about pain and to endure hardship silently. An individual asking for help could be stigmatized due to these cultural restraints. It is said that this is one of the primary reasons why psychotherapy is not very popular in Japan, as opposed to Europe and the United States. Doctors in Japan prefer to treat depression with medication, as opposed to alternative methods.[38]

As one can see, the damaging economic burden of pain and depression are about the same in all the case studies reviewed. Indirect workplace-associated costs present great damage to economies, yet the total share spent on treatment is increasing. The findings noted above suggest that no one is immune to the hampering effects of pain.

ANALYSIS

The objective of this chapter has been to present an overview of damaging personal, social, and economic impacts of pain. However, pain as such cannot be blamed for all of the world's problems. Rather, it is the externalities associated with it that complicate people's lives, increase tension in society, and inflict economic damage. Measures need to be taken for identification and elimination of painful disorders while they are in early stages of development because, untreated in the long run, the disorders have greater damaging effects on individuals and society as a whole. In summation, the damaging consequences of pain, such as (1) low self-esteem, (2) diminished academic performance at school, (3) social decline, (4) loss of productivity and absenteeism in the workplace, and (5) disruption of interpersonal relationships, can all be reduced if pain is resolved effectively by the right caregivers.

12

ROLE OF INTERNISTS AND FAMILY PRACTICE PHYSICIANS

In contemporary societies when a person experiences serious pain or has concerns about disease, he or she often meets with a physician. In many instances these visits lack a proper framework, and are usually left to the discretion of the doctor. This chapter will discuss this issue as it applies to internists and family practice physicians—the two major categories of primary care specialists in the United States. It will thus hopefully provide a way to ease the process of patient-physician interviews. The chapter will also include historical and educational backgrounds of medical specialties, and information on typical routines of physicians to provide a multilevel exploration.

INTERNISTS

Brief History

The concept of internal medicine as a method to treat pain and other medical conditions can be found in texts dating back to 400 BCE; referred to as *kayachikitsa*, it was part of Ayurveda, the ancient system of Indian medicine that encompasses multiple disciplines aiming to cure the diseased, reduce pain, preserve health, and prolong life.[1] The term *internal medicine* was derived from the German phrase *Innere Medizin* which was used in the 1880s to describe physicians that integrated laboratory research with patient care. At the beginning of the twentieth century, American doctors who completed their medical studies in Germany brought these practices to the United States.[2]

The first institutional appearance of internal medicine as a primary care specialty came about with the creation of the American Board of Internal Medicine (ABIM) in 1936 through the contributions of biologists, company administrators, businessmen, doctors, and scientists.[3] The vision of these founders was to institute a non-surgical, academic board of internal medicine that could competently provide the certification and intercommunication required by physicians practicing this newly "imported" branch of primary care. A strong trend for specialization made its way into the medical field during World War II, with an increasing number of funds allocated for medical research, and a growing number of physicians that placed their focus in the analytical study of pain and the human organism.

A primary division between general internists and sub-specialties of internal medicine was most evident at the beginning of the twentieth century because of scientists who involved themselves in laboratory research. This led to a boom in the 1940s and 1950s with increasing numbers of research and residency programs that allowed both clinical and academic physicians to share their findings.[4]

Education and Specialization

In the United States, the life of an internist involves extensive training and education. After the completion of a medical degree, graduates are expected to spend one or two years of supervised practice before they can be licensed. This is just about the time when they are exposed to pain patients whom they can treat as a working doctor, as long as supervision is present. Subsequently, they are expected to enroll in a training program for internal medicine, and, if desired, one of its sub-specialties. Only after this stage can a physician get certified by an organization responsible for the certification of trained internists. There currently are three organizations that certify internists in the United States:

- American Board of Internal Medicine (ABIM);
- American Osteopathic Board of Internal Medicine (AOBIM); and
- American Board of Physician Specialties (ABPS).

Internists who treat patients in pain may be classified as either general internists or specialists. General internists deal with all parts of the body and a broad range of diseases. They provide their services in ambulatory and inpatient settings, and they are experts in diagnosis, treating chronic diseases, promoting health, and preventing illness.[5]

Sub-specialists of internal medicine usually add two to three years to their medical residency training, or what is known as a fellowship, and they specialize in one of the core sub-specialties of internal medicine. We will look at each of these below.

Adolescent Medicine

Also known as *ephebiatrics*, this specialty is centered on providing support in the *psychobiological* (mind and body) and social development of adolescents. In addition to the training required to get a board certification in internal medicine, specialists in this field have to spend years learning about conditions that affect individuals in the age spectrum between thirteen and twenty-one years of age. Experts in adolescent medicine are trained to deal with a variety of medical and behavioral issues, and they can consult the pain patient on a variety of topics ranging from sexuality to growth and development.[6]

Allergy and Immunology

Solid clinical evidence proves that allergies are associated with pain.[7] An allergist-immunologist is prepared to handle a variety of inconsistencies affecting the human immune system, including allergy, which represents a peculiar condition where the immune system acquires sensitivity to particular substances and their presence in the digestive tract, the respiratory tract, or on the skin. Experts in this field mainly deal with asthma and other allergic conditions. The most commonly used test for determining allergens is a scratch exam, in which the physician punctures the patient in the forearm or back with very small quantities of the suspected allergens and then evaluates the reactions.[8]

Cardiology

This field deals with various disorders affecting the heart, such as congenital heart defects, heart failure, coronary artery disease, and valvular heart disease.[9] The residency program in cardiology is *years* long after medical school and it takes into consideration the diagnosis, treatment, identification, and research of all kinds of diseases and injuries affecting the heart.[10]

Endocrinology

With the emergence of hormonal imbalance, an *endocrinologist* is the specialist that is consulted. It takes years of additional training (on top of a medical degree and an internal medicine certification) to get into this field and it deals with various conditions such as diabetes, osteoporosis, infertility, obesity, hypertension, and *lipid* (fat) disorders.[11]

Gastroenterology

The focus of this medical specialty is the digestive tract. An internal medicine board certificate and a fellowship lasting from two to four years are required to practice in this field. Specialists in this category treat painful conditions such as gastrointestinal cancers, esophageal problems, gastro esophageal reflux disease (GERD), ulcer, Helicobacter pylori (a type of bacteria) infection, gallbladder bile duct diseases, and pancreatic disorders. Common tests used as part of the process of addressing gastrointestinal pain include colonoscopies and endoscopies.[12]

Geriatrics

Geriatrics is the one part of internal medicine that, like adolescent medicine, provides its services to individuals who fall into a certain age group. Much like all other specialties, geriatrics practice requires further training after the completion of a board certification in internal medicine. Physicians trained in geriatrics care for and treat elderly patients, so there are often issues regarding pain. Important practices include, but aren't limited to, (1) determining the effects of drugs on the patient's body, (2) making sure that the patient has appropriate familial and social support, (3) identifying the effects of past diseases on the patient, (4) helping choose a suitable environment and lifestyle for patients, and (5) curing the various disorders that affect elderly patients.[13]

Hematology

A derivative of the Greek terms *haima* and *logos*, hematology is the science that studies blood: that mysterious liquid substance that flows throughout the body to transport life-giving oxygen and other nutritive substances. The role of the hematologist is to deal, with dysfunctions related to blood and the structures that produce it.[14] Among hematologists' areas of expertise are [15]

- *hematinics* (these increase red blood cells);
- *immunosuppressants* (these prevent hyper-reactivity of the immune system);
- derivatives of blood;
- antithrombotic agents; and

- anticoagulants.

Infectious Disease

These specialists deal with viruses, bacteria, parasites, and fungi, which can all be spread to large numbers of people.[16] They are trained to treat infections of the sinuses, heart, brain, lungs, urinary tract, bowel, bones, and pelvic organs. Many experts in this field choose to focus on the *human immunodeficiency virus* (HIV), which is the main culprit for AIDS. Training in this specialty also includes a penetrating knowledge of antibiotics, immunology, and epidemiology.[17]

Nephrology

A nephrologist is an expert in the diagnosis and treatment of disorders related to the kidneys. After the completion of a basic medical education and a certificate in internal medicine, two to three years are required to complete a specialization in nephrology. Experts in this field can deal with a variety of painful renal conditions, such as kidney stones, chronic kidney disease (CKD), polycystic kidney disease (PKDs), and acute renal failure.

Oncology

Oncologists are specialists that deal with cancer. There are three main sub-branches of oncology: (1) medical oncology, dealing with the application of various types of chemotherapy to kill off cancerous cells; (2) radiation oncology, the use of high-energy X-rays to target affected cells; and (3) surgical oncology, involving the surgical removal and biopsy of cancerous tissues that may be actively causing pain. The role of these specialized internists consists in[18]

- proposing and explaining plans of treatment;
- caring for the cancer patient from the moment the diagnosis is made; and
- mitigating the pain and side effects developed during the period of treatment.

Pulmonology

An internist specializing in the lungs and pulmonary tracts is known as a *pulmonologist*. Training includes a minimum of two years besides a medical degree, and an internal medicine board certification. Experts in this field learn to approach a variety of chronic and acute pulmonary disorders by taking appropriate tests and working out suitable treatment plans.[19]

Rheumatology

Arthritis and other painful disorders involving the muscular and the skeletal body systems are usually confronted by a subspecialist of internal medicine known as a *rheumatologist*. These experts usually deal with painful problems affecting the joints, muscles, and bones. A fellowship program in rheumatology takes two to three years to complete. Conditions usually treated by these professionals may include osteoporosis, some cases of defective immune system, tendinitis, osteoarthritis, gout, and lupus—all of which can be painful. Diagnosis usually involves some physical tests and a review of the patient's history.[20]

Sports Medicine

Internists in this field specialize in treating musculoskeletal disorders affecting athletes and other physically active individuals. Specialization takes one to two years after the completion of all tertiary-level courses in medicine and a certification in internal medicine. Commonly treated painful injuries include ankle sprains, groin pulls, hamstring strains, shin splints, knee injuries, tennis elbow, and shoulder injuries. Although most professionals in this subspecialty choose to focus on treating painful sports-related conditions, some actually involve themselves in the prevention of injury and the conditioning of athletes to reach peak performance through the appropriate techniques, training regimens, and dietary guidelines.[21] Sports medicine doctors usually work with pain patients referred to them by general internists.

Special Characteristics

Internists, whether general or subspecialty, have a series of distinguishing characteristics that include the following:

- They treat patients in the context of their individuality.
- They have a thorough knowledge of the human body, and are capable of dealing with multiple painful disorders occurring at the same time.
- They only treat individuals who are above thirteen years of age.
- Relations with patients are usually regarding the onset of disease or the prevention of a particular illness.

- They know when to refer to appropriate specialists when a particular case of chronic pain goes beyond their expertise.

International Presence

Organizations such as the International Society of Internal Medicine (ISIM), the Royal Australasian College of Physicians (RACP), the European Federation of Internal Medicine (EFIM), and World Health Organization (WHO) have allowed for the emergence of global networks of internists, each located in different continents. These global networks, theorize how the specialties can adapt to cope with the ever-changing structure of society. They also allow for a far-reaching exchange of technologies, techniques, and knowledge that contribute to the ever-growing expansion of internal medicine.

Initial Appointments with Internists

Most specialized internists choose to work in a clinic that deals exclusively with their branch of internal medicine. Commonly, patients first need to consult a general internist and consider whether they need to go to a specialist or not. If it is determined that the patient needs a specialist, he or she will be referred to an appropriate practitioner. The most common conversations between an internist and a pain patient usually revolve around a detailed description of the patient's symptoms. An experienced internist is usually prepared to identify most painful disorders without having to order any laboratory tests, but the skill to know when it is appropriate to refer their patients to specialists also plays a very important role in the success of their endeavor.

FAMILY MEDICINE IN RELATION TO PAIN CARE

Brief History

The general practice of treating illness, or what is sometimes called family medicine due to the growing obsoleteness of the "general practitioner" in the United States, originated well before the establishment of the American Academy of Family Physicians (AAFP), previously known as the American Academy of General Practice (AAGP). The tendency of some physicians to maintain continuous and comprehensive relations with their patients led to the extension of the practice for the patients' family nucleus. In the mid 1960s concern over the declining number of generalists operating at the time provided the necessary foundations for the emergence of a unified organization that could maintain the various societal, political, and academic needs of the specialty. Recent attempts to strengthen the specialty have been made through projects such as the Future Family Medicine (FFM), an attempt to transform the specialty so that it might more efficiently meet the needs of its patients in the changing environment of the twenty-first century.

Education and Work

In the United States, family physicians are required to complete an accredited three-year family medicine residency before they may attend an examination to get a board certification, which is preferred by many hospitals and health plans. The exam needs to be renewed every seven to ten years, depending on the board.[22] Although family medicine residency programs may differ from university to university, the curricular orientation is very similar in that they all aim to develop general medical skills to be applied in the context of a community of patients that need to trust the physician(s) to treat their health-related issues by getting to know their environmental and familial contexts. This could involve, in spite of the fact that it's poorly advised in medical literature, the gradual emergence of a strong emotional rapport between the patient and physician. Family doctors are sometimes entwined in communal activities. Their role is to understand the societal contexts of their patients so to treat the whole person rather than separate maladies and diseases. Contrary to popular belief, this is one way by which family physicians do in fact "practice" holistic medicine.

Special Characteristics

Physicians under the category of family medicine are easily identified by some of their basic characteristics:

- They treat patients by taking into consideration their family and community.
- They specialize in the treatment and prevention of diseases among various members of a familiar and communal cycle.
- They can handle patients from gestation to death.
- They are involved in their patients' life and family, and usually maintain a good rapport whether a disease is present or not.
- They have good socialization skills.

International Presence

Family practice doesn't only exist in America. Although the AAFP is an internationally renowned family practice institution, other institutions such as (1) the South African Academy of Family Physicians (SAAFP), (2) Academy of Family Physicians of India (AFPI), (3) Portuguese Association of General and Family Medicine (APMGF), and (4) the World Organization of National Colleges, Academies and Academic Associations of General Practitioners/Family Physicians (WONCA) also play an important role in the global presence of physicians that focus on providing holistic, continuing care and assistance to their patients. The global presence of residency programs in family medicine opens up a range of possibilities to students wishing to extend their experience to specific cultural and environmental contexts academically as well as professionally.

Initial Appointments and Questions

Initial meetings with a family physician frequently occur at the onset of the birth of a child. Other instances might include couples that need consultation on their sexual life. Appropriate questions from pain patients should primarily focus on the reason of their presence and on an explanation of the approaches being proposed by the doctor as a solution to the problem. Physicians should be asking about the patient's medical history, family composition, and any question that might stimulate feedback about the proposed approach on how to confront the pain-related issues at hand.

Typical Session with a Family Physician

A meeting with a physician practicing family medicine usually includes the measurement of heart rate, blood pressure, and weight by a trained nurse, and the reporting of these measurements on a chart containing all the details known about the patient. This will be passed to the doctor as the patient enters the exam room to discuss his condition. Based on (1) this preliminary data, (2) the description of symptoms by the patient, and (3) the further tests that might be required to determine the patient's condition, the family physician might write a prescription, perform a small surgical operation, or refer the patient to a specialist that can better handle the case. An interesting trait of family medicine is that multiple members of the same family can actually visit the doctor and allow for a holistic approach to their problems.

ANALYSIS

It is often difficult to draw conclusions on an extensive topic such as medical specialties treating pain. Nevertheless, in order for the reader to gain a working knowledge on how to act in a medical context as a patient in pain, it is important that the role of each side be properly understood and identified by individuals who have developed chronic pain conditions that eventually require a specialist, or people who want to keep doctor-patient rapport at a personal level. Family medicine is a holistic (i.e., mind and body), community-based specialty of primary care best suited for family contexts, in cases where people of all ages might have a chance of contracting certain infectious diseases that can't be treated unless the whole family is taken into account, or situations where the age of the pain patient doesn't allow consultation with an internist.

13

ROLE OF PHYSICAL MEDICINE AND REHAB IN PAIN CARE

Physical medicine and rehabilitation (also known as rehabilitation medicine or *physiatry*) is a segment of medicine that restores function and quality of life to those who are impaired physically. Physiatrists, the physicians who've completed training in this field, are often called *rehab medicine specialists*. People with painful injuries to the tissues, muscles, nervous system, and bones can be treated and have their optimal functions restored by physiatrists.

INTRODUCTION TO PHYSICAL MEDICINE AND REHABILITATION

The term *physiatry* was first coined by Frank Krusen in the late 1930s. This specialty field expanded in reaction to the need for innovative recovery techniques for the vast number of hurt military personnel returning from World War II.[1] Nerves, muscles, and bones are the major concerns of rehabilitation physicians, who treat injuries or illnesses that affect how a person moves. A recovery physician's goal is to cure pain and increase overall performance without surgery. The physician first tries to figure out the source of the painful illness, and then develops a course of action that can be carried out by the sufferers themselves or by a health care group. This health care group may include other doctors and health care professionals, neurologists and physiotherapists. Physiatrists offer an appropriate course of action to stay as active as possible, given the patient's age.

CHAPTER 13

Scope of the Field

In essence, the physiatrist specializes in a branch of medicine that focuses on the diagnosis, treatment, and management of health problems
through utilizing physical means, effectively combining medications,
and physical therapy. The physiatrist usually focuses treatment on disorders of the musculoskeletal system, made up of the body's muscles,
bones, nerves, tendons, ligaments and their peripheral structures. The
rehabilitation aspect of this specialization targets the aspects of these
disorders that cause pain and interfere with normal functioning. Although physiatrists don't perform surgical procedures, their line of
treatment always begins with the end in mind. The aim of the treatment
plan is to enable patients to regain functional independence through
achieving a pain-free existence. This becomes the crux of everyday therapies in the implementation plan. After years of training, physiatrists
further hone their expertise by zeroing in on specific areas and forms of
treatment. While others focus on spine medicine, sports medicine, and
brain and spinal cord injuries, physiatrists take on the coordinating role
and continue to further their knowledge in other areas of this ever-
changing field.

Physiatry and rehabilitation combine pharmacological and non-pharmacological approaches in order to come up with a multifaceted plan to
address issues of injury. This approach includes the use of medications
while exploring the benefits of active and passive physical therapy
alongside massage therapy.[2] This approach also gives credence to the
power of the mind to manage pain through the inclusion of psychology
into the equation. Physiatrists and rehabilitation medicine practitioners
also often suggest the use of assistive devices and body braces to aid
patients in accomplishing activities of daily living. In effect, physiatrists
are often called to take on the role of the pain management specialist
(see chapter 14) because of their ability to see cases from a holistic
vantage point. Although this approach focuses on rehabilitation, the
physiatrist also solicits the expertise of various practitioners in the medical and allied health fields to achieve a truly sound and effective treatment plan.

Physical medicine and rehabilitation includes the management of
disorders and optimization of physical, pain-free function through the
combined use of

- flexible equipment and assistive devices;
- resistance and healing exercises;
- foot orthotics (braces);
- medications;

- movement and activity modification;
- prosthesis; and
- experimental exercising techniques.

Physical medicine and rehabilitation doctors may also execute *electrodiagnostics*, which are used to provide neurological system information for analysis regarding various neuromuscular conditions. A typical electrodiagnostic assessment conducted by physiatrists is hooked-wire electromyography (EMG). This nerve conduction study involves (1) electrical stimulation of peripheral nerves, (2) measurement of nerves' responses, including signal amplitude, (3) latency of onset, and (4) conduction velocity. Needle electrodes are advanced into the muscles to evaluate the electrical potential coming out from muscle fibers. Irregular electrical potentials, detected by EMG needles, indicate the presence of muscle fibers that have abnormal nerve supplies.

Musculoskeletal pain syndromes such as fibromyalgia, low back pain, and severe head injury, which are common conditions of amputation, spinal cord injury, and sports injury, are treated by physiatrists. Cardiopulmonary rehabilitation involves boosting functionality of heart and lungs. This is sometimes accomplished through a multidisciplinary strategy involving physical therapists, psychologists, and occupational therapists.

Physiatrists at a Glance

Types of Treatments Physiatrists Offer

Physiatrists provide a vast array of treatments. However, they don't do surgery except for very minor wound injuries (on occasion). They recommend medications, prosthetics, and assistive devices. They also recommend physical rehabilitation with cold and heat treatments, electrotherapies, massage, physiological traction and healing exercise, as well as work-related and speech treatments. Some physiatrists receive additional training in techniques to address pain, while some perform Botox treatments and *intrathecal* (brain and spine) medication administration to cure spasticity.[3]

Major Areas of Focus

A physiatrist is qualified to handle a variety of disorders and diseases, but practitioners will often focus on specific types of injuries. Because of the wide variety of conditions handled and the extensive characteristics of their training, physiatrists are uniquely positioned to adapt to new technology and changing trends in medical care. Areas of focus include the following:[4]

- Pain management: Examples include long-term pain approaches, *complex regional pain syndrome* (previously named *reflex sympathetic dystrophy*), severe back pain, arthritis, and carpal tunnel syndrome.
- Neurorehabilitation: Here there is specific focus on spinal cord impairment, brain injury, brain hemorrhage, multiple sclerosis, and Parkinson's disease.
- Musculoskeletal care: Topics of attention include osteoarthritis; osteoporosis or fragility of the bones; rheumatoid arthritis; fibromyalgia or long-term, body-wide pain; back pain; and sacroiliac joint impairment.
- Injuries associated with sports: Examples include stress-associated fractures, tendonitis, injury to the knee, *turf toe* (sprain of the toe joints, including the big toe), medial and lateral inflammation of the *epicondyle* (covers the end part of bones), *tenosynovitis* (a tendon inflammation), separation of *acromioclavicular joint* (one of the shoulder joints), tendonitis of the biceps, and concussions.
- Health care during the postoperative period: Examples include bone replacement, organ transplantations, assistive gadgets for left-ventricle, or cardiac or pulmonary rehabilitation.
- Pediatric disorders: Examples include motor nerve dysfunction, muscle weakness, and loss of muscle tissue, developmental or congenital disorders, or Down syndrome.
- Distinct rehabilitation: Examples include stress-reduction (music, dance, vocals), cancer of various organs, cardiac impairments, pulmonary diseases, pelvic pain, or palliative care.

Standard Treatments and Other Procedures

In an inpatient establishment, physiatrists offer general therapy similar to essential medication to maintain health care balance and deliver secondary protection of impairment. Physiatrists don't perform major surgery, but they have many stepwise approaches for analysis and therapy:[5]

- Electromyography (EMG): Entering fine needle electrodes into muscle tissue and monitoring muscle potentials when the muscular tissues are stimulated to help differentiate whether a weakness is due to muscle tissue or nerve malfunction (i.e., myopathy vs. neuropathy).

- Nerve conduction studies (NCS): Electrodes are used to monitor muscle and nerve feedbacks that are disseminated by electrical current. This test can help identify the location of a neurological system sore (radiculopathy, peripheral neuropathy, motor neuron impairment, or neuromuscular junction).
- Injections into peripheral joints: Injections are used for the diagnosis and treatment of bone and soft tissue impairments, which are common in rheumatologic, orthopedic and sports-associated disorders such as osteoarthritis of the knee, *tendinopathy* of the rotator cuff muscles, and *epicondylitis*.
- Spinal therapeutics: Diagnosis of and injections into the spine that are image-guided. These methods are being used as a non-surgical pain-relieving technique for back pain and radiculopathy.
- Point injections: For the treatments of trigger points, an adjunct such as lidocaine or dry needling, a technique similar to acupuncture, can be used.

Physiatry vs. Physical Therapy

Physiatrists and physiotherapists treat patients with the same types of circumstances. However, physiatrists are specialized doctors who have finished medical school, plus four years of residency training. A typical misconception regarding physiatrists is that they are the ones actually performing *all* therapies. In general, *physiotherapists* are qualified in the bone and joint pathology and musculoskeletal examination. They create a course of action and practical methods, including heat, cold, and *transcutaneous electrical nerve stimulation* (TENS). Physiatrists handle medical findings and suggest the treatments that physiotherapists will perform. Despite these variations, both therapists and physiatrists work together to ensure that pain sufferers are receiving appropriate therapy.[6]

The role of the physiatrist is to control a person's medical issues as they take part in the rehabilitation process. A physiatrist will evaluate the affected person and assure that the affected person is medically stable to get involved in therapies. Medical topics pertaining to recovery include pain control, the bowel and renal system, spasticity control, and disease education. A physiatrist will handle other comorbid conditions, high blood pressure, diabetes, coronary artery disease (CAD), and chronic obstructive pulmonary disease (COPD), to avoid further medical complications.[7]

PHYSICAL MEDICINE AND PAIN

Physical medicine is a division of medicine using an interdisciplinary strategy to work toward total well-being of individuals.[8] The typical physical medicine group involves doctors and other medical professionals, physiotherapists, therapists, and scientific health professionals.[9] Pain may be eliminated quickly once the underlying stress or pathology has been cured and is treated by one member of the team with medications such as pain killers and sometimes anxiety-reducing drugs. In case of long-lasting pain, however, the combined effort of all members of the team is required.[10]

When (1) an agonizing damage or pathology is resistant to therapy and persists, (2) discomfort continues after the damage or pathology has been cured, or (3) medical technology cannot recognize the cause of discomfort, the approach of physiatry is to reduce suffering. The pain management specialist's options for treating long-lasting pain, aside from obvious painkillers, include

- antidepressant drugs and anticonvulsants;
- interventional procedures;
- actual rehabilitation;
- workout;
- application of ice or heat; and
- psychological techniques, such as attitudinal treatment.

The psychological therapy approach is instrumental in increasing the quality of life for people who have a history of chronic pain conditions. Another focus of physical medicine and rehab is the potential of being able to discontinue pain medicines, and this is sometimes a sector of major emphasis. Physical rehabilitation is basically the process of regaining and reestablishing physical ability and functionality, so it can be used to handle anything from a simple ankle strain to helping a stroke survivor to walk, talk, and eat.

Physical Rehabilitation Process

The rehabilitation process varies from person to person, but a typical rehabilitation might progress as outlined below.

Physician Care: To Stabilize the Pain Patient's Condition

For severe accidents and health-related disorders such as stroke, injury to the brain, or multiple shocks, inpatient rehabilitation health care systems use an acute-care hospital accommodation. For accidents such as pains from minor stresses, strains and fractures, a visit to a doctor will be the first line of approach.

Inpatient Rehabilitation: To Restore the Ability and Recovery

At a rehabilitation facility center, pain patients receive various occupational, speech, physical, and recreational therapies. A team composed of therapists, physicians, and other health practitioners build and monitor a treatment plan to reach a specific goal.

Outpatient Rehab: Maintain and Improve the Methods

After discharge from an inpatient rehabilitation center, a pain patient has to be treated in an outpatient facility. Improving physical and mental function on an ongoing basis may include use of a fitness center or support group.

TYPICAL DAY FOR A PHYSIATRIST

A physiatrist's typical schedule varies widely from doctor to doctor depending on their specialization. Six to eight hours of examining and prescribing patients in an office-based environment is common. Also, there may be one or two visits to patients in the medical center or hospital. Physiatrists at times have to work very closely with the surgery department. Additionally, the doctor will also spend time with management responsibilities such as upgrading individual information. Physiatrists may also spend time on various research studies related to their specific expertise. Emphasis is given to theorizing methodologies as well as developing existing methods to get maximum output from their work.

Physiatrists are usually involved in a lot of problem solving and analysis, especially at the diagnostic stage. Upon determination of a suitable pain management and treatment plan, the physiatrist focuses on rehabilitation through providing opportunities for physical and occupational therapy, primarily concentrating on gross and fine motor skills. Apart from the usual active physical therapy activities, the physiatrist also facilitates passive physical therapy sessions that may include the use of ultrasound equipment to help alleviate pain. Injections may also be undertaken in the physiatrist's clinic, but this usually requires close coordination with other specialists because of the use of special medications. Focus on nonpharmacological approaches is usually preferred by most physiatrists and they revert to the use of pain medications and injections only when there is a pressing need to bring severe pain under control. Once the pain has become more manageable, the physiatrist can then encourage the patient to begin rehabilitation.[11]

APPOINTMENTS

A visit to a physiatrist may last only a very short time and what the doctor wants the patient to do may not be explained well. Often it is up to the patient to take measures to get the most out of the visit. It should be kept in mind that not all physiatrists suit all pain patients perfectly. Of utmost importance, is to focus on the goal for the appointment, whether be the need for a diagnosis, advice on coping with an existing condition, referral to a specialist, or a change in treatment. This goal will guide the patient's communication with the physiatrist, who will generally first listen to the pain patient's history and then perform a physical examination. If the pain sufferer feels any general health issues are relevant to the case, such as diet, weight, sleep, and so on, he or she must discuss them with the physiatrist. Patients can also find out what screening tests might be appropriate for their age, such as a mammogram or colonoscopy. It is important not to be embarrassed to discuss sensitive topics with the physical medicine specialist, as there is probably nothing the patient could say that an experienced physician would not have already heard.

Upon leaving the physiatrist's office, the patient should be clear about (1) what should or should not be done at home, (2) required approaches, (3) how to receive treatment, and (4) the length of time the treatment may go on. If the patient needs more information about his or her condition or treatment protocols, the doctor should be able to provide resource options such as the library, medical resource centers at hospitals, or other alternatives. Pain patients should feel comfortable entrusting their health to their physical medicine and rehab specialist.

Questions for the Patient

The first appointment with a physical medicine specialist is much like a visit with other physician. Although there are many similarities, the focus is on pain, the cause or contributing factors, and the pace at which the pain is corrected. Physiatrists perform a physical and neurological examination and review the pain sufferer's medical history, paying particular attention to his pain history. Factors the patient may be asked about include[12]

- pain rating on a scale from zero to ten;
- pattern of change during night and day;
- any instances that relieve the pain;
- the physical condition of the patient when the pain started;
- the consistency of the pain;
- trends of spread of the pain to other body parts;
- starting time of the pain;
- events that make the pain more severe;
- efficacy of measures that have been taken to reduce the pain; and
- instances of medicinal overdose.

Some physiatrists use an illustration of the front and back of the body to allow the individual with pain to point out where the problem lies, as well as to indicate pain propagation. The patient may or may not be requested to complete the form at each appointment. The appropriate analysis may include acquiring an X-ray, CT scan, or MRI to validate the cause of discomfort. When healing spine-related pain, other assessments such as discography, cuboid assessments, nerve system assessment (electromyography, sensor transmission studies), and *myelography* (spinal canal imaging) may be conducted. Some spinal injuries and treatments require participation by other professionals, including the patient's primary doctor, neurosurgeon, and professionals in[13]

- radiology;
- psychiatry;
- oncology;
- nursing; and
- related alternative health care.

In the case of spine-related pain, the physical medicine specialist might refer the patient to a neurosurgeon to determine if the pain necessitates back surgery.

Questions to ask the Physiatrist

Some sample questions are listed below that can serve as effective guidelines. Sometimes, it is helpful to write down particular questions to prepare for the visit to the physician. The answers may help the patient make informed decisions about treatment.[14] Questions about the physiatrist can include the following:

- Any board certification?
- Open to a second opinion?
- Fellowship trained?
- Are family members or friends allowed during visits?

A trip to the physiatrist should be a flow of interaction in both directions. The physician often has a lot of concerns, but it is also in the individual's interest to ask as many questions as is required to completely comprehend the situation. The first queries would probably be to find out the exact medical disorder the patient really has, what triggered the situation, and whether it can be verified. An individual in pain will also need to know if more assessments are required. He or she should ascertain (1) whether any planning is necessary for the checkup, (2) what the checkup requires, and (3) how long the additional assessments are and (4) what the outcomes of the assessments mean. During the visit, it is essential for the patient to let the physician know if he or she is confused by the details or if the physician is using too many medical terms. If the patient is disappointed with the physiatrist's analysis, it is within the patient's privilege to request a second opinion. Diagnostic topics for the physiatrist include

- severity or degree of illness and how it will affect personal and work life;
- the long-term and short-term prognoses;
- a source that is responsible for the painful condition;
- indications of symptoms worsening;
- whether an examination for a certain condition is needed;
- how the diagnosis can be confirmed;
- additional symptoms the pain sufferer should look for;
- how a specific painful condition can be determined;
- what specific tests will be included in diagnosing a specific painful condition and what the results will indicate; and
- the degree of safety and accuracy of the specific tests.

A pain physician, after verifying the tests, might then offer the affected person one or more treatments. These alternatives may range from drugs to natural techniques. The ultimate choice about what therapy to take is obviously the patient's. After being informed about treatment options, the patient may want to find out about each—such as where the treatment is available and how much time the treatment plan will take. Clearly, treatment plans vary for different people depending on their condition, thus even the expense of the treatment may influence which one is chosen in the end. Other factors that may influence the decision are what side effects or risks are associated with the treatment, and what the positives and negatives are of each remedy. Furthermore, the pain patient may want to know what will happen if he or she (1) refuses treatment, (2) delays the onset of treatment, or (3) fails to complete the full course of the treatment. If the treatment is complicated, the client may want the physiatrist to provide a written treatment plan.

Another important question to ask the doctor is whether the patient should avoid anything or should undertake any lifestyle changes during treatment. If the treatment causes unexpected or unwanted side effects or doesn't seem to be working, the pain sufferer should inform the doctor immediately so the latter can look into possibly changing the diagnosis or treatment. Questions regarding treatment should include:

- What are the treatment options for the patient?
- Where is the treatment available?
- Is any generic form available?
- What happens if a dose of drug is missed?
- Is there way of knowing whether the medication is working?
- What are the effects of delaying the treatment?
- What is the most common treatment plan for this kind of condition?
- What is the expense of the total treatment process?
- What side effects may the patient face?
- What should the patient do if any side effects occur?
- What are the associated risks to the treatment plan?
- How long is the treatment procedure?
- Is there any need for change of lifestyle?

The pain sufferer should be relaxed with the physiatrist. Asking questions is the best way to keep the interaction open and alive.

ANALYSIS

Physical medicine and rehabilitation are always evolving in medical science, providing pain patients with a vast array of new treatment plans and developing techniques and methods to serve more effectively. For

guaranteed effectiveness of the treatment of a pain patient, the physiatrist, patient, and laboratories are all necessary.

14

ROLE OF THE PAIN MANAGEMENT SPECIALIST

Pain management, also known as pain medicine or *algiatry*, is a branch of medicine utilizing an interdisciplinary method for reducing the suffering and enhancing the quality of life of individuals coping with pain.[1] A pain management specialist (PMS) is typically a physician who is board certified in pain management, whether or not he or she is a physiatrist. The role of the pain management specialist is pivotal in ensuring that holistic (mind and body) care is given to patients who are in need of highly personalized medical attention. Since this branch of medicine is extremely multifaceted, it requires a unique skill set. Apart from medical expertise, physicians who specialize in pain management need to have the aptitude to approach patients as individuals, taking into account the psychology that goes hand in hand with the physiology of the various aspects of pain. PMSs are also team players, recognizing the need for coordination among members of an interdisciplinary group of experts, all focusing on the common goal of achieving a better quality of life and level of functioning for patients who suffer from chronic pain.[2]

HOW PAIN MANAGEMENT SPECIALISTS CONTRIBUTE TO PATIENT CARE

Pain management as a clinical discipline puts significant focus on the holistic care of patients through ensuring that a comprehensive medical history is taken prior to the commencement of a more long-term plan.

Furthermore, PMSs are primarily focused on a patient's quality of life, treating individuals as a sum of multiple parts rather than just focusing on a particular part of the body that may have been identified as the source of pain. To achieve a holistic approach, PMSs are keen on formulating an accurate diagnosis. This can be achieved through establishing significant rapport with the patient. The PMS usually needs to go beyond the apparent, especially in cases where chronic pain is the chief complaint. The patient-doctor rapport established while going over patient history becomes a keystone in this professional relationship.

The involvement of several experts in the pain management team also ensures that a patient is provided with comprehensive care. For instance, PMSs may come from a variety of backgrounds such as physiatry (see chapter 13), physical therapy, neurology or psychiatry, anesthesiology, and interventional radiology.[3] The pain specialist may stand as the coordinating physician in the team, playing a vital role in keeping the treatment plans on track. The coordinating physician must also work toward keeping communication lines open to ensure that the patient's voice is given credence. Ultimately, care and treatment must be patient-centric.

Pain management specialists can guide patients toward finding an optimal combination of treatments and approaches that will cater to their dynamic and evolving needs. Many pain sufferers find consultation sessions frustrating and confusing because of the availability of numerous options that can be explored.[4] Patients need to feel "cared for" as they participate in the search for a pain management program that suits their unique and individual needs. The PMS becomes a fundamental point of contact even after patients find the approach that they agree with most. It is important to remember that this specialty is a process, and it involves "hand holding," especially for patients enduring severe pain. Pain management specialists also need to consider the level of commitment that goes into treating patients who suffer from chronic pain. Pain management plans can be very demanding in terms of time and resources invested by the patient, physicians, and caregivers. The desire to communicate and see the treatment plans through must come primarily from the pain management specialist.

DIFFERENCE IN APPROACHES

Pain management challenges experts to come up with combination therapies in the management of acute and chronic pain. Since the discipline is dynamic, there is no single field of health care that can be considered as the preferred approach. In fact, a multidisciplinary approach is considered optimal in pain management, and as such, many pain management specialists are *unofficial* members of a variety of disciplines, both in the medical field and its ancillary services. These disciplines include anesthesiology, interventional radiology, occupational and physical therapy, and even neurology and psychiatry. Expertise coming from these disciplines makes it possible to come up with a more elaborate pain management treatment plan for patients. Pain sufferers should also acknowledge that because of the wide array of options available, the process of determining a suitable approach integrated into a pain management treatment plan requires a lot of time and patience. It is imperative that patients seeking relief from acute and chronic pain work closely and cooperatively with health professionals until the best approach is established. All the hard work and time invested in seeking a suitable approach will be well worth it once improvement in quality of life and level of function are achieved.

Inpatient versus Outpatient Settings

Inpatient care is essentially extended to a patient admitted to a hospital, hospice, nursing home, or any care facility. The initial step in inpatient care requires a stringent multi-disciplinary evaluation to determine possible pain management approaches that may be undertaken. The patient's medical history, properly supported by medical records and actual X-ray films and MRIs, is obtained through proper dialogue between members of the clinical team and the patient or his next of kin. The pain management specialist's recommendations are made based on conclusions drawn from the collation of data, and these include whether inpatient care is indeed the best option. If it all leads to an inpatient pain rehabilitation program, patients are admitted into a care facility for a predetermined period of time and are advised to participate in the prescribed multidisciplinary regimen.

Inpatient care is also often provided to hospitalized patients experiencing pain as a result of their illness or the treatment or procedure they underwent to treat their primary illness. These procedures may have been necessary to treat the illness such as a surgical procedure, colonoscopy, endoscopy, intubation or even chemotherapy. Such necessary procedures may cause patients to experience pain. In instances such as these, inpatient care becomes a preferred approach.

Inpatient care also becomes necessary for pain sufferers who have already undergone a rehabilitation program but have shown little to no progress. Patients who have not managed to regain a significant amount of functional movement, despite undergoing an outpatient rehabilitation program, are also good candidates for inpatient care. Outpatient care, on the other hand, usually involves follow-up programs that support an established pain management and treatment plan. Comprehensive outpatient programs cater to (1) individuals who have completed an inpatient program, (2) clients who are able to function and perform activities of daily living with chronic pain, and (3) those seeking supportive therapy options to address their long-lasting pain. Outpatient care may be availed at a clinic, treatment facility, doctor's office, hospital or the patient's home, especially for those who have limited mobility and have difficulty traveling. Therefore, the PMS needs to "stay on top of everything" to ensure that everyone in the team carries out the aspects outlined in the pain treatment plans. Coordination is a key factor, and the PMS plays a major role in both inpatient and outpatient care scenarios.

QUESTIONS TO ASK THE PAIN MANAGEMENT SPECIALIST

It is important to recognize that pain management in all of its complexity tends to be extremely patient-centric. Individuals in pain should be open-minded when discussing their condition, needs, and apprehensions with their PMS or with the members of the pain rehabilitation team. Pain sufferers also need to be able to set their own expectations regarding the treatment based on the available resources of their chosen treatment center. Treatments in the management of pain tend to be quite varied, especially with the involvement of multiple disciplines. Therefore, when in dialogue with several pain management specialists, it is imperative to note differences in approaches and ask questions that will help lead the team and the patient toward the appropriate treatment plan.

When formulating questions to ask the PMS, the pain sufferer may also need to keep his or her own expectations in check. What are the goals and objectives for seeking treatment from a particular pain management clinic? Through managing expectations, the patient will be able to compare these with what the pain management clinic has to offer. Since information is now more widely available, the patient may also opt to do prior research to review existing therapies and modalities of treatment and then decide on an option based on personal preferences and needs.

Typically, there is some common ground among experiences offered by pain management clinics. Going through the different options can help patients formulate appropriate questions for each step along the way. Patients should consider preparing a list of questions to serve as a guide, while highlighting major points during the discussion. Clients are also encouraged to take notes during the initial and succeeding meetings or perhaps ask a companion to do this so as to be able to fully attend to what is being said.

Step 1: Evaluation and Diagnosis

It is imperative that patients ask about what evaluation and diagnostic procedures are utilized and followed by the team. Questions to ask at this stage could include the following:

- Who will conduct the medical history and physical exam?
- Who will be the coordinating physician? What is that person's specific area of specialization?
- Do I need to bring results of previous tests as well as other documentation? What specific paperwork do I need to bring?
- What sort of tests do I need to expect as part of the diagnostic procedure? Which of these are invasive and which are noninvasive?
- Will there be a need for imaging or lab tests?
- Will I be able to request a comprehensive summary of the assessment results?

Step 2: Referral to Other Doctors and Specialists

- Will there be other doctors and specialists in the team? What will be their role?
- What test results would merit the participation of other doctors and specialists?

Step 3: Determining a Treatment Plan

- How much involvement am I allowed to have as far as participating in the determination of my pain treatment plan is concerned?
- What invasive techniques are necessary in the treatment plan? What are the alternatives to these invasive techniques?

- What are the specifics of the pharmacological approach that will be used? What are the medications that might be prescribed? Are there any side effects that I need to watch out for?
- What are the specifics of the nonpharmacological approaches that will be used? Will the PMS consider alternative medicine options as well?
- Is there a need to enroll into an inpatient program or is it more beneficial to visit an outpatient clinic?
- What is the prognosis for the chosen treatment plan? What are the best and worst-case scenarios? What timelines are in place to gauge efficacy or failure of the treatment strategy?

Step 4: Getting into the Specifics

- What sort of preparations do I need to make in line with insurance requirements to be able to enroll in this pain management treatment?
- What is the usual waiting or observation time where I can measure the efficacy of the treatment plan? When is it fair to say that we can move on to an alternative treatment plan?
- What are your expectations of me as a patient in terms of the level of compliance to ensure the success of the treatment plan?
- What specific Current Procedural Terminology (CPT) codes related to pain management do I have to seek from a health insurance provider, if required?[5]
- How will this illness and its accompanying treatments affect my daily activities? Will my family be affected as well?
- What sort of preparations do I need to look at in case some complications or special needs arise from my illness or the treatment plan?

Ultimately, an honest dialogue is the key to achieving a treatment plan that will work. Patients seeking help are encouraged to be open about therapies and medications they have already tried in the past, with or without advice from a medical professional. This level of honesty is integral in building a working relationship that benefits all parties involved. The first consultation will set the tone of the patient's relationship with the pain management specialist handling the case. It will also give an initial indication of how comfortable he or she will feel about discussing other aspects of his painful condition during future visits. Devising the right questions to ask pain management specialists can help patients make more informed decisions in the long term. Patients also need to be proactive in making suggestions based on what they feel may be the best route to take to manage their pain effectively. However, the pain management specialist may or may not approve of suggestions from the pain patient.

QUESTIONS THE PMS MIGHT ASK THE PAIN PATIENT

It is important for the pain management specialist to possess effective questioning techniques and to be armed with questions that can isolate critical details from patients' anecdotes and experiences. Here are some inquiries that pain management specialist may ask patients during medical visits:[6]

- Aside from the obvious, why are you seeking treatment?
- Can you describe how the pain feels? Is it piercing, stabbing, shooting, throbbing, sharp, burning, tender, or simply unbearable?
- Does the pain follow a "feeling" or warning signal that you feel consciously?
- Are there other symptoms that preempt or accompany the pain that you feel? For instance, do you feel lethargic, nauseous, or do you have difficulty sleeping or eating?
- Does your pain interfere with activities of daily living, whether you are at home or at work? Does your pain affect your mood? In what way?
- Where do you feel pain? Is it localized or do you feel pain in several parts of your body at the same time?
- On a scale of zero to 10, with zero being the lowest level of pain and 10 being the highest level of pain, how will you rate the last pain episode that you experienced prior to this visit? Do you keep a pain diary? Are you open to the idea of keeping and maintaining one?
- How often do your pain episodes happen? Will you describe the occurrences as periodic, occasional, or continuous? Do you notice that your pain episodes are connected with specific times during the day? Could the pain episodes be connected to the seasons and temperature changes?
- What specific actions or activities seem to trigger the pain? These can include simple activities of daily living such as reaching for a soup can in an overhead cupboard or bending a knee to pick up the morning paper.

ANALYSIS

The specialty of pain management has evolved further through the years, requiring more of highly specialized practitioners who are in tune with their patients' needs while in possession of the necessary knowledge, aptitude, and skills to address pain. Today, pain management specialists are encouraged to further hone their skills through advanced certification programs—specifically in the field of pain management and pain medicine.[7] All in all, the PMS focuses on keeping the balance between the many faces of pain itself.

III

Many Faces of Pain

15

CONGENITAL INSENSITIVITY TO PAIN

A world where the sensation of pain does not exist in any form and where hot and cold are indistinguishable is difficult to imagine. It may be appealing at first instant, but on reflection, it is a shuddering thought. From the time a baby is born, pain is a crucial in communicating to the brain any instability of the body's homeostasis. The brain activates the proper defensive mechanism for receiving this signal. The perception of pain is a protective mechanism for realizing an impairment and for aligning activities toward restoration. The consequences of failure to realize the impairment could culminate in life-threatening, permanent damage.

OVERVIEW

The rare disorder characterized by the inability to sense pain or any nerve-related sensation with all other sensory modalities remaining intact is called *congenital insensitivity to pain* (CIP), or CIPA when *anhidrosis* is present. Anhidrosis is a malfunction of sweat glands. CIP is caused by genetic mutations that prevent the production of nerve cells for transmission of pain.[1] The exact origin of this disorder and the cure for it are being researched. First recognized in the 1930s as a condition warranting due medical attention, various descriptions have been forwarded along the way.[2] Patients exhibiting manifestations of this disorder were said to be suffering from (1) *congenital general pure analgesia,* (2) *congenital universal insensitiveness to pain,* (3) *congenital universal indifference to pain,* or (4) *congenital universal absence of pain.*[3] The various names indicate the myriad of responses experienced by CIP patients. Some patients do not exhibit a response to injury, do not suffer from involuntary responses to pain, or have difficulties in distinguishing various types of pain stimuli. Others display a lack of responsiveness to pain, but have the ability to identify the presence of pain and modality. Modality in this context refers to a sensory identification of pain using hearing, smell, taste, touch, vision, or cold.

Real Meaning of Congenital Insensitivity to Pain

The multitude of terms, when used loosely, can be consolidated into (1) congenital insensitivity to pain, and (2) congenital indifference to pain. Although these definitions are sometimes used interchangeably, there is a distinct difference. Patients diagnosed with congenital insensitivity to pain seem to disregard sensations of pain. They have the pronounced inability to perceive the type, intensity and quality of pain stimuli. Meanwhile, in patients diagnosed with congenital indifference to pain, even though pain is perceived, there is a complete absence of a response to it. Patients experience sensations of pain, but despite an absence of neurological abnormalities in the pain pathways, show no emotional response, such as aversion or withdrawal action from the stimuli.

The term *congenital* pertains to anything inherited genetically from birth. Impairment of pain perception caused by mental retardation, infection, trauma or toxic agents is excluded from the definition of congenital insensitivity to pain. Peripheral neuropathy related to the degenerative state of the nervous system is considered a criterion for diagnosing CIP. Researchers have focused on channels and the genetic abnormalities within the channels, which could possibly have implications toward the cause of CIP. Although an accurate estimate on the number of CIP patients is unknown, the New York University School of Medicine, which specializes in the treatment of CIP, has on average thirty-five patients, of whom seventeen are from the United States. Globally, there are an estimated three hundred people suffering from CIP.[4] The extremely low number of patients could be due to various factors, including the high mortality rate resulting from the nature of the disorder, as most die before the age of three.[5] It could also be due to the fact that manifestations of the disorder might not be considered a disease, but a simple abnormality. This is the general opinion in the developing and underdeveloped world. Case studies conducted in particular areas of the developing world indicate that the disorder is accepted as an anomalous behavior by society.[6] In Pakistan, a ten-year-old boy who had CIP was a street performer who would cut himself with knives and walk on flames. The society was aware of his abnormal qualities, but unfortunately, he was not diagnosed as a CIP disorder victim. He finally died by jumping off a building, apparently unaware of the dire consequences.[7]

Another factor to be taken into account in developing countries is the lack of monitoring required by victims of CIP in preventing harm to themselves. The potential for similar occurrences in many parts of the world cannot be overruled. In North America, the paucity of CIP cases, the lack of simple diagnostic tests, and the variable presentations of CIP have also made it difficult to identify victims of this disorder.[8]

Research has been conducted within multiethnic groups to determine whether ethnicity is a contributing factor to getting CIP. Toward this end, a study conducted with CIP patients from Spain, Japan, Italy, Kuwait, United Arab Emirates, and Canada concluded that gene mutation could cause CIP in various ethnic groups.[9]

CATEGORIES OF CIP

Exhibited as a recessive trait, CIP is transmitted down through families, and if only one parent has the corresponding gene, then the chances of it passing on to their children are greater. CIP has a recessive genetic characteristic and occurs more often among families with close blood ties with the disorder. Clinical studies are still ongoing for CIP, as it is difficult to find cases unless brought to the attention of medical authorities. CIP testing involves accurate diagnosis of the physical and biochemical characteristics determined by genetic makeup and environmental influences.

Classifications of CIP

CIP itself falls within the genetic *hereditary sensory and autonomic neuropathy* (HSAN) class of neuropathies. Three subclassifications of HSAN, which manifest as CIP with slight variations, will be the focus of interest below.

HSAN IV

HSAN IV is a subclassification of HSAN caused by mutations in the *neurotrophic tyrosine kinase receptor Type 1* (NTRK1) gene and localized to *chromosome 1q21-22*. HSAN IV is sometimes classified as CIP with (1) anhidrosis, (2) severe degeneration in the nervous system, (3) mental retardation, and (4) absence of *unmyelinated* (uncovered) fibers and loss of small myelinated fibers. The NTRK1 gene, which is also known as the TRKA gene, provides encoding for the making of a protein or *nerve growth factor* (NGF) that is critical for certain neurons. A mutation in NTRK1 does not permit NGF to function normally, thus causing problems in the growth of pain receptors. Skin evaluations of HSAN IV patients reveal a distinct lack of nerve stimulation within the skin epidermis. An absence of sweating or anhidrosis is due to the loss of nervous stimulation of sweat glands by neurons.

A person must inherit two copies of the defective NTRK1 gene (one copy from each parent) for the disorder to appear. People who inherit a mutated gene from only one parent are called "carriers" of the disease.[10] Children of a parent who is a carrier, or has only one copy of the defective gene will have a 50 percent chance of inheriting one defective gene and also being a carrier. When both parents are carriers, about one out of four children have CIP. As with many other inherited disorders, CIP occurs more often in closely related or consanguineous families that share a bloodline. Consanguineous families are a common cultural trait in traditional homogenous societies.[11]

HSAN V

HSAN V is categorized as two different types, based on mutations in the genes causing the disorder. The first is the NTRK1 gene. The second is the *nerve growth factor beta polypeptide* gene (NGFB). HSAN V is classified as CIP with mild anhidrosis and no mental retardation. Pain and temperature insensitivity is evident in childhood accompanied by painless fractures, ulcers and burns. However, sensitivity to touch, pressure, and vibration and subconscious sensations of the body and limb movement are unaffected, which is a similar situation to congenital indifference to pain. Involuntary manifestations vary from minimal to the extreme of skin blotching, abnormal sweating, and high temperatures. There is a severe loss of small myelinated fibers with a possible decrease in unmyelinated fibers.

SCN9A Channelopathy

This is considered by some experts to be the third classification of HSAN. As far as *channelopathy* (defects in cellular channels) is concerned, there have been research studies on the *sodium-channel-voltage-gated-type IX-alpha-subunit* gene (SCN9A). The SCN9A gene's primary role is to ensure the proper functioning of one part of *nav1.7 sodium channels*, for transporting of sodium into cells. The nav1.7 channels are found at the end of nerve cells called nociceptors located near the spinal cord. CIP occurs when there is a mutation in the SCN9A gene resulting in impairment and production of short nonfunctional nav1.7 channels, which in turn suppresses the transmission of pain signals.[12]

Further research was conducted on nine families from several different nationalities. DNA was collected and testing for CIP was narrowed to chromosome 2q24-q31, a region known to contain a cluster of voltage-gated sodium channel genes. The genetic data supported the evidence that nav1.7 plays an essential role in mediating pain in humans and that SCN9A mutations underlie congenital insensitivity to pain. SCN9A is characterized by CIP with *hereditary erythemalgia*, a disease of the hands and feet characterized by purplish coloring accompanied by a burning sensation. As compared to HSAN IV and HSAN V, the central nervous system appears unaffected in the candidates.[13]

RECOGNITION OF PAIN IN AN INFANT

Historically, infants were believed to not experience any pain. Considered to be sub-human, pre-human, and even "a lower animal in human form," infants were unfortunately discriminated against in more ways than one.[14] The traditional view expressed in medical journals during the nineteenth century was that the defensive mechanism observed in infants is attributed to mechanical movements but not to neural connections of the brain. Operating on babies in the absence of anesthesia was a widespread practice in the 1940s and 1950s due to the commonly held view that anesthesia was too strong for them.

In reality, newborn infants do have functional nervous systems capable of perceiving pain. With repeated painful procedures, infants develop an increase in signs of discomfort. Unmanaged pain during the neonatal period can bring about long-term complications. It was falsely presumed that infants lacked memory of pain and so they would have no means of interpreting it (see chapter 6) the way adults do. Even the drawing of blood without any form of analgesic should be considered a practice that could have long-term physiological and behavioral consequences.

The effects of pain experienced by infants can be categorized into (1) physiological impacts, (2) behavioral cues, and (3) hormonal or metabolic responses. Physiological effects relate to changes in physiology, such as dilation of pupils, heartbeat, blood pressure, intracranial pressure, oxygen requirement, and change in complexion and muscle tone. Behavioral cues include crying, facial expressions, body movements, and emotional state. Hormonal responses relate to internal chemical reactions such as hormones and secretions. The changes in the hormone levels effect changes in the composition of fats and proteins with far-reaching implications on the development of the infant.

Neglected pain in the infant can form abnormal pathways in the brain with the potential to affect social cognitive skills and cause self-destructive behavior. Premature infants have unpredictable responses to pain stimuli. They are more vulnerable to the effects of pain, as they have been thrust abruptly into an environment for which they might not be ready, physically and emotionally. For assessment of pain within a structured and standardized framework, pain assessment scales have been formalized.

Scales

There are various pain scales used as benchmarks for assessment of pain in newborns, which are used in procedures such as pain medication administration. The determinant factors in formulating a pain scale include behavioral signs such as quality of cry, breathing pattern, facial expression, muscle tone, and changes in oxygen requirement. The behavior-based *face-legs-activity-cry-consolability (FLACC) scale* is used for children ranging anywhere from two months to seven years old and for others unable to communicate pain messages coherently.[15] Scores for each variable are rated from zero to two, with a sum total of ten. A total of four or greater indicates pain. The CRIES scale is used for accessing infants up to six months old for all neonatal pain assessment except surgery. CRIES is the acronym for "*c*ry, *r*equires oxygen, *i*ncreased heart rate and blood pressure, *e*xpressions, and *s*leeplessness." Similar to FLACC scoring, a score of four or greater on the CRIES scale implies the infant is experiencing pain and intervention is required. There is also the neonate and infant pain scale (NIPS), which assesses the pain experienced by infants based on criteria such as facial expression, crying state, arm and leg movement, breathing patterns and state of arousal.[16]

Stopping the Problem before It Happens

As with adults, pain signals in an infant send an alert for attention due to an unstable condition that requires management. Symptoms of CIP can be observed from the embryonic stage, birth, or early infancy. Irregular development in the outer layer (or ectodermal layer) of an embryo can signal the start of CIP. The ectodermal layer develops into (1) the skin and epidermic tissues, such as the nails, hair, and glands of the skin, (2) the nervous system, including pain receptors, external sense organs and mucous membrane of the mouth, and (3) the anus. An early detection of CIP will enable correct management of the disorder. However, CIP infants will not manifest physiological or behavioral responses to the above-mentioned assessment scales due to the absence or mutation of nerve cells. *Hypotonia* (diminished muscle tone) and delayed developmental milestones are frequent in the early years of CIP patients, while strength and tone normalize with age.

Close and frequent observation of the infant is carried out by the parents and formal caregivers to determine any anomalies such as self-inflicted wounds and scratches. Due to the habit of scratching the cornea, an ophthalmologist might routinely check such infants. For other forms of self-mutilation, expert evaluation is required on a routine basis. Young CIP sufferers are normally recommended to have their baby teeth removed so they cannot chew through their tongue, lips or fingers until their full set of adult teeth grow through. Ensuring a safe and secure environment and taking preemptive measures in alleviating harm will provide a higher level of confidence in the safety of the CIP infant. In reality, most patients rarely live longer than three years and the maximum age of most adults is twenty-five.

TRUE DANGERS OF INSENSITIVITY TO PAIN: INFANCY VS. ADULTHOOD

Since infants are not physically and mentally capable of protecting themselves in full, internal injury within or outside of the body will go unnoticed, leading to infection and ultimately death.[17] Infants are vulnerable to serious risks of injury, as in self-biting of the tongue or fingers, rubbing of eyes, and bruises on the body. During childhood, medical incidents, such as a ruptured appendix, can go unobserved with serious implications. Due to the inability to sweat in CIP victims, infants are unable to regulate their body temperature.[18] The heat contained within their bodies can result in high fever with dire consequences such as hypothermia. It can also weaken the immune system, making the body susceptible to further implications such as cell damage and virus infections. Death from hyperpyrexia or extremely high temperature occurs within the first three years of life in 20 percent of patients.[19]

Susceptibility to Heat

In hot-climate regions, extra precaution should be taken to ensure that infants and small children do not suffer from contact burns. Protective clothing and appropriate footwear should be used at all times. There should not be any contact with sun-exposed objects. Hot water taps should be regulated to prevent burns from scalding water. Similarly, children and infants should be kept away from any objects that could cause a burn, such as heaters, irons, matches, and so on. Burns and trauma can be prevented by ensuring a safe and secure environment. Educating and instilling these habits in caregivers and parents will reduce the suffering experienced by infants and young CIP victims.

Examples of CIP

To illustrate an example of a young CIP patient, one could consider the case of a five-year-old CIP patient from the United States.[20] As a baby, she chewed her hand, bit through the skin, and continued on to the bones. This was resolved by having all her teeth extracted. She poked one eye, resulting in blindness and has second-degree burns due to grabbing a light bulb. Another case is of a seventeen-month-old British baby whose parents took the preemptive measure of extracting all his teeth before he could do further damage to his oral cavity.[21] The initial observation of the parents was that they had a son who was a "real tough baby," an observation that later translated into a diagnosis of CIP.

SCREENING TECHNIQUES AND NEW ADVANCES IN CIP

In the event that a family member has been identified with CIP-causative mutations, carrier testing for at-risk family members, such as prenatal testing for pregnancies, can be conducted. General diagnosis should include a complete physical exam with a detailed study of the family history, focusing on the patient's receptivity to pain and history of injuries. Furthermore, biopsies are carried out to determine the degenerative condition of nerve fibers as well as the absence or presence of sweat glands. Tissues are extracted from CIP patients and family members for this examination.

Prenatal DNA genetic evaluations can now be performed by *amniocentesis* (analyzing the blood or the amniotic fluid) surrounding the fetus at fifteen to eighteen weeks gestation. *Chorionic villus sampling* (CVS) is another form of testing where placenta tissues are extracted from the fetus at ten to twelve weeks gestation. Due to risk of miscarriage in prenatal testing, it is highly recommended that genetic testing is there only when identification of CIP-afflicted family members are confirmed.

Pre-implantation genetic diagnosis (PGD) is a relatively new procedure that tests embryos created by artificial fertilization for NTRK1 gene mutations that could cause CIP. This test is done before implantation and it provides parents with the requisite knowledge on the health of the embryo. There is no definite cure for CIP, although there are medications still at an experimental stage, such as *naloxone*.[22]

Current Approaches

Due to the ongoing research for a definite cause and cure for CIP, the current focus is on the management and prevention of injuries and infections. Behavioral therapies recommended include counseling and education on the implications of CIP. By studying the structure of the mutant genes for CIP, researchers also hope to find ways to reduce the pain suffered from chronic disorders such as back pain.

Anesthetic Approaches

While CIP patients do not feel pain, sufferers who undergo surgical operations still require anesthetic management.[23] According to a study conducted on Bedouins, cardiovascular complications following anesthesia are common in patients with the Israeli variant of CIP. A similar study done in Japan concluded that when it comes to anesthetic management of patients with CIP, anesthesia is a necessary component and that sufficient sedation must be given during operations since CIP patients are sensitive to touch sensations. Temperature management should likewise be given due consideration.[24]

ANALYSIS

Prognosis for HSAN disorders such as CIP is improving with current research methods, and these disorders can no longer be viewed only as childhood medical conditions. With greater understanding of CIP, an increasing number of patients are reaching adulthood. Because CIP is extremely rare, centralization of its care would undoubtedly boost the ability to (1) diagnose pain patients in general more accurately, (2) understand the natural progression of painful disorders, and (3) recommend appropriate interventions for professional caregivers.

16

ACUTE VS. CHRONIC PAIN

Acute pain is a sudden pain caused by an ailment or a hazardous condition in the body. It is typically defined as intense, shocking, or severe in characteristic but can also be trivial depending on the cause. The duration of the pain can vary from a few moments to a few months, though not longer than six months in general.

Chronic pain is endured by the body, even after the causative ailment is cured. It persists to affect the body physically or mentally for weeks, months, or years. Chronic pain can as well be described as the pain with no exact duration. It usually persists beyond the anticipated period of recovery.[1] Chronic pain isn't entirely dependent upon its origin, and it can evolve into new stages with time. This dynamic behavior makes chronic pain difficult to treat.

A recent market research report revealed that more than 1.5 billion individuals across the world suffer from chronic pain and that almost 3–5 percent of the worldwide populace suffers from neuropathic pain.[2] The prevalence of chronic pain increases with the increase in the age of the people. Another research report indicated that chronic pain afflicts around one hundred million U.S. adults. The yearly nationwide financial cost associated with chronic pain is assessed at $560–$635 billion.[3] The cost of treatment for chronic pain is particularly high because it is an ongoing problem and can also involve spending on psychological damages caused by the chronic pain. Geographical area might also be a factor if proper medical resources are not locally available and thus minor illnesses possibly turn into more painful, chronic ones.

ACUTE VS. CHRONIC PAIN: UNOBVIOUS DIFFERENCES

Pain Management

The management protocols of the two types of pain differ. Acute pain can be alleviated by treatment from one practitioner, whereas the management of chronic pain generally involves the combined efforts of a team that includes a medical or clinical practitioner, a psychiatrist, and a physiotherapist, depending on the nature of the pain.[4] Acute pain is usually treated with analgesics and painkillers, and the main focus of the doctor is to eliminate the origin of pain. The treatment of chronic pain is generally not focused on its origin, and instead of analgesics and painkillers, physical therapy can play a major role in the remedy.

In addition, the management of acute pain is more direct and physical in nature, while the treatment of chronic pain involves physical as well as mental factors. Patients dealing with chronic pain usually have a tendency to be worried more regarding their pain, and they are also susceptible to suffer from conditions such as depression and anxiety more immediately. Emotional conditions can distinctively affect the way pain is experienced, and can even hinder the organic pain-inhibiting processes of the brain. People with acute pain may also experience emotional trauma, but it generally ends once pain is diminished or eliminated. Formal caregivers such as physicians understand that the pain tends to *last* when it is chronic. This can have a significant effect on the way pain is felt and experienced and how patients react to it.

Aftereffects

Acute pain can result in severe suffering for the patient, but it does not last as long as chronic pain. Chronic pain is known to have caused psychological depression due to the pain lasting for prolonged periods of time. Chronic pain can also change forms after the initial source of pain is addressed, thus making it more challenging to rectify in the long term.

Socioeconomic Differences

Pain can be a major cause of reduced work ability and well-being. A questionnaire was distributed from 2000 to 2002 to find out which forms of pain are more common among employees: acute, chronic, or disabling chronic pain.[5] The questionnaire was targeted at workers in

Helsinki, Finland, aged between forty and sixty. It included (1) demographic and socioeconomic elements of present pain, (2) time intervals of pain, and (3) disability related to pain. The parameters for defining pain were that if the pain lasted a maximum of three months, it was acute, but chronic when carrying on for more than ninety days. Disabling chronic pain was verified with the use of the disability subscale of the *Von Korff Chronic Pain Grade* survey. Fifteen percent of the women reported acute pain, about 30 percent were suffering from chronic pain, and 7 percent were affected by disabling chronic pain. The comparative statistics for men were 12, 24, and 5 percent. Disabling chronic pains were more frequent in senior citizens of both genders. The secondary-educated women tended to be more likely to suffer from chronic or disabling chronic pain as compared to those with higher education. Low-skilled non-manual employees and manual laborers were more exposed to disabling chronic pain than managers. Separated, divorced, or widowed men were more likely to suffer from acute pain than married men, and labor-intensive workers were more likely to complain of chronic pain than executives. Chronic pain was fairly widespread in this populace, and the ones who were older, with lower education, and working class appear to be at extra risk of chronic pain, particularly for the disabling type.[6]

Difference in Drug Therapy

The kind of pain, whether acute or chronic, should be taken into account when dealing with pain pharmacologically. The category of pain can suggest different medications or therapies being used. Certain medications or therapies may be more effective for acute pain, others for chronic pain, and some might work well on both. Acute pain medication is usually for quick onset of pain, such as from forced trauma or postoperative pain. Chronic pain medication is generally for removing long-lasting, ongoing pain.

Abdominal pain can further demonstrate the difference. A quick diagnosis is essential in emergency situations of acute abdominal pain. Analgesia has to be given as soon as possible. The different classes of painkillers should be applied according to their recognized effects, side effects, and incompatibilities. Postoperative pain after abdominal surgery is also deemed as a unique case of acute abdominal pain. Main treatment choices are chiefly comprised of non-opioid painkillers and opioids. Opioids can be processed into the circulatory system through patient-controlled analgesia mechanisms. *Neuroaxial (surrounding the nerves) painkillers* provide ideal pain relief with constructive influence on gastrointestinal movement and the cure for patients when preferably dispensed through an epidural catheter in major abdominal surgery. Fundamental medication often turns out to be tricky because of difficulties in assigning chronic abdominal pain to a specific organ. Co-analgesics such as anticonvulsants and antidepressants are also used in order to lessen sensitization and recover the endogenous pain-reducing process. Nondrug tactics and substitute treatment methods may be beneficial, and the treatment of chronic cancer pain through oral or transcutaneous opioids is an effective method of treatment.[7]

There are also dissimilarities among chronic pain patients themselves, with at least three recognized chronic pain patient groups. The first type of patient suffers from a chronic disease with chronic pain very much dependent and related to the pain-causing illness. Their pain can also be contingent on a previous injury that has caused other unresolved issues. The second type of patient suffers from a chronic sickness in which new nervous system processes coincide with those connected to the causative disease. Of the third type are patients affected by chronic pain in which the relationship between pain and the original tissue injury is nowhere to be found anymore, and the pain persists due to newly developed pain mechanisms in the body. Patients can be differentiated according to these types into sufferers from painful chronic disease or independent chronic pain.[8]

WORKINGS OF ACUTE PAIN

How Acute Pain Turns into Chronic Pain

Whether acute pain can always become chronic is not entirely clear, but some types of stimuli and constant nociceptive processes may change the nature of acute pain. The mechanisms are complicated and depend on various factors.[9] Effects of factors such as damaged tissues and injuries diminish and other influences gain more importance as the pain transforms from acute to chronic. The efficiency of a specific treatment for chronic pain will usually vary from patient to patient. For example, a specific therapy or injection for a herniated disc might give sufficient pain relief to some patients but not to others.

Not all patients with identical disorders develop chronic pain, and it is not known why some people can develop chronic pain while others do not. Caregivers should realize that a disorder that may appear considerably minor can transform into severe chronic pain, and a severe medical condition may not be painful at all. The term *chronic* is commonly used in everyday clinical practice in order to specify a type of pain that persists over time and is complemented by diagnostic and medicinal complications. Consequently, the health expenditure for the treatment of chronic pain patients is becoming consistently higher. There are many patients with ambiguous pain disorders that are considered to be chronic and incurable only because it persists for a long time, though they achieve full pain relief after correct analysis and treatment.[10]

Many pain sufferers who go through surgery will need drug therapy to manage the acute postsurgical pain. Efficient control of acute postsurgical pain is necessary for the patient not only in the short run, but also in the long run so as to eliminate the chances of developing chronic pain, which can arise if initial acute pain is prolonged. At the moment, opioid painkillers are used worldwide for dealing with acute postsurgical pain. Aphids give effective postsurgical pain relief, but their use is associated with a vast number of dangers, including—in particular—the growth of opioid-related side effects.[11]

Acute pain could be the origin of the chronic pain in case of injuries caused by accidents. These mishaps could be caused by trauma, collision, or a sudden movement in the body. This pain can result in chronic pain due to many factors, such as a complex wound that may not heal back to its original state, lack of awareness and ignorance of the patient, and inappropriate diagnosis and treatment by the physician. Acute pain may not be severe in some cases and may come across as trivial and insignificant, in which case it may gradually turn chronic.

Prevalence of Acute Pain

Very little is known about the prevalence of acute pain in pre-hospital emergency medicine compared to the case of emergencies. A study was conducted to find out the pre-hospital prevalence of acute pain and to pinpoint the elements related to ineffective treatment.[12] The patients in the study were age sixteen or older and were able to self-assess pain. These patients were involved for a period of eleven months in 2007, and 947 among the 2,279 participants had acute pain. Pain was reported to be anywhere from intense to severe in 64 percent of the patients. Trauma was partly responsible for acute pain in the under-seventy-five age group. Strong pain was specifically linked with pain of cardiac (heart-related) or traumatic derivation, and 48 percent suffered from acute pain among the 1,364 patients who were transported by mobile units. A sedative was given to around 70 percent of the participants. Fifty-one percent of the patients found pain relief and the percentage of pain relief was lower in patients who were affected by trauma or a gyneco-logic or obstetric ailment. Pain in pre-hospital emergency medicine influenced more than 40 percent of patients included in the studied population. The rate, however, differed greatly depending on the source of the pain. Pain management was inadequate considering the fact that only one in two patients experienced relief overall.[13]

EXAMPLES OF ACUTE PAIN

Endometriosis

Endometriosis, occurring when the lining of the uterus grows beyond its natural boundaries, is one of the significant sources of acute pain. Several theories have tried to describe the growth of such tissue. The biological incident of endometrial reflux in the fallopian tubes during menstruation sometimes may oppress native immune systems, embed, and multiply. This is the most commonly mentioned hypothesis and is known as the *implantation theory*, although this theory doesn't clarify the reason why endometriosis only develops in roughly 10 to 15 percent of women, while the reflux of endometrial tissue through the fallopian tubes during menstruation is a very common phenomenon. The endometrium of women suffering from endometriosis is usually abnormal compared with the endometrium of fit women.[14]

Diagnosis of endometriosis is usually late, and the signs are commonly normalized despite the fact that the patient suffers from pain often reported as intense and overwhelming. That, along with the inadequate efficiency of treatments makes women experience problems with friends, work, family, and sexual relations.[15]

Complex Regional Pain Syndrome

Complex regional pain (CRP) syndrome is another important example of acute pain. This is a type of neuropathic syndrome signified by intense, ongoing pain and reaction, autonomic dysfunction, and motor symptoms and signs. Complex regional pain syndrome is twofold. CRP syndrome Type 1, often labeled *reflex sympathetic dystrophy*, is associated with injury to minor sensory nerve branches. CRP syndrome Type 2, formerly known as *causalgia*, is related to damage and disorder of the major nerve trunks, such as median or sciatic nerves. Complex regional pain syndrome is most commonly observed after trauma and surgery, but it can also appear after conditions such as heart attack or stroke. Sensory symptoms of CRP syndrome include acute pain, normally described as "burning" in character, and hypersensitivity, which can be associated to touch, pressure, and any temperature change. Cold conditions affect most of the patients. A large number of patients experience numbness and tingling, which are known as *negative sensory phenomena*, in addition to pain and other positive physical occurrences. *Sensorimotor neglect* (inability to measure motor functions) is a phenomenon that was discovered recently. CRP syndrome patients who go through this phenomenon report that the body part feels as if it does not belong to the body and that they struggle to use that body part. Autonomic symptoms involve *thermoregulatory* (temperature control) problems such that the affected body part is either warmer or cooler as compared to the remainder of the body, even at room temperature; skin color changes, as the skin may come across as "blotchy and light," or "dark blue and brown"; *hyperhidrosis*, or excessive sweating, due to changes in glands; and weakness and exhaustion as well as tremor and *dyskinesia* (movement impairment). Patients with CRP syndrome generally also suffer from muscle spasms.[16]

Early identification and treatment increases the chances of a successful cure, as in most medical conditions. Patients with physical signs and symptoms of CRP syndrome after an injury should instantly seek medical assistance. Physical therapy is the fundamental and basic way to treat complex regional pain syndrome. Mild conditions can be cured through physical therapy and physical modalities. Patients with moderate to severe pain may need regional anesthetic blockage in order to participate in physical therapy. A small number of patients may suffer from chronic pain and may require long-term, multidisciplinary treatment, which may include a combination of physical therapy, psychological help, and pain-relieving measures. Pain-relieving techniques may include medications, sympathetic or somatic blockade, spinal cord stimulation, and spinal analgesia.[17]

Groin Pain

Groin pain is another common example of acute pain. It can be a disturbing and displeasing injury, especially for athletes who play such sports that involve kicking, rapid accelerations and decelerations, and swift direction changes. The most usual problems are adductor muscle strain, *osteitis pubis* (inflammation of a bone called *pubis symphysis*), and sports hernia. Other important causes include nerve pain, stress fractures, and intrinsic hip pathology. Multiple problems frequently co-exist and thus make the condition complicated at times. Correct diagnosis helps to streamline the treatment, with therapy focused on purposeful reinforcement and stability.[18]

Groin pain may actually be caused by other factors, such as

- kidney stone traversing through a ureter;
- a urinary tract infection;
- hip problems in children and older adults in particular;
- inflammations, bumps, and swelling in the groin region caused by the infection;
- seizure, infection, inflammation, or low blood flow in the large intestine;
- female pubic complications, such as pelvic inflammatory disease, ovarian cyst, or ectopic pregnancy;
- male pelvic complications, such as a skin infection of the scrotum, a prostate infection, or torsion of a testicle;
- a hip fracture, diseased hip joint, or strain fracture of the hip;
- arthritis;
- spine problems in the back close to the lower ribs; or
- tweaking of nerves that pass through the groin area, triggering groin and thigh pain.

When it comes to infection, groin pain is often confused with testicular pain, although *groin* pertains to a much larger area and has many organs in it. Testicular or scrotal pain is usually acute in nature, but depending on the cause and nature of the pain, things can turn chronic.

EXAMPLES OF CHRONIC PAIN

Cancer Pain

Cancer pain is among the most significant forms of chronic pain. The prevalence of cancer pain is extremely unpredictable and incompletely understood. Research is not populace-based and samples only represent vague data on the etiology of pain, pain pattern, and medical or demographic elements in relation to cancer. Furthermore, the dynamic nature of pain has not been thoroughly clarified, but cancer-related pain is usually caused by (1) direct tumors, (2) diagnostic or therapeutic techniques, or (3) toxicities of medication. Patients may suffer from more than one kind of pain simultaneously that may be related to cancer. Some researchers have concentrated only on particular causes of cancer-related pain in specific patient populaces, and only a few of them have identified groups at greater risk of pain, such as the senior citizens or the underserved. Researchers have not always surveyed cancer-related pain to find its course of attack, intensity, effects on quality of life, and other associated factors.[19]

There are four basic methods of controlling chronic cancer pain: (1) altering the origin of pain, (2) amending the main perception of pain, (3) lessening transmission of pain to the central nervous system, and (4) limiting the advancement of pain to the central nervous system. General pharmacological management is usually targeted at the first three of these approaches, and the three collectively serve as the fundamental technique for treatment of the majority of cancer patients with mild to severe pain.[20]

Fibromyalgia

Fibromyalgia is another critical example of a chronic pain disorder. It is described as prolonged, widespread pain with *allodynia* (excessive pain when the stimulus is normally painless) or *hyperalgesia* (excessive pain when the stimulus is normally painful), and is categorized as one of the prime groups of tissue pain disorders. The pathogenesis of fibromyalgia is not completely known, although it is believed to be the result of a central nervous system malfunction. There are no examinations to prove the diagnosis, but most alternative possibilities for the pain can be eliminated through a general medical examination and from the past medical history of the patient. It would appear best to accept the whole range of sensitivity and distress in order to adapt treatment on an individual basis.[21]

A Word or Few on Chronic Pain Approaches

Long-term pain does not subside eventually. This disorder can affect a specific part of the body, as in low-back discomfort or complications, or involve many areas simultaneously, as in fibromyalgia or arthritis. Chronic pain is more than an indication of an illness or injury. It is almost as if it becomes a sickness in itself. Regardless of the affected organ or cause, chronic pain influences the daily routines of many people who may experience work-related problems, depressive disorders, drug-related issues, and decline of the quality of life. When all is said and done, pain-reduction approaches such as medicines, injections, and surgical operations provide little to reduce the severe pain and long-term strife that can develop.

THIN LINE BETWEEN ACUTE AND CHRONIC PAIN

Occipital Neuralgia

Occipital neuralgia is a medical condition that is an example of both acute and chronic pain. It is defined as a *paroxysmal (sudden) stabbing pain* in the cutaneous circulation of the superior or inferior occipital or third occipital nerve. The pain is generally labeled *sharp, jabbing,* or *shocking,* especially one-sided and remitting, exuding to the occipital and frontal areas of the brain with related signs indicating a pain source in the neck. Types of occipital neuralgia include (1) shocking (72 percent), (2) deteriorating (14 percent), and (3) oncological or idiopathic (14 percent).[22] Most instances result from a flexion-extension injury to the neck, which usually arises from a posterior motor vehicle accident. Treatment modalities for occipital neuralgia differ from traditional procedures, which are generally the main treatments for injections and surgical involvements. Injections such as regional sedative nerve blocks are primarily useful in most of the situations and are also beneficial as a diagnostic device. [23]

Sacroiliac Joint Pain

Sacroiliac (SI) joint pain is another of those pains that can be either acute or chronic in nature. The sacroiliac joint is a common origin of pain in the lower back and buttocks in nearly 15 percent of people.[24] Identifying sacroiliac joint pain can be difficult because the signs and symptoms are identical to those of other sources of back pain. People with sacroiliac joint pain rarely complain of pain above the lumbar 5 (L5) region of the back. Many identify their pain to the region close to the *posterior superior iliac spine.* Radiographic and laboratory examinations mostly assist in excluding other origins of low back pain. Magnetic resonance imaging, bone scans, and computed tomography, of the sacroiliac joint are not dependable when it comes to figuring out whether the joint is the origin of the pain. Moreover, regulated analgesic injections of the sacroiliac joint are crucial tools in the diagnosis. Treatment modalities for SI joint pain, whether chronic or acute, could include medications, bracing, physical therapy, radiofrequency denervation, manual therapy, and *arthrodesis* (fusion of the joint).[25]

ANALYSIS

There is no absolute medicinal approach to acute or chronic pain, and most of the time, successful treatment is achieved through a medley of strategies. Caregivers should note that while the time intervals of acute and chronic pain are different, both types of pain result in damage to the health of the pain sufferer, if not addressed promptly.[26]

17

OCCUPATIONAL PAIN

Every profession has its own health risks. Working individuals can easily suffer from occupational hazards in their workplace. The first indication of serious health problems at work is often occupational pain, which is strictly connected with the *type* of job at hand. For example, IT specialists, accountants, and managers spend much time at the computer desk where they work all day long. A continuous seating position may lead to

- extra load on the spine;
- degenerative disorder of vertebral discs;
- muscle spasm of shoulders and neck;
- impaired blood and lymph outflow in the legs;
- damage of neuronal cellular parts; and
- rise of specific pains.

It is important for pain patients and caregivers to know the health risks of the kind of work being done in order to prevent disease, to start treatment immediately if any occupational pains surface, or to select a profession less harmful for their individual health. This approach is much more efficient, faster, and certainly cheaper than treatment of chronic suffering arising from occupational pain that has been ignored during early stages due to lack of knowledge, time, or attention.

DISCUSSION OF THE VARIOUS TYPES OF WORK-RELATED PAIN

There are three categories of occupational hazards: chemical, physical, and biological. Chemical hazards can be found in substances used in the manufacturing industry, agriculture, construction, or transport. Physical factors associated with work involve the lack of mechanization, lack of ergonomic equipment, or overestimation of the *psychophysiological* (mind and function) capabilities of an individual. Biological hazards are those connected to exposure to living organisms such as bacteria. Based on these broad categorizations, occupational pains can be divided into three groups: (1) thermal pain, caused by temperature factors, (2) mechanical pain (i.e., injury to limbs), and (3) chemical pain (irritation from aggressive chemicals). These may involve pain accompanied by vomiting and nausea (visceral pain), pain from minor wounds or burns (superficial pain), and pain from stimulation of the nociceptors in bones (deep somatic pain).[1]

In the chemical category there are occupational pains caused by jobs *directly* involving strong chemicals. Those who work in chemical plants or factories and are in contact with chemicals or their by-products during manufacturing processes could suffer from symptoms of chemical poisoning or chronic toxicity. Even the smallest daily exposure of chemicals may lead to the accumulation of toxins and serious destruction of health. This kind of toxicity can happen with either isolated or combined lesions of various organs and body systems. Work-related pain in such cases differs from general chemical intoxication, which could manifest as weakness, headache, and vomiting within just a few hours of inhaling the substance, for example fine dust or metallic vapor during casting, cutting or welding certain metals. Skin disorders that could also result are *paronychia* (skin infection around the nail) or *folliculitis* (infection of hair follicles) caused by the direct impact of chemicals on the skin.

Among the most harmful dusts are those containing silica (quartz drillers, coal miners, sand tone polishers are among those typically injured), and fine dust (dust particles with a diameter of less than five microns), such as flour, cement powder, or plastics-related dust. The dust enters the lungs and causes respiratory disorders known to manifest with pain in limbs. However, the severity of pathological process, its terms, and development are dependent on the nature of inhaled dust and its concentration. This occupational factor can lead to different manifestations of lung disease such as silicosis, chronic dust bronchitis, or alveolitis. In the initial stages of these work-related disorders, patients usually just suffer from minor somatic pain caused by pathological changes such as dry cough, shortness of breath on exertion, and chest problems.

Becoming at Risk of Occupational Pain

Occupational pain can result from conditions that involve

- vibrations from machinery (e.g., while drilling or tractor driving);
- contact with ultrasound;
- exposure to electromagnetic radiation;
- scattered laser light (e.g., hospital workers or doctors can be exposed);
- atomic radiation while working with radioactive substances;
- fluctuations in atmospheric pressure (e.g., in airplanes); and
- adverse weather conditions (e.g., agricultural field work in very warm climates).

Occupational pain in the physical category can afflict office workers, IT professionals, teachers, barbers, and even cash register operators, who often have to sit or stand at work for long periods. Continuously retaining a stagnant position can result in muscle spasm, slow blood circulation in strained limbs, and pain and diseases of the musculoskeletal system. Disorders of the vocal apparatus and vision problems (in the case of eye strain) may also occur in these occupations. There can be neuropathic pain, or pain from the damages to the nervous system, as well as psychogenic pain (i.e., headache, back pain, stomach pain, and pain from work-related stress).

In the third group, there are jobs involving biological factors. These include bacterial infections, parasites, and *candida*, a type of fungus. Farmers, agricultural workers, veterinarians, furriers, and other professions related to constant contact with biological material are most at risk for occupational pains and diseases of this type. Work-related pain will mostly be symptoms of the inbound disease. Visceral pain from tuberculosis and brucellosis serves as an example of this.

Acute versus Chronic Occupational Pains

Occupational pain can be divided into acute and chronic.[2] Acute occupational pain occurs suddenly, for example, after exposure to relatively high, concentrated chemical substances in the air, a dose of radiation, or contact with other harmful substances during one work shift, but not longer. Chronic occupational pain is caused by prolonged systemic exposure to harmful factors in the workplace. Chronic diseases and their varying symptoms are the gradual features of chronic occupational pain.

PREVALENCE AND STATISTICS

According to reports from the International Labor Organization, there are around one hundred sixty million victims of occupational diseases registered yearly worldwide.[3] Since the vast majority of diseases are painful, this number can relate to the prevalence of occupational pain. In a sense, every employee has suffered from occupational pain in the workplace, whether psychological or physical.

Occupational Pain Statistics

Chronic pain disorders account for 98 percent of work-related cases, while acute pain disorders are responsible for only 2 percent. However, strong acute pain after accidents, which injure the main limbs and body systems, accounts for the most cases of immobility and morbidity.[4]

Among the occupational pains, those caused by physical factors such as sore muscles and broken bones take first place statistically. In 2011, the main reason for occupational pain was poor organization of the workplace together with deficiencies in the production process. The highest prevalence of occupational pains and disease was observed among the physically demanding professions, while the best health and working abilities are found among men who do not have jobs that require physical labor (e.g., office workers).[5] Unfortunately, nowadays the lack of occupational physical labor for many professions also means a lack of physical activity, leading to other problems.

Occupational Pain Statistics for Age Groups

The statistics for different age groups show that younger and older individuals are the most vulnerable to occupational pain. Furthermore, general aging of the population in developed countries, along with extended pension age requirements, boosts the overall number of older employees. According to research, the incidence of occupational pains and diseases rises in the forty-five-and-above age group, and having job experience of more than twenty years in a profession is linked to harmful effects.[6] The representatives of this age group are mostly suffering from variable nociceptive occupational pains that occur from (1) heavy use of muscles, (2) tensed or poor work postures, and (3) damaging physical environments such as rooms with chemicals.

Besides the elderly working class, increased susceptibility to harmful chemicals with corresponding occupational pains is also observed among adolescents and young workers, especially during the first years of contact. The adjustment to heavy labor and overworking is also more difficult for young employees and adolescents. Nociceptive, *psychogenic* (originating from the mind), and neurological occupational pains surface faster and injure this age group more often. Clinical symptoms are also more severe. Young workers can even have various types of allergic reactions and their related occupational pains, which don't normally take place among older adults with similar conditions of labor.

Occupational Pain: Males vs. Female Statistics

The female body is more sensitive to harmful elements of a manufacturing process and to the occupational pain caused by it in comparison with the male body. The difference is related to anatomical and physiological characteristics as well as by social conditions such as major household duties. The main occupational hazard for women is strenuous physical labor.

Moreover, disorders such as silicosis, develop earlier in women's organs than in men's, even if a man and woman are working in the same conditions and are exposed to equal concentrations of silicon dust. Women are also generally more sensitive to the effects of ionizing radiation than men working in similar conditions. The greater overall sensitivity of women to vibration can be explained by greater vulnerability of the woman's nervous system. The higher levels of tenderness and permeability of a woman's skin causes susceptibility to dermatitis (including allergic) and to conditions that derive from the penetration of toxic substances through the skin, such as pain from *toxic polyneuritis* (multiple nerve inflammation) caused by organic solvents.

Acute occupational pain is harsher for women, and if it transforms into chronic pain, it can lead to more serious aggravations. Additionally, women have more problems with thermoregulation in both hot and cool climates, as well as increased sensitivity to electromagnetic fields. Generally speaking, ovarian-menstrual function is also very sensitive to toxins. A female's resistance to chemicals and other occupational hazards is reduced during pregnancy, even possibly causing functional anomalies for a newborn's genes.

DISTINGUISHABLE CHARACTERISTICS OF PAIN FROM WORKPLACE ENVIRONMENTS

The impact of undesirable labor conditions and workplace environments can lead to adverse consequences for employees such as tiredness, illness (sickness), trauma, and death.[7] Each of them are either supporting or predicting factors of occupational pains.

Occupational Pain and Fatigue

Physical fatigue is a physiological condition of the human body resulting from overly intense or prolonged activity. It is manifested in a temporary decline in functional capacity. Physical fatigue, usually from intense and prolonged physical labor, leads to the impairment of muscle tissue and consequently diminished strength, accuracy, and consistency of movement.

Mental fatigue can also result from overwork, reducing productivity during intellectual labor. The symptoms include difficulty concentrating and decreased interest in work. This form of fatigue occurs in jobs that require intense intellectual activity. Emotional fatigue can also arise from occupational stress. It is marked by a decline in emotional response caused by a lack of leisure time and excessive workloads experienced in the workplace.

Fatigue and the occupational pain often arising with it can be adverse effects of even simple labor. However, the employee's body can be rejuvenated after appropriate rest. Scheduled breaks, lunchtime, rest days, and vacation—all the traditional, widely used, and often mandatory measures to prevent stress—can relieve occupational pain. Unfortunately, the modern pace of life has increased the number of people suffering from occupation-related pain.

The relationship between occupational pain, occupational disease, and workplace conditions is very complex and ambiguous. The set of environmental factors that create the general conditions of labor, its severity and intensity, can have a specific and direct pathological impact on workers (such as acute pain) as well as more nonspecific indirect harm (for example, accumulation of chemicals in the body over time). Nonspecific effects lead to reducing the overall protective functions of organs and to the development of disorders signified by chronic pain. As these disorders are triggered by labor conditions, they're called occupational or work-related disorders.

Distinguishing occupational pains from disorders caused by natural diseases can be difficult. The vast majority of occupational disorders and pains (around 98 percent) are chronic.[8] Pathological changes in a pain patient can advance unnoticed for many years and then suddenly emerge as a serious occupational disorder. However, pain can be the principal indicator of this pathological process and it is important to know its connection with occupation. The level of mortality among people with occupational medical disorders that develop either from harmful factors in the workplace or eventual disintegration of health and immunity later in life is higher than that seen in the general population. The diagnosis of occupational pain may require specialized medical facilities that employees can use in case of suspicious symptoms or pains traceable to work-related conditions.

Occupational Pain and Trauma

Another painful effect of poor working conditions is trauma. In the case of trauma, the distinguishability of the pain is dependent on the type of exposure. Traumatic occurrences can include

- falls;
- bruises;
- bites;
- punctures;
- burns;
- wounds;
- crushing;
- cuts;
- electric shock;
- stroke;
- shock (such as from *sepsis* or blood infection); and
- *asphyxia* (suffocation).

Depending on the severity of injury or trauma, the pain may require medical treatment.

Occupational Pain and Death

The most serious traumas can lead to occupational disability (inability to work within the scope of their expertise), or total disability (complete inability to perform occupational duties), or even death. The occupational pains from minor cuts, sprains, and other relatively minor injuries are considered to be micro-traumatic pains.

Social Characteristics of Occupational Pain

All forms of occupational pains, including those from fatigue, trauma, and their respective consequences, are together a purely medical phenomenon. If the occupational pain and its aggravations are sustained while on the job, things can quickly escalate into a social matter. If the person is unable to work due to occupational pain or poor health caused by undesirable working conditions or because of trauma, the patient's income source may be insufficient to cover living expenses. Therefore, sufferers of occupational pain may receive financial assistance and worker's compensation from social (taxpayer) funds. Occupational injuries are thus distinguishable according to their significant social consequences.

AVOIDING OCCUPATIONAL PAIN

There are many approaches to avoiding occupational pain. One method is ergonomic organization of the office.[9] Ergonomics is a way of evaluating the optimum conditions for worker capability and effectiveness, thus aiding in the prevention of muscular or skeletal pains and disorders. While there are specific injuries for every industry, the most common occupational pain occurs in bones, muscles, and nerves. The symptoms related to occupational pains in the hands, back, neck, or nerves do not completely disappear after resting. That is why it is not all about tiredness or overstraining. If an employee has noticed continuous or repeated occupational pain, he needs to analyze his workplace to correct the harmful factors there.

For employees suffering from occupational pain caused by repeated movements during work, ways to avoid further harm include

- adjusting the workplace by using different mechanical tools or working instruments to increase comfort and unstrained positions of the body;
- substituting manual labor with technology;
- following the work schedule properly (no overtime when in pain); and
- rotating the tasks and types of work with colleagues.

Use of properly working tools and gloves or other protective materials, as well as limitation of lifting heavy objects can prevent occupational pain. It is also possible to reduce the load for pain sufferers by lifting or carrying objects using special mechanisms such as rollers or powered belts.

It is essential that employees and employers actively work together in this process, since occupational pain affects both parties—physical suffering for the former, and economical loss for the latter. Self-education for preventing and distinguishing occupational pain, training programs for employers and employees about ergonomics at the workplace, and simply creating a safe working environment can all help to avoid occupational pain.

ANALYSIS

Work is an important part of people's lives, as they devote thousands of hours to it every year. In most cases, occupational pain happens from physical labor, especially if there are repeated movements or strains in posture. Approaches to occupational pain can include ergonomic reorganization to minimize exposure to harmful factors, and educational workshops. In the end, preventing occupational pain in the first place is much more efficient than treatment or having to compensate workers for immobility later.

18

SPORTS-RELATED PAIN

When it comes to sports, sustaining injuries is inevitable. Injuries have always been part of athletics. Athletes learn from their injuries and try their best not to make the same mistakes again. When painful injuries are left untreated or overused the body is not given time to rest, the damages may have lasting effects. Before playing a sport, athletes must be mentally prepared for the possible injuries that they might sustain. Sports often challenge a person's ability physically and mentally, and therefore athletes require a lot of effort to reach a specific goal. When injuries come into the picture, they are often disappointed with themselves for not being able to participate.

NATURE OF PAIN ARISING FROM SPORTS

Pain is actually normal for athletes. One cannot consider oneself an athlete without having gone through *some* pain. This is where the phrase "no pain, no gain" comes in handy. But pain from sports injuries is actually deeper than what is perceived through the naked eye. From a mental standpoint, athletes often strain themselves to please their trainers and often end up frustrated because they cannot meet the goals they set for themselves. In short, pain in sports isn't just physical; there is also psychological pain associated with it. But usually athletes focus on getting back to what they do best—playing the sport that they love.[1]

Short-Term Effects of Painful Injuries

Short-term injuries take little time to fully heal. Injuries such as a broken rib cage may take a few weeks or months to heal completely. It is important to be aware that when sustaining such injuries, one must always make sure to check with a doctor. If left untreated, the result may be a longer-term injury and, possibly, the end of a career in sports. Repeated short-term damage to the same area may bring about serious injuries in the future.

Long Term Effects of Painful Injuries

Long-term sports injuries occur when an athlete's body can no longer sustain the constant wear and tear. Boxers, for example sustain injuries not only during matches, but even when they are in training. Intense training without proper supervision, knowledge, and equipment can result in losing a fight or worse, damage with far-reaching consequences. For instance, boxers often suffer from brain injuries.[2]

DANGER, NATURE, AND FACTORS OF PAIN IN SPORTS

The danger of injuries when it comes to sports is actually quite frightening. Athletes have even ended up paralyzed for life or dead. Boxers have died due to head injuries that led to a coma.[3] Even if athletes survive such an injury, they may not be their old self anymore. Professional boxers also sometimes have to deal with swelling on the left side of the brain. Recovery is possible, but authorities may refuse to allow further fighting.[4]

Factors of Sports-Related Pain: Age and Decrease of Performance

Age is a crucial element when it comes to sports-related injury. Athletes' performance is always based on what their body can do physically, and the peak of their prime in general is usually during their twenties. At this age, the athlete is already physically and mentally trained for the game and his or her entire body has developed fully, anatomically and physiologically.[5] They incur short-term injuries, such as a broken arm due to a fall during game play, but recovery is typically faster than for older athletes. In the thirties, performance will start to dwindle, as will the body's rate of recovery from painful wounds. Athletes from ages seven to seventeen who sustain an injury also heal rapidly.

Factors of Obtaining Injury: Type of Sport

Statistics about the rate of injury in sports really depend on the *type* of sport in question. The more contact an athlete has with other players, the higher the risk of injury. Men are more aggressive by nature, and this always shows when it comes to contact sports. Studies show that most male athletes suffer from acute injuries and that it usually happens during warm up, exercise, and/or playing the game itself. Examples of sports that involve a high risk of injury are basketball, football, rugby, boxing, and mixed martial arts.[6]

COMMON SOURCES OF INJURIOUS PAIN IN SPORTS

Sprains are caused by the stretching or tearing of the ligaments around the joints. This happens when an athlete falls and lands on his hand or foot, or twists his knees. A person suffering from this injury can feel pain, swelling, bruising, or the inability to use the affected joint. Sprains range from mild to severe. It is best to seek medical help to assist in easing the pain and help the joint to fully recover. To prevent getting sprains, play or exercise should never be done when tired, and the necessary protective gear should be worn at all times for the sport.[7]

Broken bones are caused by falling or receiving a heavy blow to the affected area. A person will feel intense pain throbbing from the area and may not be able to move it. In some instances, a bone will protrude from the area. The athlete must be taken to the nearest hospital to help prevent infections and further injury.[8]

A concussion is caused by severe head trauma. This happens when the brain moves vigorously within the skull. If vomiting, sudden dizziness, and unusual sleepiness occur, it is best to seek medical help so professional caregivers can conduct tests.[9]

Muscle cramps, on the other hand, have no direct cause. Usually, they are caused by various factors such as lifestyle and activity in sports. When a professional athlete suffers from a cramp, he is unable to move the affected area and is in great pain. This happens often within the leg. Swimmers often experience this type of injury if they are not careful. People who frequently suffer from cramps must always drink a lot of fluids, eat the right foods, and pay attention when playing sports. The duration of this injury usually lasts only for a few minutes. Athletes can stretch for the excruciating pain to cease. [10]

Muscle pain in general is the pain felt when a particular muscle is overused or stressed. It is common among athletes who strain themselves while practicing, warming up, or playing. It is advisable to seek medical attention when it persists for more than three days or if there is something unusual, such as infection. To prevent muscle pain, athletes should always warm up before exercising and do stretches before playing the game. It is best to drink lots of fluids from start to finish. [11]

Fractures are also common to those whose sport involves physical contact. Most require medical attention to prevent further injury to the affected area. Giving the body plenty of rest will help the injured part to fully heal. [12]

Neck injuries are very common in sports. Most are just muscle-related pains, but on a rare occasion, neck injuries can also do serious damage to an athlete's nervous system due to effects on the spinal cord or irritated nerve roots. When such an incident happens, an athlete must be consulted by a doctor to check whether the injury is serious or not. If a neck injury is serious, it is quite complicated to recover and treat. When the injury seriously damages the spinal cord, it may result in disability, paralysis, or even death. There are sports that often involve this injury, such as American football. [13]

Side stitches are common with swimmers and runners, this is the discomfort usually felt in the right lower abdomen. There isn't any concrete cause for it, but there are medical theories that mention the type of food eaten before exercise or game play that could be responsible. To lessen the pain, a runner must stop running and place the hand to the right side of the belly while pushing up and inhaling or exhaling. When such incident happens to a swimmer, he or she must try and take even, deep breaths. In general, the athlete has to stretch to lessen the pain. Prevention will be more likely if enough time is allowed to digest food and drinking sodas or juices before or during exercise is avoided. If it happens often, it is best to consult a doctor. [14]

A jammed finger is a painful injury that sometimes occurs. Basketball players are susceptible to this injury. A player will have a tendency to experience finger joint pains or swelling due to impact. Immediate attention from professional caregivers is needed in order to help heal the affected area faster. While the duration of this injury is very quick, the athlete must allow some time for the affected joints to rest. This can take from just a few weeks to a few months, depending on the depth of the injury. [15]

Deep thigh bruising is often a result of a direct blow. Players who often experience such an injury are in contact sports such as football and rugby.[16] Pain will range from mild to severe, depending on the impact received by the affected body region. The athlete must always seek medical attention in this circumstance, as it may lead to permanent complications. Treatment for this painful injury requires (1) plenty of rest, (2) application of ice, and (3) elevation of the leg. Once the pain is lessened, the player must then try to stretch the area, but not to the extent where the pain is unbearable.

Stress fractures happen when an athlete repeatedly causes stress to the reparative ability of the skeletal system. Runners, for example, should find ways to decrease the amount of shock the tissues receive on impact. It is also important to wear the right shoes, cross train in other sports that strengthen muscles, maintain proper posture, and listen to what the body is "trying to say" when in pain.[17]

Heat exposure is also quite common with athletes who spend a lot of their time under the sun. Since most sports are played outside, a large number of athletes end up experiencing this injury. The factors involved here are dehydration, heat exhaustion, and heat stroke. In order to prevent heat exposure, athletes must always drink enough fluids to replace the ones lost during exercise or sports. The right clothing must also be worn. Professional athletes can wear lightweight, loose-fitting clothes for the heat to dissipate properly. Sunscreen is advised to reduce the risk of getting painful sunburns. Sunblock (SPF25 or higher) is commonly used for such activities. The athlete should limit going out under the influence of alcohol or recreational drugs and should take time to rest following consumption of large meals. If an athlete feels there is something wrong during play, he or she is advised to slow down and gradually stop. The idea here is to give the body adequate rest in order to regain what is lost.[18]

Whiplash is a painful sport-related injury wherein a forceful impact (usually from behind) causes an individual's head and neck to snap forward and backward in a violent motion. This injury is also commonly seen in car accidents. The recovery from pain usually lasts weeks. Injuries such as this should always be checked by a doctor in order to receive proper treatment and to prevent the pain from lingering on and leading to serious injuries in the future. Close attention should be paid for the first twenty-four hours after experiencing a whiplash injury. Symptoms may include

- dizziness;
- headaches;
- difficulty concentrating or remembering;
- pain over the shoulder or shoulder blade;
- neck pain and stiffness;

- pain or numbness in the arm or hands;
- ringing in the ears or blurred vision;
- irritability;
- sleep disturbances; and
- fatigue.

If two or more symptoms are being experienced, it is best to check with a doctor immediately. The treatment for whiplash will always depend on the extent of the injury and the pain associated with it. This injury often damages the cervical disks, muscles, and ligaments around the neck and shoulder. Proper treatment must be received in order to fully recover.[19]

Shoulder separation is a painful injury that occurs when ligaments stretch or tear where the collarbone and the shoulder blade meet. This happens when an athlete experiences a fall or strong impact in the shoulder region. A person who has suffered from this injury will have mild to intense pain around the shoulder. There are times when a slight deformity can be seen around the infected area as well.[20]

Rotator cuff tendinitis is a painful event caused by inflammation of the tendons of the shoulder. The cause of this damage is because the rotator cuff, a group of muscles that join the *scapula* and *humerus* bones, partially tears off. This happens when the arm is required to move over the head repeatedly in sports such as baseball (especially pitching), tennis, weightlifting, and swimming. When an athlete is over forty and is involved in the sports mentioned above, the risk of getting injured is high. If there is pain when moving the arm, discomfort in sleeping on the affected side, or extreme weakness when reaching for something above, it is advised to check with a doctor and verify the extent of the rotator cuff tendinitis. During the treatment, the athlete must avoid activities that may cause the affected area pain. An ice pack is to reduce swelling and anti-inflammatory drugs that don't contain steroids can be used to lessen the pain from rotator cuff tendonitis. Physical therapy is also given to gain full functionality in the shoulder area.[21]

ALTERED KINETICS FOLLOWING FRACTURES AND JOINT REPLACEMENT

Sometimes an athlete is required to undergo a surgery in order to aid with the healing process. The operation will have a great effect on game play if the injured part is replaced. After the operation, the knee or joint itself will be quite sore for weeks; doctors give their patients painkillers to ease the pain. While in the recovery process, the area may get infected and the patient may need to take antibiotics. If the balance between the two knees or joints is not as it used to be, a second surgery may be needed. There is also a risk of getting blood clots in the veins of the legs. A stocking specially made for this is given to the patient to prevent such a complication. When an athlete has fully recovered from surgery, the ability to play sports will be quite difficult in the beginning. The reason behind this could be that the joint replaced is not perfectly aligned with the other joints or the athlete is still getting used to stress that the sport places on the replaced part. This only applies in the months following successful replacement.[22]

SCREENING TECHNIQUES FOR SPORTS-RELATED PAIN

Athletes should undergo prescreening tests in order to make sure they are still physically fit to play the sport and to help reduce the risk of future injuries. This is also done to satisfy the legal requirements imposed by athletic boards. Physical tests are given to determine the current level of pain and the medical condition of an athlete. Using such techniques will reduce the risk of repeating a past injury or having limitations due to the injury. Physical attributes are also recorded to check if there is any change in weight, muscle formation, and pain relief.

Formal caregivers such as sports medicine physicians can check the measurements of muscle strength, joint flexibility, gait, and posture with functional specific and neuromuscular assessment. Skin sensitivity and illness is also evaluated in order to determine if an athlete has skin-related diseases that can also harm other players. Allergies are reviewed to pinpoint an athlete's specific sensitivity. Eye coordination is checked to make sure that there are no complications when it comes to an athlete's vision.

Drug testing is widely done to make sure the player is not under the influence of illegal drugs during or prior to the game. Athletes are also assessed for psychosocial issues that have been clinically linked to pain and pertain to alcohol, tobacco, and steroid use.[23] Sexual practices are included in this stipulation. Menstruation is also checked in female athletes in order to determine *amenorrhea* (absence of menstrual cycles), eating disorders, and *osteopenia* (loss of bone mass) that could contribute to the absence of their monthly period.[24]

NEW ADVANCES IN SPORTS-RELATED PAIN

When it comes to advances in sports-related pain, science is accumulating findings and discovering other ways to treat injuries. For example, an athlete no longer needs to undergo some surgeries as there are more natural ways of rehabilitating musculoskeletal injuries that cause pain. There are also technical advances and improved imaging methods to better diagnose and treat an athlete in pain and stronger understanding of proper nutrition when it comes to specific sports and for the pain recovery process. Tissue engineering is another great addition to the advancement in treating athletes with painful injuries. There have been studies for this kind of treatment with the view to make it ordinary as proper treatment as far as bone-mending is concerned.[25]

ANALYSIS

Accidents and pains may surface together, but full prevention of the pain is always better than having to treat a sports injury. In terms of treatment of sports-related pain, medical science is "getting there." Furthermore, seeking medical attention for even the slightest injury an athlete experiences must always be done. If an injury happens, it is also advisable to give the body enough rest for it to be able to fully recover. Pain patients and caregivers should understand that a focused mind and a calm persona must be exercised to meet the painful challenges one faces on the professional sports stage.

19

PAIN FROM EXCESSIVE MOVEMENT

Pain from excessive movement can affect any number of joints and tissues, but this chapter will focus on the knee, which is a very common locus of pain from overuse. Pain in the knee greatly restricts mobility and it may cripple the pain patient if it becomes permanent. These pains are often associated with actual or potential tissue damage due to overuse.

INTRODUCTION TO PAIN FROM EXCESSIVE MOVEMENT

Pains in the knees are caused mostly by injuries, degeneration, arthritis, and infection. Knee pain alone is responsible for about a third of musculoskeletal problems handled by primary care practitioners annually. In fact, each year, about 55 percent of athletes who participate in active sports suffer from some kind of knee pain.[1] The reason for this is the fact that the knee joints are almost constantly at work, being essential for body movement. Therefore, knee pains have the ability to restrict someone from working or performing daily activities in order to earn a living.

The knee joint, considered a type of "hinge joint," is very complex and intricately designed to allow extensive movement. The complexity of the knee design is one big factor that puts the knee joint constantly at high risk of being injured. Two disks, known as menisci, separate the *femur* (bone above the knee), and *tibia and fibula* (bones below the knee). These bones meet at the knee joint where they are connected by ligaments, tendons, and muscles. A tough cartilage known as *articular cartilage* covers the surface of the bones inside the knee joint. It is this surface that helps the knee joint absorb shocks and makes for a smooth gliding surface during movement. To reduce wear on the knee joint, a secretion from the membrane around the joint called *synovial fluid* flows over and lubricates the bones at the joint.

The knee joints are the largest hinge joints in the body and are considered to be the most active weight-bearing joints, since the muscles and tendons around the knee joints hold the legs relatively straight and bear most of the body weight. Because the knee joints carry almost the full weight of the body, they are particularly susceptible to injuries when overused. Once any of the tissues such as the tendons, muscles, ligaments, or bursae surrounding the knee joints is injured, pain sets in. Other pains in the knee joints occur when the cartilage, menisci, and bones forming the joints are injured. Some of these pains come about as a result of excessive use of the knee joints, while others may take place due to ageing, traumatic injuries, and mishaps in athletic activities.

CHARACTERISTICS OF PAIN DUE TO EXCESSIVE MOVEMENT

Knee injuries developed through excess movement of the joints may occur when people engage recreational activities, work-related tasks, and home projects. Knee injuries can be serious. In the United States alone, it is estimated that roughly 1.3 million people visit the emergency rooms of hospitals as a result of knee trauma.[2] The first noticeable sign of overuse of the knee joint is pain, followed by swelling. The acute pain ranges from mild to excruciating in magnitude. Ironically, the symptom is often experienced after a long period of just sitting or standing in place. Another symptom of knee joint overuse may be a recurring pain around the kneecap, especially at the place where the kneecap and thighbone meet. The pain gets more intense when the knee joint is used, especially during exercises, walking, running, kneeling, or squatting. The pain may worsen when climbing or descending stairs or walking uphill or downhill. Sometimes there may be a popping or grinding sensation experienced within the knee. All these injuries can be classified into two types: sudden or acute injuries, and injuries due to long-time overuse.

Acute Pain from Excessive Movement

Sudden or acute injuries mostly occur when (1) the knee suffers a direct blow, (2) a person falls on the knee, (3) the knee is bent excessively, or

(4) the knee is abnormally twisted. Symptoms that result may be in the form of bruising, pain, or swelling that occurs within minutes of the injury. Sudden or acute injuries may also cause damage to the blood vessels such that the person experiences numbness in the knee or lower blood vessels. Weakness, coldness, a tingling sensation, or the color turning pale or blue may also occur. Below are some particular acute injuries of the knee joint.

Knee Strain

This is an injury that influences either the muscle or the tendon (fibrous cords that connect muscle to bone) of the knee joint. Such an injury usually occurs when these muscles or tendons located near the knee become overstretched or awkwardly twisted or when subjected to unnecessary force. A strain may be a simple overstretch of the muscle or tendon, depending on the severity of the injury. Sometimes a strain happens as a result of a partial or complete tear of the muscle or tendon.

Knee Sprain

A sprain is an injury that occurs when there is a stretch or a tear of the ligament (a band of fibrous tissue that connects two or more bones at a joint) around the knee joints. Injuries of the ligament are usually painful and worsen when (1) the injured knee bends, (2) weight is exerted on the injured knee, or (3) the knee is used for walking excessively. In a sprain, one or more ligaments may be affected, and an acute sprain may be partial or complete, depending on the extent of the injury and the number of ligaments involved. Painful ligament tears are of three types. The first occurs on the inner portion of the knee, known as the *medial collateral ligament*. This is the ligament of the knee joint most commonly injured from overuse. The second ligament tear occurs in the outer part of the knee, the *lateral collateral ligament*. When the injury of the lateral collateral ligament is felt deep within the knee, the location of the pain is usually the *anterior cruciate ligament*. This third type of injury of the ligament usually occurs as a result of trauma.

Knee Tendinitis

This occurs when the tendon suffers an inflammation as a result of strain, such as from jumping. Tendinitis comes in two forms. When it takes place just below the patella or kneecap, the tendinitis is called *patellar tendinitis*. When the inflammation is in the popliteal tendon in the back of the knee, it is *acute popliteal tendinitis*.

Meniscus Tear

A common injury that damages the rubbery cushion of the knee joint, this happens as a result of a twist of the knee when the foot is firmly on the ground. People who play tennis or ski are prone to suffer from this injury. The *meniscus* is a crescent-shaped tissue with two disks: the medial meniscus and the lateral meniscus, which both act as shock absorbers, distributing weight evenly across the knee. A meniscus tear is common among the elderly due to the normal wear and tear associated with aging, and can result from everyday activities such as walking, squatting, sitting, and rising from a chair or bed.[3] A meniscus tear usually involves acute pain that results from swelling and damage of the tissues. When this pain occurs on the inside of the knee, it indicates that the tear is in the *medial (inner) meniscus* while the pain experienced at the outer side of the knee means the tear is in the *lateral (outer) meniscus*.

Knee Dislocation

When the bones that comprise the knee region are out of position it is a dislocation. There are two types: dislocation of the *patella* (the kneecap bone that lies at the end of the *quadriceps tendon*), and dislocation of the knee joint. When dislocation occurs, nerves and blood vessels may get damaged. Soft tissues around the knee joint, such as ligaments, tendons, muscles, and cartilage may overextend or tear in a very painful manner, and excessive movement obviously does not help the situation. Dislocation of the kneecap is the more common of the two, and is likely to happen when the knee is bent in such a position that it is turned outward, or when the side of the kneecap is hit by a blunt force that pushes it out to somewhere within the leg. Kneecap dislocation is more common in females between thirteen and eighteen years of age.[4] Once a kneecap is dislocated, it is more likely to dislocate again when hit by the type of force that dislocated it the first time or when another injury affects the kneecap.[5] The symptoms of a kneecap dislocation are pain and swollen knee. Dislocation of the knee joint is rarer than a kneecap dislocation, and may sometimes be associated with serious vascular injury.[6] A diagnosis of knee dislocation is often difficult to make since a multisystem trauma or spontaneous reduction may be present.[7] Knee joint dislocation is much more serious than kneecap dislocation and thus requires immediate medical attention even if the bones return to their normal position, as there may still be pain and swelling.[8]

Knee Fracture

This is a more serious acute injury of the knee joint that can happen due to excessive movement. It occurs when the kneecap or any of the knee bones (including the tibia and femur) is cracked, broken, or fractured. Symptoms of knee fracture include bruising, severe pain and swelling, twisted and bent leg, or a malformed or malpositioned knee. A knee fracture also results in *locked knee*, wherein the knee cannot bend or straighten. When an individual's knee is fractured, the skin usually becomes cool and pale with numbness or a tingling sensation at or below the knee. These symptoms are more common when nerves and blood vessels are injured or pinched. Knee fractures may result from excessive movements such as atypical twisting of the knee, bending the knee the wrong way, and sports-related activities. Knee fracture is also quite common with elderly people who suffer from osteoporosis. The fracture usually results in some sort of trauma, and such trauma may vary according to the type of fracture involved. Examples of knee fractures, some from extensive movement and some from trauma, are:

- *Patella fracture*—occurs when the knee suffers a direct hit such as in vehicular accidents. It may also happen if the knee is in a semi-fixed position during a fall.
- *Femoral condyle fractures*—occurs when the knee is stressed.
- *Tibial eminence fracture* is a fracture that is common with children aged between eight and fourteen years, although it can also happen to adults in some occasions.[9] This injury usually comes in cases of sports accidents or in bad falls during cycling or horseback riding.
- *Tibial tubercle fracture* is an injury that is rare in adults but more common with physically active adolescents between the ages of fourteen and seventeen years who engage in sports that involve powerful contraction of extensor muscles.[10] These active sports involve sprinting, hurdles, and jumping movements that may result in *avulsion fracture*, which happens in the area where a tendon or ligament attaches to the bones.
- *Tibial plateau fracture* is a fracture of the tibial plateau (one of the most critical load-bearing areas in the human body), which affects knee alignment as well as the stability and motion of an individual. Early detection is very important for this painful injury in order to avoid disability or complication that may result in *posttraumatic arthritis*.

Runner's knee is a common ailment that affects runners, jumpers, skiers, cyclists, and soccer players because of the excessive movement they exert on their knees. A number of factors are responsible for runner's knee. These may include partial or complete dislocation of the knee joint or kneecap; injury, tightness, imbalance or weakening of the thigh muscles; and flatfoot. Many victims of runner's knee suffer from anterior knee pain syndrome (a pain that occurs at the front and center of the knee). This comes as a result of overuse of the knee, strained tendons, muscle imbalance, and inadequate stretching. Runner's knee may cause pain and irritation of the soft tissues around the front of the knee. Some individuals who suffer from runner's knee may experience misalignment of the kneecap from cartilage overuse that takes place during vigorous exercise, thus leading to the softening and breaking down of the cartilage on the patella, causing pain in the underlying bone and irritation in the knee joint lining. Sufferers may also experience a dull aching pain, both under and around the kneecap, especially where it connects with the thighbone. The pain becomes more intense when the individual walks up or down stairs, kneels, or squats or sits for a long period of time with the knees bent.

More on Pain from Overuse of the Knee Joints

The excessive movement of the knee joint may cause irritation and inflammation. Prolonged repetitive activities include stair climbing, cycling, jogging, and jumping. Injuries due to overuse of the knee joints may lead to the following:

- *Bursitis*: This is caused by the inflammation of the knee bursa. The bursa is a saclike cavity situated in the tissues of the knee joint where fluid is produced that lubricates and cushions the knee to avoid unnecessary bone friction during movement.
- *Tendinitis*: This is the inflammation, irritation, and swelling of the tendons as a result of overuse, injury, or ageing. The affected tendon may burst during severe cases of inflammation. Symptoms of tendonitis include pain, especially at night, and tenderness along the affected tendon. This pain worsens with movement of the joint.
- *Arthritis*: This is a result of inflammation.
- *Chondromalacia patellae*: This occurs when the cartilage at the back of the kneecap is damaged due to the overuse of the knee joint and softening of the cartilage.

- *Pathellofemoral pain syndrome*: Pain in the front of the knee caused by the inflammation of the patellar tendon as a result of overuse, injury, excess weight, or other problems in the kneecap.
- *Plica syndrome*: A joint ailment caused by the thickening or folding of the knee ligament due to remnant embryological cells that differentiate into the knee during fetal development. Plica syndrome is accompanied by swelling coupled with pain when bending the knee—especially after a prolonged exercise.

Screening Techniques and New Advances

Any pain in the joint could be an indication that a ligament, tendon, bone, or muscle is ailing due to excessive movement. In order to adequately treat and prevent further deterioration, it is important that a competent medical practitioner conduct a proper diagnosis. In some cases, treatment might immediately begin after a careful visual observation, but further screening and tests are often be required to confirm the diagnosis or to rule out other possible causes of the pain. Supplementary tests may later be needed if the symptoms do not show signs of improvement.

The doctor's first visual screening test is to look for signs of knee dislocation or fracture. When this is ruled out, other screening procedures begin. One of the first areas that a physician treating the painful joints would look into is the diagnosis for *chondromalacia patellae*. The first screening may come in the form of blood tests as well as standard knee X-rays to help rule out inflammation or some types of arthritis.

If inflammation and arthritis are ruled out, the medical practitioner can then proceed with other screenings:

- Magnetic Resonance Imaging (MRI) is a type of scan that uses magnets and radio waves, eliminating any exposure to X-rays or other damaging forms of radiation. MRI would show details of the knee joint, thereby exposing any case of *chondromalacia* (softening of cartilage).
- Arthroscopy is the use of a minuscule camera inserted inside the knee to give the medical practitioner a clearer view of what the cartilage looks like. Screening with arthroscopy techniques requires anesthesia and thus the patient runs a small risk of developing complications.

One important tool used for screening dislocation and fracture is X-ray. The X-ray will determine the condition and position of the bone before treatment proceeds. In knee dislocations and fractures, more often than not arteries surrounding the knee joints become injured as well. A physician would first search for the location of the arteries in the knee to ensure that pulses in the affected foot exist. After this procedure, the *arteriogram* (X-ray of the artery) is conducted to make sure that no artery has suffered any injury or damage. Some caregivers might assess the blood flow in the affected arteries by using special ultrasound or *Doppler* (sound wave) machines. In cases of *tibial eminence fractures* where children are involved, the anterior cruciate ligament may be injured. Moreover, CT scans are occasionally required in serious fractures in order to delineate the extent of tibial plateau fractures as well as other complex knee fractures fully.

A standard practice of screening knee injuries from excessive movement is by the use of *plain radiographs* (X-rays that show only two-dimensional images) to have a clearer image of the fracture, even though only 6 percent of knee injury patients worldwide suffer fracture. The Pittsburgh Decision Rules and the Ottawa Knee Rules, the latest rules for the use of radiographs in knee trauma, have made it possible for physicians to clinically identify knee fracture and determine whether radiographic evaluation is needed, thereby reducing unnecessary radiographs.[11]

ANALYSIS

Pain is inevitable in times of injury or sickness caused by excessive movement. The knee joint is particularly susceptible to excessive movement, being central to moving the body through space and bearing most of the weight of the body. Several kinds of injuries due to excessive movement of the knee can be observed in people of all ages. These have given rise to various techniques and therapies to temporarily alleviate the pain or resolve the painful condition.

20

PAIN FROM SEDENTARY LIFESTYLE

In this age of advancing technology, sedentary lifestyles continue to expand. Years of working in offices, playing video games, and watching television take a toll on general health. A sedentary lifestyle is defined by the lack of physical activity. There are various health problems connected with this kind of lifestyle, including obesity, cardiovascular diseases, arthritis, high blood pressure, diabetes, and many others that frequently cause a great deal of pain.

PAIN FROM LIMITED USE OF THE BODY

Back Pain, Hip Pain, and Arthritis

One of the most common forms of pain caused by sedentary lifestyle is back pain, especially that of the lower back. Sitting in place for long hours is the worst possible position for the health of a person's spine. In that position, the weight of the whole upper body pressures the lower part of the spine, leaving the legs to carry no weight at all. Sedentary office workers most commonly suffer from lower back pain and have a high rate of back muscle fatigue.[1]

Hip pain is another type of pain connected to this kind of lifestyle. It mostly affects persons over sixty years of age and is more often reported by women than men. The pain can be additionally increased if a person is obese.[2] Obesity is a side effect of limited use of the body because a person can never spend the amount of calories digested if there is very little or no physical activity present. It can lead to numerous painful diseases and conditions and it is sometimes very difficult to treat, so the pain can continue for years or even end in death.

Sedentary forms of lifestyle can also cause arthritis. Patients who suffer from it have joint infection, which is extremely unpleasant since, sometimes, even medicine does not help. Painful, inflamed joints become disfigured, as they are worn out, swollen, or stiffened.[3]

High Blood Pressure

High blood pressure is problematic for many people who lead slow, inactive lives. If blood pressure is extremely high, it can cause severe headache and chest pain among other uncomfortable symptoms. High blood pressure can be controlled by medicine, but when left untreated, it can lead to a heart attack or stroke.[4]

It is important to have regular medical checkups because people who have a sedentary lifestyle rarely pay enough attention to their health problems and cannot see how damaged their lives have become. Whether the main reason is office work, work from home, unemployment, or general attraction toward computer games, online surfing, or television, the consequences are the same: obesity, arthritis, high blood pressure, and other potential disorders. Strong will and some persistence can go a long way in battling consequences of a sedentary way of life.

SEDENTARY PAIN VS. HYPERACTIVITY PAIN: DISTINGUISHING CHARACTERISTICS

With the rise of the awareness connected to obesity and a sedentary lifestyle, the opposite problem of hyperactivity emerges, and it can be a cause of a lot of pain. It is also referred to as exercise disorder. People experiencing this problem are those who overindulge in fitness routines, jogging, bodybuilding, and other physical activities. In trying to lose weight or get into shape, they sometimes become addicted to exercise, which has some adverse consequences. Nowadays, activity is considered as a way to get slimmer and look better and gives the sense of accomplishment. Hyperactivity is often connected with eating disorders, and ironically it is (to a certain extent) linked to a sedentary lifestyle. This is because when people who are normally sedentary suddenly become very active, they end up overusing their muscles (see chapter 19) in an attempt to compensate.[5]

Muscle Soreness

One of the most usual and immediate consequences of hyperactivity is muscle soreness, which happens when (1) a sedentary person is not fully prepared for exercise, (2) intensity and duration of exercise is increased, or (3) when the exercise routine is changed. It is caused by microscopic tearing of muscle fibers and manifests as severe muscle pain, which is very uncomfortable and can limit one's use of the muscles. The total amount of the tearing (and soreness) is dependent on how rigorously and how long a person exercises and what type of exercise they do. The muscle then heals and is more fit and prepared for further physically demanding exercises. To ease soreness, one can rest and let the body recover on its own, try sports massage, perform muscle stretching, or do yoga and warm-ups before exercise. If the pain fails to pass in over a week, the patient should seek assistance from a physician.[6]

Cramps

Another frequent form of pain that can occur when a sedentary person becomes overactive is a cramp. It can be defined as an involuntary and forcibly contracted muscle that refuses to relax. Muscles that can be controlled voluntarily, such as the muscles of the legs and arms, alternately contract and relax as a person moves. Muscles that support an individual's head, neck, and trunk contract similarly in a synchronized movement to maintain posture. A muscle, or even a part of a muscle that involuntarily contracts is in a spasm, and when the spasm is strong and continuous, it becomes a painful cramp. Muscle cramps very often cause a tangible or visible hardening of the involved muscle.

Hyperactivity can cause many other pains. Some of the most common forms are those of the knee, ankle, neck, shoulders, elbow, and wrist pain. They can be temporary and pass quickly, but they can also be indicators of larger problems that cause much more pain and result in surgery.

APPROACHES TO PAIN FROM SEDENTARY LIFESTYLE

The easiest way of preventing pain when sedentary lifestyle is concerned is activity. Sedentary pain sufferers and caregivers should gradually become more active to make their health better. To prevent back pain, people should maintain healthy movement patterns. The spine needs to move properly and the musculature that supports it should be strong and stable. Appropriate exercise is the right way to keep one's back healthy.

Drinking plenty of water does wonders for the sedentary pain patient. This includes the back. Since the body is more than 60 percent water, most pains go away or are relieved due to hydration because water-based fluid cushions the muscles, tendons, ligaments, and disks in the spine. A few glasses of water a day are usually suggested, but for every cup of coffee or black tea, a person should drink an additional glass of water. Paying attention to posture is an important aspect of preventing back pain, especially when a person spends their days sitting at a desk. It is also highly important to have a good chair that follows natural curves and supports the back.[7]

To prevent high blood pressure and the potential pain it causes, the sedentary pain patient should maintain a healthy weight. This can be very difficult for someone who leads an inactive lifestyle and is involved in little or no daily activity. Further tips include (1) avoiding salt, drinking only moderate amounts of alcohol or none at all, reducing stress, and introducing a higher amount of nutrients such as potassium, calcium, magnesium, fish oils, and garlic into the diet.[8]

ANALYSIS

Some people lead sedentary lifestyles by their own accord, while some lead it because they are confined by illness. Such a lifestyle is dangerous and can eventually lead to major health problems. Whether pain arises from a sedentary lifestyle or hyperactivity, it may warrant immediate medical assistance.

21

AGE-RELATED PAIN

Old age is usually accompanied by a high incidence of generalized pain. As their bodies deteriorate, elders begin to experience headaches and back pains more often than usual. Joints are severely affected, as are the ligaments and bones. Wrists, knees, hips, and heels begin to swell and crack, and a higher incidence of arm and ankle pains is usually reported. The backbone and vertebrae start to become brittle and somewhat frailer and are more likely to shatter or break when *geriatric* (elderly) patients fall or suffer other accidents. Old age therefore has a substantial, painful impact on the musculoskeletal system.

The natural immune system's response to harmful stimuli, known as *inflammation*, starts to become more active at old age as well. Normally, this response is very useful for addressing infections and for promoting wound healing, but chronic inflammation has an adverse effect on the aging, as it both heals and destroys tissue concurrently. Thus, inflammation becomes one of the most common sources of pain for seniors, and one of the major hurdles that caregivers need to overcome to treat pain sufferers.

HOW PAIN INCREASES WITH AGE

Osteoarthritis

Clinical studies have shown a direct correlation between old age and an increased incidence of pain.[1] The most significant sources of pain in seniors are degenerative spine diseases, which cause a progressive or sudden loss of structure and function in the spinal cord. These are followed closely by osteoarthritis, which is caused either by the normal aging process, or by wear and tear of the joints. Former athletes and manual laborers have a higher incidence of osteoarthritis when they become old-aged, as their current occupations involve extensive usage of the joints. A 2004 finding supported by the World Health Organization shows that around 40 million people experience moderate or severe disabilities caused by this disease.[2] Osteoarthritis is the most common form of arthritis, and one of the leading causes of disability for seniors in the United States and other developed countries. In 2005, nearly 27 million American citizens suffered from this condition, and by 2020, experts estimate that osteoarthritis will become the fourth leading cause of disability in the world.[3]

This higher incidence will primarily be caused by a sharp increase in life expectancy and by an aging population. Studies have determined a positive correlation between old age and the onset of osteoarthritis, especially in women. The syndrome acts on articular cartilages, causing localized loss of hyaline tissue. Simultaneously, new bone formations called *osteophytes* (bone spurs) are produced on the bones adjacent to the affected cartilages. The process affects all joint-related tissues including ligaments, muscles, bones and cartilages. This defines an osteophyte as dynamic and metabolically active.

A number of scientists think of osteoarthritis as the repair process that fixes synovial joints. When trauma affects these tissues, the effects of osteoarthritis can mend the initial damage to some extent by promoting the formation of new tissues. This makes the condition very hard to detect earlier on because its onset is masked by some benefits. However, the structure of the bone-cartilage system affected by osteoarthritis is different now than it used to be, and this can raise a "red flag" on a medical scan. Experts prefer to think of painful osteoarthritis in seniors as a common complex disorder, meaning that it has a large set of risk factors, including genetics. Though scientists have yet to discover any gene or gene complex responsible for this condition, they have established that heritability for osteoarthritis can range between 40 and 60 percent.[4] Constitutional factors refer to aspects such as age, gender, the density of bone tissues, and other risks, including obesity. The third category of risks, primarily biomechanical ones, refer to preexisting (and possibly painful) conditions such as the poor alignment of joints, the amount of muscle strength available, occupation-related damages, or past injuries affecting the joints. Treating osteoarthritis is a very complex process. The disorder doesn't affect all joint tissues in the same way, and a course of treatment that is suitable for mending hips may not work for the knees. Additionally, patients experience a wide variety of symptoms, which are never identical. It falls upon professional caregivers to figure out the particularities of each case and to determine the best treatment for each individual.

Polyneuropathy

This neurological disease occurs when multiple nerves in the body malfunction simultaneously. Some of the symptoms include a burning pain, weakness, as well as a feeling of losing sensations in the arms and legs. A similar condition of the nerves, called *post-herpetic neuralgia*, often affects seniors with a compromised immune system. The disease is largely a result of bodily damage produced by the *varicella zoster virus*.

A neurological condition of the nerves, *polyneuropathy* is one of the most significant sources of pain for geriatric patients. The disorder can be caused by a wide variety of factors, ranging from autoimmune reactions and various infections to the use of specific medication and the onset of cancer. Its symptoms vary, since polyneuropathy types are classified by their underlying cause, their progression speed, as well as the parts of the body that they primarily affect. Experts often catalog the condition according to which part of the nerve cells it affects as well. Some types of polyneuropathy go after the myelin sheath that coats axons; some attack the axons themselves, while others affect the cell body.

While polyneuropathy develops alongside other medical conditions, it is often a direct effect of the latter. For example, a form of polyneuropathy called *distal axonopathy* accompanies the onset of metabolic illnesses such as renal failure and diabetes. It may also occur in individuals who suffer from malnutrition or who are exposed to the effects of certain drugs. The medications used in chemotherapy for treating cancer patients are known to produce this variation of polyneuropathy as one of their many side effects.

The symptoms associated with polyneuropathy are weak, burning pain in the most severely affected areas of the body, pins-and-needle sensations, and loss of sensation. Often the condition affects the hands and feet first, and does so in a symmetric manner. This means that the effects felt on one part of the body are exactly the same as those felt on the opposite side. Certain types of painful polyneuropathy in the elderly can affect the autonomic nervous system, an integral part of the peripheral nervous system described earlier. The former is responsible for controlling digestion, respiratory rates, perspiration, sexual arousal, heart rates, and other visceral functions.

Medical disorders that usually accompany old age aren't always the cause of painful polyneuropathy. Excessive alcohol intake over prolonged periods of time favors the development of this condition. Symptoms usually start to manifest themselves in the feet and lower leg, and may include loss of position sense, and a reduced ability to perceive vibrations. Usually, this occurs in the form of generalized weakness before the onset of motor symptoms. Though alcohol-related polyneuropathy develops gradually over time, professional caregivers such as physicians also encounter cases wherein the disorder sets in rapidly, then later, is accompanied by acute pain. This is why seniors who were or still are alcoholics are at greater risk of painful nerve disease.

Degenerative Spine Diseases

There are several medical disorders classified as *degenerative joint disease (DJD)*, but *degenerative spine disease (DSD)* can be broadly considered a DJD due to the location of the spinal cord in the vertebral column. DSDs share traits such as irregularities in the normal structure and function of the spinal cord. Most often, they are caused by undue pressure applied to the spinal nerves, or the spinal cord itself. There are multiple ways this can happen. The normal aging process is the primary method, but disc displacement or herniation can play an important role as well. Elders affected by tumors, various infections, and arthritis are more at risk of developing degenerative spine disease, as are those who suffer from muscle strain. Conditions favoring pressure on the roots of nerves and on the spinal cord itself, can also catalyze the development of these diseases. Finally, the conditions can be brought about by the narrowing of the spinal canal, called *spinal stenosis*, as the patient ages, and by the slow breakdown of spinal joints.

There are several ways to detect these painful conditions once the first symptoms are reported. Physicians can choose to subject their patients to a spinal X-ray, a technique that doesn't reveal any damage to the discs themselves, but detects changes in the overall structure of the spine. The X-ray can be followed sometime later by an MRI scan that shows the disks and spine more clearly. This is the most common medical tool used to set a permanent diagnosis of DSD. Furthermore, degenerative spine disease has a significant impact on pain patients' quality of life. Their overall mobility is reduced, especially when their spinal cord is hurt. Chronic pain usually accompanies this type of bone and cartilage degeneration, requiring constant supervision by health care professionals and other caregivers. As far as treatment is concerned, doctors begin by prescribing painkillers taken orally and bed rest to seniors. Physical therapy can also help strengthen aged muscles and bones, reducing the speed—and therefore the pain—at which these conditions usually progress. In more severe cases, surgery becomes the most suitable option. This is especially true for patients experiencing chronic, severe pain, as well as for seniors suffering from nerve deficits and loss of bladder or bowel control.

Post-Herpetic Neuralgia

Another source of pain in seniors is *post-herpetic neuralgia*, a condition whose symptoms largely come in the form of nerve pain caused by the varicella zoster virus. When the infectious agent first enters the body, it causes an acute condition known as *varicella*, commonly referred to as chickenpox. Varicella usually affects children and young adults, and it lasts for a few weeks at the most. Though the disease subsides after this interval, the virus is not eliminated from the human body, and can easily take up residence inside neurons. Safely tucked away, the varicella virus can lie dormant for years or even decades. In many elderly individuals, the pathogen manages to escape the nerve cells and produces a painful secondary infection called *herpes zoster*, also known as shingles.

This viral disease has different symptoms and properties than chickenpox. It produces painful rashes and blisters on the body, which usually subside within a few weeks. But the infection can result in lingering pain lasting anywhere from a few days to several years after the blisters heal. Research studies have shown that the incidence of herpes zoster is higher in aged people.[5] The only vaccine against the condition works for individuals above the age of sixty, and the lifetime risk for developing herpes zoster is 50 percent for seniors above the age of eighty-five and roughly 25 percent for the general population.[6]

In old-age patients, infection can cause lasting damage, also resulting in *post-herpetic neuralgia*. Nerves in the areas affected by the blisters and rash send unusual electrical signals to the brain, even in the absence of specific stimuli. In many cases, these signals are converted by the *somatosensory cortex* (specialized area of the brain) into severe pain. The pain is both persisting and recurring, as it can last for a few years after the patient developed herpes zoster or linger on for life. Some individuals experience stark pain that does not respond to medication at all.

Cancer Pain

Cancer is another important source of pain in the senior age group. Elders experience pain not only from the tumor itself, but also from chemotherapy and radiotherapy—two prevalent courses of treatment for cancer. Additional pain is experienced from diagnostic procedures as well as from the reactions of the patients' own immune systems. The tumor can release hormones that interfere with natural biological processes, causing more pain. Physicians in developed nations have a respectable track record when it comes to managing cancer-related pain in the elderly, but in Third World regions, this is seldom the case as adequate pain medication is limited.

The incidence of pain arising from cancer is steadily growing worldwide, as an increasing number of people develop one or another of the many forms this disease takes. Unfortunately, seniors are no exception to this trend. The number of deaths caused by cancer in 2007 accounted for around 13 percent of all deaths registered globally. That's the equivalent of approximately eight million people.[7]

The World Health Organization has published guidelines covering the treatment of cancer.[8] While the evidence suggests that 80 to 90 percent of all cancer-related pain can be reduced or eliminated entirely through the use of appropriate medication, surveys conducted by other national health organizations suggest that only about half of all cancer patients receive the pain moderation they need. The situation is even worse for elders, who are notoriously either undertreated or overmedicated for the painful conditions they already suffer from. As such, older cancer patients experience a lot of pain from tumors *and* the treatments they undergo. Medical procedures associated with investigating the nature of the cancer being treated also cause significant acute pain.

The tumors are a primary source of chronic pain for these individuals, since they may press against organs or directly on nerve endings. Cancer cells also produce various toxins and hormones, which may elicit other types of pain. This is one of the main reasons why a correlation exists between the development of cancer and depression, anxiety, fear, and anger in patients. Nearly three-quarters of all cancer patients report chronic pain, usually associated with the effects of the actual tumors.[9] If properly used, specific medication can keep most of these pains in check, but bouts of *breakthrough pain* (sudden pain after cancer medication) can occasionally occur.

Chemotherapy—the "cocktail" of active drugs used to destroy tumors—often acts indiscriminately; that is, both cancerous and healthy cells alike are killed. This killing of healthy cells causes peripheral neuropathy, a condition similar to polyneuropathy that affects anywhere between 30 and 40 percent of all chemotherapy recipients.[10] Chemotherapy causes hypersensitivity to cold and intense pain primarily in the hands and feet, but these sensations can sometime progress to reach higher in the legs and arms. Tingling and numbness oftentimes accompany the onset of painful peripheral neuropathy in older cancer patients.

Tumor radiotherapy can cause even more harm to the brain and spinal cord of senior cancer patients since its primary mode of action damages the connective tissue that surrounds nerves. The extreme radiation can also damage white and gray brain matter, thus contributing to the reduction of brain volume. If radiotherapy is applied to the spinal cord, it may cause intense pains, which become obvious a few weeks to a few months *after* the treatment concludes.

Geriatric pain patients can experience all these types of pain more intensely than younger patients do. This is why great efforts are being taken by physicians to address the painful side effects of cancer as early on as possible. Cancer is undoubtedly one of the primary sources of pain in the elderly, especially in the developing world, where cancer detection rates are very low and the treatment options available are rather limited by Western standards. Great efforts are being undertaken in these areas to bring medical capabilities up to par with those in more developed countries.

HOW PAIN DECREASES WITH AGE

While studies indicate that seniors generally experience more pain, much of that pain originates from the conditions that often accompany old age. There are no investigations to clearly suggest that "getting old" must be painful. In fact, many authors have shown that individuals tend to experience a reduction in pain as they age. This reduction is primarily because neuron numbers dwindle in the brain with each passing year, causing a diminishing of all forms of perception, including pain perceptions.

In essence, seniors may easily detect or recognize a painful stimulus they feel, but the sensation may not bother them as much as it would a younger adult. The interpretation of painful stimuli changes. Besides the loss of neurons in the brain, reasons why this happens in old age, include exposure to brain surgery, nerve damage and degradation, confusion due to dementia and other mental illnesses, and various medications. The internal organs, joints, tendons, muscles, and skin all have receptors for detecting pain. The way these receptors operate changes with time, but studies have yet to demonstrate whether this shift is due to old age, or some of the medical conditions that usually accompany it. This change isn't limited exclusively to pain, since it also affects heat, cold, vibration, and touch perception.

One possibility experts speculate upon is that pain receptors become less sensitive due to naturally occurring vitamin B1 deficiencies. Another reason could be the steady decrease of the amount of blood flowing to these receptors. While the detection of painful stimuli becomes more difficult for seniors as a result, there are also some advantages. Studies suggest that *somatosensory* (body sensor) thresholds tend to increase as people age. In other words, it gets harder for seniors to detect pain originating from pressure stimuli. The studies suggest that aging causes no changes in somatosensory thresholds that detect pain produced by heat.[11]

Other scientists indicate that the intensity of pain stimuli is largely responsible for how seniors experience pain.[12] These researchers found that the frequency and intensity of pain associated with certain medical disorders decreases as people age. Disorders include musculoskeletal diseases, infections of the viscera, as well as some conditions affecting the *myocardia* (inner layer of the heart). Indeed, pain perception can decrease in old age based on the type of painful stimuli individuals are subjected to. *Cutaneous* (skin) pain has been determined to be a smaller problem for seniors than for younger adults. However, this advantage is countered by the fact that seniors' tolerance to deep pain decreases considerably as they get older.[13]

SPECIFIC APPROACHES FOR THE GERIATRIC PAIN PATIENT

Prevention

Pain can be managed in a wide variety of ways, but the best way to handle it is to keep it from occurring in the first place. Over the past few years, health care providers have placed a heavy emphasis on preventive medicine, an approach that seeks to avert or delay the development of chronic ailments. The process basically begins from birth, but not many geriatric patients are capable or willing to adjust their lifestyle so that they minimize the risk of disease. Painful disorders affecting seniors, such as cancer, diabetes, obesity, nerve damage, and so on, are often the result of a hectic lifestyle during their midlife years. The human body can take a great deal of abuse before it starts degrading, but once that process starts, severe pain becomes a common occurrence.

In addition to reaching for a healthier life, seniors who are informed that they are at risk of developing certain conditions can take preemptive action to ensure that the severity of their symptoms is kept in check. For example, individuals who experience back pain can engage in a variety of physical exercises that boost the strength of joints and muscles, thereby helping to delay the onset of very severe pain. This preemptive approach is also more affordable, and it allows older pain patients to avoid taking medication that may cause damaging side-effects.

Approaching Painful, Age-Related Spine Disorders

For treating degenerative spine diseases, doctors have an array of options of both the invasive and noninvasive types. The physician might choose to begin treating a patient with a combination of oral medications aimed particularly at combating pain in seniors. They also prescribe a lot of bed rest and physical therapy. The latter is meant to strengthen the back so that the progression of the disease is slowed or stopped entirely. In older patients with severe pain, physicians tend to administer steroids and pain medication via epidural injections, which enables them to alleviate the painful area directly and enhance the effectiveness of physical therapy.

While most pain patients can be provided with care in this manner, the most severe cases require additional attention. If a senior is suffering from debilitating pain that does not succumb to the usual methods of treatment, doctors may recommend surgery. This approach enables them to correct structural abnormalities in the bones, thus restoring some function back to the affected regions. If much tissue is removed during these procedures, an approach called *spinal fusion* will enable surgeons to use metallic inserts to cover the gap. The main advantage of using these metallic inserts is that new bone can be encouraged to grow on them, closing the gap left by the removed tissue.[14]

Managing Painful Osteoarthritis

The effects of osteoarthritis on patients' quality of life are very severe, especially if the disease is allowed to progress unchecked. Doctors prefer to start addressing it as early as possible, primarily through recommending lifestyle changes, including exercise and weight loss. Obesity is a complication for osteoarthritis patients who are elderly, yet it is a problem that can be removed from the equation using natural techniques. In addition to these changes, analgesics are commonly used to help ease joint pain.

Those who have more severe symptoms are prescribed non-steroidal anti-inflammatory drugs, which are more effective at quelling pain than basic analgesics. Surgery is required in more severe cases, or when the disease has already progressed to an advanced stage before doctors have a chance to begin treatment. Joint replacement surgery is performed relatively often on the hips in older pain patients, as the bones and surrounding cartilages become increasingly brittle. Knees are often a target for replacement surgery as well, since the procedure contributes to improving mobility and also reduces the amount of pain an aging knee generates.

Polyneuropathy Treatment Options

The medical guidelines currently in use for treating pain arising from polyneuropathy are not meant to treat this disorder directly. Doctors usually concentrate their efforts on treating the underlying disease that causes the damage to the nerve. But if the nerve pain is caused by chemotherapy. and discontinuation of the medication would result in death, the pain must be treated directly with painkillers.

Vitamin deficiencies, diabetes, immune diseases, nerve entanglement, and shingles can be addressed before they result in different types of polyneuropathy. Treatment options specific to each of these conditions are normally applied and any residual pain is eliminated through common pain relief medication, but only at the doctor's discretion. Tricyclic antidepressants, ibuprofen, vitamin B6, and aspirin are used for this purpose.

Managing Post-Herpetic Neuralgia Pain

One of the first steps health care providers take to prevent post-herpetic neuralgia is to stop *herpes zoster* (shingles) from developing. This can be achieved by promptly administering sympathetic nervous system injections to senior patients. Alternatively, *capsaicin* and *pregabalin* might be prescribed to eliminate this type of pain in the elderly. Painkillers, tricyclic antidepressants and anticonvulsants are also used for treating the symptoms associated with herpes zoster. Topical treatments, such as special creams, can be used instead of oral medication, though their effects are not as strong or thorough. In more severe cases of post-herpetic neuralgia, patients may choose to undergo *transcutane-*

ous electrical nerve stimulation (TENS). The artificial nerve stimulation provides temporary pain relief by saturating the painful areas of the skin with low-intensity electrical currents. The interference takes place between the signals passing through the nerves, thereby reducing the painful sensation. A permanent solution for eliminating the pain that comes from a single nerve or set of nerves is nerve *ablation*. This irreversible procedure involves the removal of a small portion of the nerve that transmits the pain stimuli to the brain, and it cannot be reversed. However, the issue with this type of surgery is that it does not produce effects that last over time.

Handling Cancer Pain

Treating pain attributable to cancer is a very complex procedure. Physicians first need to assess the stage of the disease as well as the source of the pain. The pain can originate in any number of locations, and tracking those down is made difficult by the fact that the sensation itself is compounded. This means that seniors may have a difficult time pinpointing any one source of pain, since they experience a form of generalized pain. This is especially true for those in the more advanced stages of cancer. Even though the World Health Organization published clear guidelines for the treatment of cancer-related pain years ago, a U.S. study demonstrates that around 26 percent of seniors in nursing homes do not receive any type of analgesics for their daily pains.[15] Others receive only weak opiates instead of the morphine they need.

The same study revealed that daily pain is felt by 25–40 percent of all seniors with some form of cancer.[16] For most of these individuals, a form of constant pain relief is required. Doctors prefer to use strong opioids such as morphine as rarely as possible, since these chemicals can be very addictive. Physicians therefore have the extremely difficult task of establishing when the pain caused by cancer can be alleviated with a drug that would normally turn seniors into addicts. Radiotherapy is also a useful tool for pain relief. It produces effects that last anywhere between two and four months, especially for seniors suffering from late-stage bone metastasis. The beneficial effects take effect around a week after the elderly patient has been exposed to the treatment. The exact mechanisms through which these low doses of radiation act on tumors are not fully understood, and the approach does not work for many types of cancer.

In some cases, even morphine will not reduce pain to bearable levels. When this is the case, a nerve-blocking procedure called *neurolysis* may be attempted. This approach damages the nerves to such an extent that the latter is unable to transmit the pain stimuli. Neurolysis is different from simply cutting the nerve strand, because it allows for the damaged scar tissue to regrow in time. This technique is not guaranteed to eliminate pain, but it often reduces it to a point where morphine and other heavy drugs can take effect. Doctors prefer to use it on terminally ill patients (such as seniors in pain), but not on those with Stage I and Stage II cancers.

Approaching Painful Terminal Illnesses

The very definition of the term *terminal disease* excludes any possibility of recovery in the medically accepted terms. However, this does not mean that seniors with such an illness are left without care. Rather than focusing their efforts on treating the fatal disease, doctors often switch their approach once the conclusion that the patient cannot be saved has been reached. Pain management becomes the primary objective, and potentially harmful treatments such as chemotherapy are discontinued.

A formal caregiver, such as a nurse or a doctor, takes care of the terminally ill pain patient until the latter dies. This is done for numerous purposes, often the most important being that too much pain is present. Many of the drugs used for end-of-life care can only be handled by qualified professionals. Usually, these caregivers also provide psychological support for their senior patients and help them perform daily tasks. When ethical issues arise, such as seniors refusing to eat or drink when they feel their death approaching, informal caregivers usually contact doctors or other health care professionals who have more extensive training in such matters. When the pain associated with terminal illnesses becomes too severe, doctors are authorized to use a variety of opioids, including morphine and diamorphine. The chemicals these medications contain are very effective analgesics.

ANALYSIS

The incidence of pain is extremely high in seniors, as they suffer from more medical disorders in comparison to other subgroups in the general population. Furthermore, geriatric patients experience pain *differently* from other age groups. While pain stimuli can be more harmful for seniors than for younger adults, sometimes the sensation of pain dulls as age increases. Caregivers should take this information into account when tailoring effective treatment options for an aging pain sufferer.

IV

Resolutions

22

TROUBLESHOOTING PAIN

Pain "troubleshooting" is an approach that deals exclusively with the alleviation of discomfort, without regard to curative benefits. It can extend to all branches of medicine; thus, it requires an interdisciplinary approach, as other symptoms and experiences are considered in the overall approach to pain. Though there is no surefire cure for pain as yet, some government bodies have proposed laws urging further pain care specialization.

IN CASE OF A PAIN-RELATED EMERGENCY

Pain is usually treated in emergency situations with medication such as anesthetics and the often misunderstood analgesics. Examples of analgesics include acetaminophen, morphine, and codeine. These are used to treat mild to severe acute pain. Chronic pain, however, requires the coordinated effort of a team of medical practitioners from different disciplines to treat effectively, even during an emergency. Patients who suffer from painful emergencies are also increasingly trying alternative treatments such as acupuncture, hypnosis, and spinal manipulation. Noninvasive pain treatment is used when analgesics are unavailable or when there is a real concern of opioid addiction.

The troubleshooting technique used in an emergency depends on the type (for example, whether the pain is chronic or acute) and cause of the pain experienced (see chapter 10) and whether the patient is comfortable with the treatment or believes that it will bring relief. Distraction techniques make the patient less aware of the pain, and can be effective for brief periods of acute pain. Emergency massage and pressure techniques are used to stimulate tactile signals that negate the discomfort felt by the patient. Applying appropriate heat or cold to the area of the body affected with pain, liniments, ointments, unguents, and menthol might work in pain-related emergencies.

WHEN TROUBLESHOOTING FAILS TO WORK

Pain Care Inadequacy

Pain is a pervasive and influential experience, as demonstrated by attempts from ancient times to cure it.[1] Human cultures have always developed clear attitudes to pain and its treatment, even if these attitudes and treatments differed greatly from preexisting troubleshooting modalities. If a case can be made to declare pain care as a fundamental human right, then a legitimate question to ask is: if pain and its treatment are a universal experience and a fundamental human characteristic, why is the prevalence of inadequate pain care on an alarming global scale?

Pain care has received significant attention only recently, despite its relevance to medical practice and the quality of life of patients.[2] Physicians have focused more on trying to treat their patients than on alleviating pain because, generally speaking, pain can be avoided to the degree that its cause can be prevented. Pain alleviation methods are viewed to be dangerous, potentially addictive, and an invitation to hazardous side effects, both by medical practitioners and informal caregivers. Some contend the marginalization of pain care is common in almost all aspects of medical care, from intensive care units to emergency wards, and among all age groups, including newborn infants, elderly patients, and the terminally ill.[3] The contention that inadequate pain care is rampant is more interesting in view of the relatively low price, cheap production cost, and widespread availability of pain medications. This is thought to be due to a number of factors that are political, cultural, societal, and religious. Examples of these factors would include the acceptance of torture as legitimate in the political scene, or the belief in some religious systems and cultures that pain is a just punishment from a deity, a consequence of sin, or simply the human condition, and is therefore not to be alleviated (an example would be the belief of some sects that childbirth is *supposed* to be extremely painful). Other factors that may result in inadequate pain care include misperceptions such as

- thinking that pain in the elderly is to be expected, or that seniors always suffer from decreased pain sensitivity anyway;
- inadequate training and personal biases such as the perception that patients belonging to a race, religion, gender, or social group that is somehow deemed inferior and need not be prioritized for pain alleviation;
- physicians' and other health professionals' fear of prescription drug abuse and possible accompanying legal charges due to over-prescription and abuse;
- focus on the biomedical and pathophysiological aspects of a disease, rather than its impact on the quality of life of patients.

The full list of factors that affect the troubleshooting of pain is too large for this study and therefore only some of these factors will be treated in detail in this chapter.

When the Doctor Disbelieves the Patient

Physicians tend to underestimate the severity of pain experienced by patients. This is in direct contradiction to the maxim that pain is anything the individual going through it says it is, and that pain exists whenever the one who experiences it says it does.[4] A crisis of mistrust between the patient and the health care provider will ensue if this maxim is not followed. This mistrust will hamper the troubleshooting of pain and will affect patients' quality of life. Physicians and other professional caregivers may also face legal consequences for inadequate pain care, as will be shown by examples later on.

Paradox of Health Care Provider's Contribution to Patient's Pain

Paradoxically, health care providers seem to contribute to the pain patients feel, or at least fail to alleviate their patients' discomfort. The most common physician deficits in pain care are: (1) failure to recognize that the patient is in pain; (2) inadequate prescription of opioid doses and treating the resultant side effects; (3) failure to reassess the pain after the initial treatment; and (4), most disappointingly, simple negligence.[5]

The health care system also has its share of barriers that hinder the effective management of pain. These include

- failure to adopt specific assessment tools for diagnosing pain;

- insufficient time and space allowed for pain assessment and documentation;
- emphasis on outpatient care and reduced access to practitioners who can effectively treat pain;
- inadequate health insurance and reimbursement policies; and
- failure to recognize pain as a disability that could severely impact a person's quality of life.

Studies point to very alarming realities. Although physicians and other medical practitioners are by no means the only cause of inadequate pain care, they seem to contribute substantially to it. While significant advances have been achieved in the various branches of medicine, including advances in the treatment of pain, the prevalence of pain experienced by patients hasn't changed significantly, nor has it been noticeably reduced for decades.[6] The same studies also indicate that patients with certain characteristics are prone to being administered inadequate pain care. These characteristics are age (with the elderly and children at more risk for inadequate pain care), race or ethnicity (minority groups are particularly prone), gender (females are treated with less-than-adequate pain care), and real or perceived impairment in the pain patient's cognitive status.[7]

Minorities and Inadequate Pain Care

Minorities frequently suffer from inadequate pain care. African American and Hispanic patients typically need to bring up the topic of pain and pain management with physicians. Pain management for these minority patients is often not offered proactively. The same studies also indicate that while pain assessment tests are performed on these minorities when the issue of pain is brought up, the results of the assessments are included in their medical records with much less frequency than their non-minority counterparts.[8]

Other findings are equally alarming. African-American and Hispanic patients are less likely to be prescribed analgesics for their pain, and are more likely to receive inadequate pain care and therefore suffer from more problems.[9] They are also more likely to take more of their pain medication prescribed by their physicians and health care providers. Comparisons of physician and patient pain ratings show that doctors tend to underestimate the pain intensity of minority patients by an average of two points on an eleven-point numeric scale; the same physicians were twice as likely to overestimate the pain levels of Caucasian patients.[10] Caucasians tend to receive higher dosages of opioid analgesics, or dosages comparable to the pain intensity they are experiencing, than their African American, Hispanic, or Asian American counterparts. For instance, comparable disparities are present in the treatment of postoperative pain for children, particularly those who are patients of *tonsillectomy* (removal of tonsils). Latino children receive 30 percent less opioid analgesic in comparison to Caucasian children.[11]

In a nutshell, physicians and nurses tend to underestimate the severity of the pain experienced by minority patients, fail to record their pain scores, and prescribe pain medication less frequently or in lower doses. To compensate, minority patients "self-medicate" and take higher dosages than prescribed to relieve their pain. Thus, the initial fear of over-prescription, exacerbated by misperceptions and cultural barriers, seems to create itself, leading to the actual occurrences of drug abuse due to inadequate pain care. It should be mentioned that the above deficits are not the only causes of prescription drug abuse, but the deficits mentioned contribute to it. On the other hand, there are also barriers to effective pain treatment coming from the minority patients themselves. Minority patients may fear aggressive pain treatment, may not be assertive in seeking troubleshooting for their pain, and may not be familiar with the clinical setting where they are supposed to receive pain treatment.

Gender and Inadequate Pain Care

Disparities in the way pain is treated on the basis of gender have also been noted by recent research.[12] It is shown that while women are more likely to seek treatment for the pain they experience, they are less likely to receive it effectively or at all.[13] There seems to be a biological basis in the gender-based differences in pain perception, pain reporting, pain coping, and pain-related behaviors. Women are more likely to receive sedatives for pain treatment, while men are more likely to receive opioid analgesics, which treat pain more effectively (when disregarding side effects).[14] The disparity between the genders in this regard seems to spread across different age brackets; women aged twenty-four to fifty-five and fifty-five and above are given less pain medication than their male counterparts of the same age groups.[15] It is ironic that those who are unjustly perceived to be of the "physically weaker" gender (women) do not receive the attention the supposed weakness demands. Still more surprisingly, this perceived "weakness" contributes to the inadequacy of pain treatment because it is assumed that women over-react, are too emotional, and simply imagine pain when none exists. The concept of women complaining of nonexistent pain is also present in medical literature, where women are portrayed as oversensitive and hysterical.[16] Thus, pain assessment and diagnosis may potentially be skewed because of this gender bias. A recent study of nurses, however, tends to view women as (1) more tolerant of, (2) less sensitive to, and (3) less disturbed, by pain.[17] The same research indicates that nurses believe women are more likely to express pain through nonverbal gestures, and more likely to report pain to their physicians and health care providers. "Healthy is beautiful" (or its reverse formulation, "unwell is unappealing") also seems to affect physicians' treatment of women in pain.[18] Attractive female patients were perceived by their doctors as experiencing less intense levels of pain than unattractive females. All of the mentioned disparities related to gender are of a similar nature to the disparities related to age and race.

Physician Responsibility and Inadequate Pain Care

Another reason for inadequate pain care is that some doctors fear being accused of overmedicating the pain sufferer. There are patients who have died as a result of over-prescription. Pain medication must not exceed what the human body can handle. If a patient asks for more pain medication, pain specialists must understand that they cannot simply prescribe a limitless amount of medications. Physicians will need a careful study of the patient's health to determine whether they can approve extra painkillers, and both the patient and caregiver must accept the risks.

Negligence and Inadequate Pain Care

Medical personnel must listen to what the patient says and render care accordingly to enhance the pain sufferer's health. If the patient is in severe agony, caregivers must respond immediately. After the patient states subjective concerns, the caregivers must confirm it through objective observation. This could be through vital sign reports. Above-normal pulse rate and irregular respiration are signs that the patient is currently in pain. Increased blood pressure is also considered a factor. Through these objective data, the physician will decide the treatment for the patient. Thus, monitoring the results is critical when troubleshooting pain the right way.

Inadequacy of Pain Care in the Elderly

Under-treatment occurs in care of the elderly due to decrease in pain sensation caused by aging. It is not possible to rely merely on a pain scale to determine the severity of pain in older people. If they have high pain reception, they could be in a severe pain, but if they have *average* pain sensitivity, it does not necessarily mean they lack enough pain to warrant attention. While certain seniors experience moderate pain, younger individuals might feel the same pain at an above-average level. The elderly also are more likely to have decreased organ function, wherein sometimes acute pain lasts less than a few minutes but chronic pain lasts for much longer.[19] Therefore regular troubleshooting measures are appropriate so that the physician can provide inadequate care. Deterioration of body function is more common in the elderly as well, which can invite disease and cause pain.

Studies show that 45–80 percent of elderly nursing home residents suffer as a result of inadequate pain treatment.[20] The reason for this comes from both the patient and the caregiver. The elderly patients tend to be more stoic, fear that they may become a burden if they complain of the pain, and accept that pain is a natural part of the aging process. Health care professionals may share the same views as the elderly patients they are troubleshooting. In addition, health care professionals are wary of the legal consequences of possible addiction due to the prescription of pain-relieving medication, despite explicit statements from several state medical boards that health care professionals need not fear disciplinary action for administering, dispensing, and prescribing opioids where and when it is appropriate and consistent with current acceptable clinical practices. Studies show that while pain is mostly underreported, fears of pain care medication addiction are grossly exaggerated.[21] The proper dosage and administering of a necessary opioid medication may be the latest casualty in the "war on drugs." The efficacy of opioid medication in the relief of many types of pain has been proven, provided it is prescribed and administered properly by medical professionals with sufficient training. Physicians may be held liable for certain cases of opioid and other drug abuses, and they may also be held responsible for failure to prescribe the right medication, including opioid analgesics where and when it is needed. The inadequate treatment of pain may have legal consequences as serious as the legal consequences of being implicated in the wrong dosage resulting in opioid addiction. A recent landmark case of inadequate pain treatment involved an eighty-five-year old terminally ill cancer patient who died in extreme pain after being hospitalized for six days. His physician was held liable for elderly abuse due to inadequate troubleshooting; the pain he experienced before he died was consistently at a seven-to-ten range, on a one-to-ten scale. The case was indeed groundbreaking; until then, pain management complaints have never been considered in the legal context of elder abuse.[22] The punishment in this case was stiff: the deceased's family was awarded over $1 million due to the doctor's negligence and reckless conduct. Physicians and other health care providers need to take heed of the fact that pain troubleshooting always needs to be taken as seriously as the fears of overprescribing that may lead to drug abuse.

Statistics seem to indicate that some nurses also have their share of inadequate pain treatment for the elderly. Nurses are two times less likely to indicate complaints of pain on their records for elderly patients than for their young patients.[23] The frequency of receiving analgesics also diminishes as the age of the patients increase. Thus, while patients in daily pain aged sixty-five to seventy-four years are approximately 35 percent likelier to receive opiates or morphine for pain treatment, this number is reduced drastically to around 10 percent for patients aged eighty-five years and older.[24] The frequency of administering pain medication decreases even more if the patient also belongs to a minority group. This trend is particularly disappointing; it appears that those who suffer from pain and need relief from it the most are less likely to be treated effectively.

Another case is enlightening in this regard. A seventy-five-year-old cancer patient was admitted into a nursing home with metastatic adenocarcinoma of the prostate, and required regularly administered opioids to troubleshoot his pain. The opioids were effective for his pain relief. However, without consulting the doctors, the nursing staff decided to wean him from his analgesic regimen on suspicion that he was addicted to morphine. This case went to court, and the judge approved a settlement in favor of the plaintiff.[25]

ANALYSIS

This chapter has introduced part IV of this book by explaining how the multidimensional pervasiveness of pain affects its troubleshooting. Pain medication and treatment is widely available, relatively inexpensive, and generally effective. Unfortunately, the troubleshooting of pain is below what is expected in most parts of the world, even in developed countries. The common barriers to effective pain treatment, such as biases related to age, race, and gender are driven by misperceptions, which can be effectively countered by

- educating pain patients, health care providers, and medical practitioners;[26]
- providing additional training or retraining, if needed, to professional caregivers, with a focus on the different aspects of pain, its experience, its different dimensions, and the barriers that hinder effective troubleshooting; and
- systems by health care providers where sufficient time, space, and resources are allotted to pain troubleshooting.

Most importantly, the flawed one-dimensional and exclusively biochemical view of pain must be modified, if not totally abandoned. The significant impact of pain on the quality of life of those who suffer from it must become a priority if proper troubleshooting is to be practiced.

23

NATURAL APPROACHES TO PAIN

The goal of any approach to managing pain is to lessen the negative effects so that the patient can still be functional. Managing pain naturally involves social, psychological, and environmental issues.[1] Sometimes a team of caregivers is needed to coordinate a natural approach to chronic pain. Members of a pain management team, whether natural or conventional methods are used, usually include physicians, occupational therapists, physiotherapists, physician assistants, clinical psychologists, and nurse practitioners.[2]

DIFFERENCE BETWEEN TRADITIONAL AND NATURAL PAIN APPROACHES

Natural pain approaches are those methods of pain management that do not include the use of drugs. It is also known as nonpharmacological pain management. Other terms used for this approach are: *nonpharmacological options* and *nonpharmacological interventions* to pain care. Essentially, any remedy that does not make use of artificial medicine can be classified as a natural approach to pain management or natural pain approach. Natural pain approaches can be used for either acute or chronological pain and either with or without pharmacological support.[3]

Special diets and exercises that target proper metabolism are usually incorporated in the natural management of pain. Studies have shown that weight plays a major role in some cases of chronic pain. Heavyset individuals put more strain on their joints, thus contributing to pain and its complications. There are also studies that point toward specific food items that can lessen chronic pain.[4]

Patients who seek out alternative ways to manage their pain often take supplements. It is best to remember, however, that supplements are just that (i.e., they usually do not have a therapeutic effect but only enhance the effect of the pain medication or drug being taken). Still, in some situations, these natural pain supplements can have a therapeutic effect over a period of time. Unlike many pain medications that take effect almost immediately after consumption, supplements take time, sometimes a long period, to have an effect on the pain. For example, anti-inflammatory plants and herbs such as turmeric and ginger offer the same kind of action as aspirin, ibuprofen, and naproxen, but they do not work with the immediacy of these drugs and their effectiveness is not as strong. However, if they are taken together with these drugs, the effectiveness of the drugs increases.

Natural pain approaches also may include techniques such as acupuncture, massage, reflexology, and *biofield therapies* (energy techniques) that explore therapeutic and healing touch. Exercise is also showing great potential in alleviating pain. Doctors may have prescribed bed rest for many chronic pain conditions in the past, but this proved to be detrimental—contributory, in fact, to the worsening of the overall pain experience. Studies have shown that people who exercise and stay mobile are able to manage pain better than those who favor lying in bed all day (see chapter 25). Physical therapists and athletic trainers can be consulted to draft and design personal exercise programs tailored to pain patients' individual needs.

Three Types

Natural approaches to pain management can be classified into three categories: (1) cognitive or behavioral strategies, such as distraction, relaxation, imagery, and breathing techniques; (2) the physical or cutaneous strategies, which include heat/cold application, vibration, massage, position changes as well as transelectrical nerve stimulation (TENS); and (3) environmental or emotional strategies like touch, reassurance, or arrangement and decoration of a room.[5]

The cognitive behavioral strategies refer to those methods that change patients' perception of their experience of pain. They offer techniques meant to interfere with the neural perceptions of pain in the brain. These natural techniques modify the intensity of the pain that the patient experiences.[6] Experts say that in order to alter the way a patient experiences pain, he or she must be distracted by directing attention away from the pain and focusing on something else.[7] These distractions include music, and movement—practices that are very effective in relieving pain because they require the patient to participate more actively in the activity. Another effective distraction method is humor, said to be one of the most effective distraction methods to allay pain and effective even ten minutes after the laughter has ceased.[8] Relaxation, which is known to reduce muscle tension, is another cognitive behavioral strategy.[9] Relaxation imagery, which involves a person imagining a pleasant or peaceful experience, music, and slow breathing, are some of the natural methods of relaxation that a pain patient can use. Relaxation decreases the heart rate, blood pressure, and respirations.[10] Evidence of the effectiveness of relaxation in relieving pain has been scientifically validated. The research proved the positive effects of relaxation techniques regardless of how they were carried out. Patients reported that they possessed a certain feeling of control over their pain when relaxation techniques were utilized.[11]

The second classification of the natural pain approach is physical or cutaneous intervention. This involves subjecting the patient to heat or cold. This strategy works according to the *gate control theory* of pain transmission. When the skin is stimulated, large diameter fibers are activated. This activation stops the short diameter nerve fibers passing on the pain to the brain.[12] Physical stimulation may be applied where the pain is located or in places close to it. Experts say that cold application is almost always more effective than heat application, and a combination of both applications is considered to be even more helpful than using only one thermal method.[13] When both thermal applications are used, they reduce the sensitivity of the patient to pain or his muscle spasms in a natural way.[14] A second type of cutaneous or physical stimulation is vibration. Vibration brings about paresthesia or anesthesia to the stimulated region of the body and alters the sensation of the pain from "very severe" to moderately tolerable. When vibration is removed, the relief from pain can last up to 30 minutes. An even better situation is the blending of the heat and vibration methods. The third type of cutaneous therapy to relieve pain is massage, especially in the back and shoulders. A study showed that when terminally-ill patients are given a three-minute, slow backrub, their blood pressure was lowered, signifying that they experienced relaxation and were therefore in less pain.[15]

The third classification of the natural pain approach involves interventions coming from family and the social environment of the pain patient. The social environment plays a very important role in natural pain management, and a healthy family interaction will be very helpful. This can be done through family therapy.

SIGNIFICANCE OF APPROACHING PAIN NATURALLY

Nonpharmacological approaches to pain management continue to evolve, as there is much demand for further research to explore its potential further. The professional caregiver's role remains important in ensuring that such options are presented to patients alongside important data that need to be considered. Caregivers can also help patients suffering from acute and chronic pain to make informed decisions regarding the natural treatment plan they wish to pursue. Natural pain approaches without pharmacological support usually fall under the nonstandard or alternative options to pain management. Standard care, or the traditional approach to pain, refers to the practice of medical doctors and other health professionals such as registered nurses and physical therapists.[16] Natural pain approaches are significant because they consider pain, whether acute or chronic, to be more than just physiological. *Psychosocial* (mind and society) and environmental factors also play a role in the emergence of pain. Such factors cannot be managed by conventional medical treatment alone. Hence, natural approaches to pain management have become popular, even if some approaches have not yet been thoroughly researched and studied in mainstream medical practice.[17] The natural pain approach can be considered to be a holistic approach to pain management, since it takes into account all the circumstances and issues surrounding the pain. The pain is part of the patient's overall human experience.

Alternatives to drug-dependent therapies continue to emerge. Natural approaches are constantly evolving and provide complementary means to effectively manage pain. Despite these approaches gaining increased popularity among patients, few studies have been completed to validate the efficacy of nonpharmacological techniques. This situation is slowly being remedied and peer-reviewed journal articles highlighting the potential of natural approaches, most especially in the realm of palliative care, continue to appear.[18] The pain management specialist needs to be well informed about natural options to be able to provide a wide array of treatment paths for patients.

BENEFITS AND DRAWBACKS OF NATURAL PAIN APPROACHES

Cost-Effectiveness

The natural pain approach has many benefits. First is cost-effectiveness. It does not take much money to ease pain the natural way. Laughter, as is often said, is the best medicine and therefore a great step in approaching pain naturally. Laughter causes the body to release endorphins, which are natural "opiates" that relieve pain immediately or make the pain disappear over a period of time. For obvious reasons, there is no financial cost to laughing. A person can enjoy a good laugh by simply watching stand-up comedy. Entertainment is something that all people, whether in pain or pain-free, can take pleasure in.

Empowerment

As a coping strategy, another benefit of the natural pain approach is that it empowers the patient to actively respond to it when it happens. Patients may not be in control of the pain, but if well-informed by a pain management team, they can control their response to it. For example, *biofeedback*, a form of stress-management, enables the individual suffering from pain to monitor the natural reactions of his body to pain. Natural methods also enable patients to hone their attention so that at the onset of pain, their mind is focused elsewhere. Practices of this kind are found in yoga and other meditation exercises. Becoming aware would let the patient be in control of the stressful reactions to pain.

Timing

A major drawback of the natural pain approach is that there may not be enough time to make them work. If the pain is acute and must be eased immediately, the natural approach would not be so practical. Relaxation exercises, aromatherapy, massage, biofeedback and some other similar natural pain approaches take time to be administered or become effective. They do not offer instant relief to the patient. Thus, in extreme cases of pain, these approaches cannot be utilized alone but only as additions to traditional medical methods. The attitudes of different caregivers vary regarding the natural pain approach. Many times it is not from the rationale of the natural way that caregivers object to, but the time such methods involve. A research study showed that the attitude of nurses and the lack of time are hindrances to offering the pain patient the best natural approach to pain. [19]

CHANGING THE SOCIAL AND LIVING ENVIRONMENT

The unpleasantness of the experience of pain varies depending on the culture and environment of each patient. What is painful in one culture may not necessarily be painful in another. Moreover, as stated earlier, a religious social environment may also affect how patients view pain. Hence, the social and living environment of the patient has an effect on his experience of pain. As such, social and living environment changes will certainly play an important role in the natural approach to pain.

Family

Family is the most important "social" environment. The severity or the lightness of the pain is affected by the family atmosphere the patient lives in. The more stressful and strained the relationship among the family members, the harsher the mental and physical pains can be. The more loving the relationship within the family is, the more tolerable the pain becomes. Pain sufferers in abusive and disorganized families may have more difficulty in treatment. Natural interventions for them may need to be further developed on an individual basis. [20]

Light, Nature, Video, or Virtual Reality

Environment can also influence pain. Scientists recently published a study of the environmental factors that influence pain. [21] They focused primarily on the effects of environmental stimuli on pain, such as light, video, nature scenes and sounds, and virtual reality (VR). Factors in the environment that can be easily controlled may help to reduce the use of analgesics, which can remove difficult side effects from medications. They can also help lessen the cost of medication and improve quality of care and results. For example, patients of spinal surgery who have more exposure to natural sunlight after their surgery and during their recovery may have less stress, reduced pain, less use of analgesic medication, and a decrease in medical expenses. [22] In order for the patient to enjoy the long-term benefits of less health care costs, treatment environments should be designed to make better use of natural light. Managers of health care facilities could make sure that rooms with many windows are allotted to patients experiencing pain. Moreover, structural elements such as skylights and large windows can be built into facilities to fetch natural light inside. Research has been conducted regarding (1) the kinds of pain, (2) levels of pain, and (3) pain conditions that will benefit from exposure to natural light, in most people.[23] Further studies could examine which parts of the body need more exposure to natural lighting.

Viewing nature scenes can generate positive emotional responses that also affect pain levels. When a pain patient views simple and unembellished scenes of nature, the blood pressure is said to decline within a few minutes, as evidenced by researchers who showed nature films to two different sets of participants.[24] One of the groups watched a scary and "stressful" film, while the other viewed a calming nature video. After the viewing, investigators reported that those who were exposed to the nature film demonstrated recovery from cardiovascular stress in about twenty seconds. Thus, it would be beneficial to pain patients to place their beds or chairs beside windows with a good natural view of the outside. It would certainly help if they could spend some time outdoors and enjoy the sights and sounds of nature.

Studies are also being conducted to determine which kinds of patients would be helped more by viewing scenes of nature and what type of nature views are more beneficial to people suffering from pain. Another relatively inexpensive strategy for pain relief would be video or positive VR presentations. Treatment facilities can be designed in such a way that there are places, such as kiosks, where portable video and VR are present. In fact, science has provided information regarding the effectiveness of implementing video and VR presentation for treatment. Video presentations should take into account different characteristics of the patient, such as age, gender and ethnicity. Future research is recommended to evaluate the effectiveness of this kind of treatment if patients are given the choice as to what they want to view. In summary, changes in the environment of the patient, such as those involving light, nature, and video presentations appear to be essential when designing natural pain approaches.

Effects of Travel on Pain Patients

Pain patients should not be constantly moved across far distances. However, sometimes circumstances compel a move or brief travel. A report on the effect of airplane travel on patients with fibromyalgia noted that altitude, atmospheric pressure, dehydration, weak air flow, and lack of movement for an extended time can worsen the symptoms. Between 40 and 70 percent of fibromyalgia patients go through sporadic or frequent nausea, which can be worsened by the movement, shaking, and weak air circulation on an airplane.[25] Migraine headaches are also a common fibromyalgia symptom, and they can contribute to extreme nausea. When sitting in a cramped position for too long, the air-travelling fibromyalgia patient may experience severe and widespread muscular pain, specifically that of the back. Long-term travelling in a sitting position can also aggravate *temporomandibular joint (TMJ) disorder*, a common side effect of fibromyalgia. In order to prevent these painful experiences, a few, simple precautionary steps must be taken. For example, the patient should bring along a lumbar support pillow or a headrest. In order to stay hydrated, the patient may be advised to drink several glasses of water per hour. Some precautionary measures and medication could help prevent nausea and pain.[26]

"NATURE" OF NATURAL PAIN SUPPLEMENTS

Enzymes

Enzymology is defined as the branch of science dealing with the biochemical nature and activity of enzymes.[27] Enzymes can be extracted from any living organism ranging from microorganisms to plants and animals, and they have many uses in an individual's everyday life. Studies for pain show that supplementary enzymes are beneficial in alleviating pain naturally.[28] Enzymes have been discovered to be an effective alternative to pharmaceutical drugs that are not only natural, but can also answer the problem of prescription drug abuse. There are two kinds of supplementary enzymes: digestive enzymes and the systemic enzymes.[29] Digestive enzymes are those used to improve digestion and are taken orally with food, whereas systemic enzymes are also taken orally, but in between meals. Some enzymes used for healing pain and inflammation include the following:[30]

- Amylase: aids in digesting carbohydrates and increases joint mobility. It also reduces muscle pain and inflammation.
- Bromelain: used to treat swelling and inflammation related to injuries, blood clots, hemorrhaging, and the like.
- Papain: used against insect stings.
- Trypsin: for treating bruises and inflammation.
- Chrymotrypsin: treats inflammations and wounds related to dental work and surgeries.

- Protease: helps in alleviating soft tissue problems caused by accidents or surgery.
- Catalase: relieves inflammation caused by injuries and functions as an antioxidant.
- Lipase: alleviates swelling and muscle spasms caused by calcium deficiency.

Like other pain medications, the use of enzyme therapy should be regulated by a physician. Previous health records are critical in this type of treatment because certain conditions such as gastrointestinal inflammations don't react well to enzyme treatment.

Fish Oil/Omega-3

Many chronic conditions produce inflammation and pain. Headaches, back pain, some nerve pain, and autoimmune conditions such as rheumatoid arthritis are treatable to a certain extent by fish oil. Omega-3 can be discovered in other sources, but it is best found in fish oil and flaxseed. Its mechanism of action is anti-inflammatory, and mild blood thinning is its side effect. Its painkilling effect is boosted if it is taken with other pain supplements such as turmeric or ginger.[31] In a 2004 study, 250 patients experiencing nonsurgical neck or back pain, were told to take a total of 1,200 mg per day of omega-3 *eicosapentaenoic acid* (EPA) and *decosahexaenoic acid* (DHA) found in fish oil supplements.[32] Results showed the same effect in this selective group, as those in another selective group, who were taking ibuprofen, in easing arthritic pain. It was also concluded in this study that omega-3 EPA and DHA in fish oil supplements seem to be a safer substitute to NSAIDs for the treatment of patients with nonsurgical neck or back pain.

Antinflammatory Plants and Herbs

Many painful conditions such as osteoarthritis and back pain are brought about by chronic inflammation. Aspirin, ibuprofen, and naproxen are anti-inflammatory medicines that function as blockers of the enzymes that set off both the swelling and the pain. Alternatives to these medicines are turmeric, green tea, ginger, rosemary, cat's claw, devil's claw, and willow bark. A physician at the Center for Integrative Medicine at the Cleveland Clinic said that her patients who started using turmeric had gotten off their use of NSAID medicines completely.[33] Turmeric can be found in standard capsules. Rheumatoid arthritis can be eased by turmeric, whose mechanism of action is anti-inflammatory.[34] In an issue of *Time*, a doctor tells of an experience of a patient who found turmeric useful. He said that his patient, a seventy-three-year-old male, had two faulty hips. His joints did not develop correctly as he grew up. The patient started to experience pain when he entered his sixties. The doctor prescribed the usual anti-inflammatory drugs to treat arthritis, but the pain did not go away. His patient stopped taking the medication and began taking eight capsules of turmeric each day—four in the morning and four in the evening—and has since been pain-free.[35]

A medicinal herb that contains anti-inflammatory agents called flavonoids, *sage* is a remedy used to relieve swelling of body parts of patients.[36] Tea from sage is also used as a spring tonic that increases blood circulation, improves memory, and promotes long life.[37] Ginger is another natural anti-inflammatory supplement. It is said that ginger can alleviate the pain and swelling that result from an arthritic condition.[38] Symptoms of osteoarthritis were significantly reduced when a well-purified and uniform ginger extract had been given to approximately 60 percent of nearly two hundred sixty patients who were examined. They reported that their knee pain was reduced when standing and after walking fifty feet.[39]

Vitamin D

Natural uses for vitamin D include painful osteoarthritis, rheumatoid arthritis, fibromyalgia, and *generalized myalgia* (muscle pain). Vitamin D is a champion pain reliever because it supports healthy muscles, bones and joints.[40] When pains in these areas are experienced, it usually is symptomatic of a lack of Vitamin D. Vitamin D is also called the "sunshine vitamin" because it is made by the skin when exposed to the rays of the sun. Indeed, it is a natural supplement. When the skin absorbs vitamin D, the liver and kidneys break it down to form an active chemical that essentially performs as a hormone. It acts all over the body in many tissues and organs, as well as in the muscles, nerves, and the brain. When vitamin D is inadequate in the pain patient's body, muscles can ache and nerves get irritated. Because vitamin D supports healthy bones, getting an adequate amount can help patients with many types of bone and joint pain. It is particularly beneficial for patients with back pain. Other natural pain supplements are magnesium, capsaicin, riboflavin (vitamin B2), glucosamine sulfate, s-adenosylmethionine (SAM), acetyl-L-carnitine, alpha-lipoic acid, bromelain, and methylsulfonylmethane (MSM).[41]

These natural pain relievers can be very effective, but traditional approaches that make use of NSAIDs such as ibuprofen and naproxen are also very effective. These drugs can be more affordable than some of the natural supplements. Natural pain relief and traditional medicine do not have to be conflicting, since the best approach to relieving pain is a combination of both. Nevertheless, the advice of a doctor must be sought first before a patient uses natural pain supplements and prescription drugs concomitantly. It would be wise to ask a good health care provider who is familiar with both the medicines and supplements that a pain sufferer can use.[42]

NATURAL BALANCE

Blending Alternative and Traditional Treatments

Every patient has the right to optimal care. Fortunately, the progress of science and medicine in recent times has made optimal care for the patient possible using a combination of therapies. These days, traditional medical treatment to manage pain is not enough. The body has natural capacity to heal itself and sometimes the best way is to let the pain pass on its own (if it is mild and nonthreatening) since the body will automatically find a way to overcome it.

For pains that are severe, medicines are readily available for the patient to take. However, several clinical studies have shown that even traditional medications, if taken without the proper guidance of a health professional, induce serious side effects, which in some cases, worsen the pain rather than heal it.[43] Alternative approaches to pain management have emerged to serve as adjuncts to potentially harmful conventional approaches to pain. It is therefore important that a patient not depend entirely on only one doctor, but rather utilize the expertise of a small team of health professionals. This team can offer a satisfactory natural pain management plan, which in most cases, consists of a combination of natural and traditional or pharmacological approaches.

Individual vs. Cooperative Approach

Each patient is unique. In order for patients to be able to find the balance between pharmacological and natural approaches to pain, they must be able to connect with a professional caregiver they can trust and depend on. It is not always easy to find this balance. If traditional approaches are working, then things are going as planned. If not, then the pain sufferer may resort to natural approaches.

ANALYSIS

Natural approaches are advisable in pain caregiving even if studies of their efficacy have not been very conclusive. This kind of approach to pain management varies according to the kind of pain a patient experiences. The drawbacks of this approach are due mainly to the lack of its knowledge in certain caregivers as well as the length of time for natural tactics to succeed. Some of the goals of the natural pain approach are: (1) minimize the fear and distress that sufferers feel before, during, and after the pain, (2) increase the tolerance of the patients to pain to normal limits, and (3) enhance their quality of life.

24

DIETS FOR PAIN RELIEF

A person going through physical *or* psychological pain could possibly be affected by the food that he or she consumes. Some believe that some foods can make one "feel good" while others can be pain triggers. Since various types of food have different chemical compositions, the patient may consider what groups of food will either aggravate or relieve pain. Developing such awareness about diet enables the patient to manage pain more effectively, thus coping with the situation easier and faster. Patients and caregivers should understand that a healthy diet does not ensure a complete cure for painful medical disorders and that it is definitely not a silver bullet. Specific diets that work on one patient may not work on another. It will always depend on the type and the level of pain being experienced.

A holistic approach to pain includes special diets and exercises that target proper metabolism, which is greatly correlated to the management of pain. Studies have shown that weight plays a major role in some cases of chronic pain. Heavyset individuals put more strain on the joints, thus contributing to pain. There are also studies that point toward specific food items that can lessen chronic pain. Examples of these include (1) salmon, which contains omega-3, (2) onions and garlic, which contain anti-inflammatory antioxidants, and (3) other antioxidant-rich fruits and vegetables such as blueberries and sweet potatoes.[1]

Dieticians may likewise recommend veering away from food additives known to contribute to or even cause chronic pain. Information regarding food additives that need to be eliminated or lessened becomes increasingly useful, especially for pain conditions where the source is not readily apparent. Painful conditions such as migraines and arthritis are increasingly common. Patients suffering from migraine headaches and arthritis are encouraged to stay away from natural and artificial sweeteners including high-fructose corn syrup (HFCS). Salt and *monosodium glutamate* (MSG), a common flavor enhancer, are both pinpointed as common culprits as well. All in all, individuals suffering from pain are encouraged to steer clear of preservatives—especially the synthetic kind. A dietary approach to pain management requires one to choose fresh food over instant or ready-to-eat items, not just to help decrease pain, but also to improve overall health.[2]

HOW WEIGHT LOSS AFFECTS PAIN LEVELS

While diet and weight loss programs are often associated with overweight individuals, they also have been regarded as major factors in reducing health risks or the severity of various medical conditions.[3] In 1990, research was conducted on 105 patients that determined weight loss as a major factor in relieving musculoskeletal pain of obese individuals.[4] The findings of this research significantly showed that about 90 percent of the total patient population who lost weight had experienced pain relief in at least one of their joints, such as back, knee, ankle, or foot. A similar study was also conducted in 2000 on twenty-four obese adults, ages sixty years or older, with knee osteoarthritis.[5] The researchers concluded that improvements in pain levels were achieved after the research participants went through a six-month diet program combined with regular exercise. In 2003, a U.S. survey was carried out among the older population (minimum sixty years old) to examine the relationship between an individual's body mass index (BMI) and the pain felt in the hip, knees, and back.[6] It was discovered that as elderly people gain weight, their pain also increases proportionally. In 2004, scientists evaluated the positive effects of weight loss on the musculoskeletal pain of almost sixty obese women who were assigned at least twelve weeks of diet regimen.[7] The study concluded that weight loss had normalized the pain, starting from the lower back and down to their feet. Since the intensity of pain decreased, most of the women's functional limitations improved and physical activity levels increased.

Aside from the studies conducted to determine the association between an individual's weight and musculoskeletal pain, there are other clinical works of research that investigated how weight loss can affect symptoms of certain painful diseases. A medical team from Princess Alexandra Hospital in Australia carried out a study to understand the long-term effects of moderate weight loss to the pain symptoms experienced by forty-three overweight patients with fatty liver disease.[8] After the patients had gone through a three-month weight reduction period followed by a twelve-month weight maintenance program, improvements in the symptoms of chronic liver disease (e.g., pain felt under the rib cage, swollen abdomen, fever, and jaundice) could be seen, resulting in increased physical activities of the patients. Another research study was conducted on thirteen individuals suffering from acute intermittent gout who followed a modified weight-loss diet consisting of complex carbohydrates, and *monounsaturated* and *polyunsaturated* fats.[9] There was a significant reduction in the frequency of gout attacks among these individuals only after four months of going through diet intervention.

SPECIFIC DIETS FOR PAIN PATIENTS IN THE SHORT TERM

Medical researchers are now trying to develop diet therapies to lessen pain for patients who are going through an unpleasant physical and emotional experience. Even if such diet therapies only provide temporary relief, some patients are willing to try them out just to improve their medical condition. Surprisingly, there are certain common foods that possibly have been used traditionally as herbal medicines and that can help alleviate physical pain.

Anti-Inflammatory and Analgesic Group

One group of foods is characterized by anti-inflammatory and analgesic properties that might provide relief from simple to major disorders such as fibromyalgia, osteoarthritis, or chronic pain.[10] Popular examples from this food group include the following:

- Apple: In herbal medicine, bandages made from apple peelings can cure skin inflammations and some eye problems. When stewed, they can relieve diarrhea. Furthermore, apples are used to treat kidney stones and liver conditions.[11]
- Celery: This contains a natural active anti-inflammatory compound that reduces the pain brought about by gout and rheumatism. It has a sedating effect that encourages a relaxing sleep and alleviates anxiety.[12]
- Chamomile Tea: Used externally as a compress, chamomile tea has anti-inflammatory and antiseptic properties that soothe minor pains, swellings, insect bites, and bruising. Cold tea bags can give

a patient relief from inflamed and itchy eyes that are commonly associated with hay fever or reduce facial swelling caused by toothaches and abscess.[13]

- Cherry: This acts as an anti-inflammatory agent by neutralizing free radicals and impeding tissue inflammation in a pain patient's body.[14] Cherry is used in traditional medicine to help prevent painful gout because it contains substances that eliminate uric acid from the blood. It also cleanses and keeps the kidneys functioning properly. Furthermore, it is a mild laxative that eases constipation and promotes regular bowel movements.[15]
- Coffee: Drinking a cup of black coffee a day can be a temporary relief from strong headaches. A sugary ice coffee drink can also act as a stimulant that could help a person suffering from heat exhaustion.[16] According to preliminary medical studies, it is possible that drinking coffee reduces an individual's risk for cancer.[17]
- Dark Chocolate: Rich in chemical compounds called flavonoids, dark chocolate can lower blood pressure and increase blood circulation. Also, it might prevent blood clots and heart attacks when consumed in considerable amounts. According to the Johns Hopkins University School of Medicine, cocoa beans have a biochemical composition that is comparable to aspirin.[18]
- Ginger: Whether used as an add-in or consumed on its own, ginger is used for a variety of painful disorders such as stomachaches and colic pains. Ginger tea also eases cold symptoms such as fever and nasal congestion. In addition, it boosts blood circulation, enhances liver function, and improves heart conditions. It also relieves a toothache when the root is chewed.[19] One remarkable discovery from clinical research at the University of Michigan is that ginger, when dissolved in a solution, can control inflammation and impede the development of ovarian cancer cells.[20]
- Green Tea: This is one of those excellent sources of an active compound called *polyphenol* that lessens free radicals known to cause inflammation in a patient's body. Green tea's medicinal properties have been widely used for centuries.[21]
- Olive Oil: Popularly known as the staple of the Mediterranean food diet, olive oil has been found to reduce the risk of strokes and the occurrence of some cancer diseases. Also, it has an anti-inflammatory ingredient that is strong enough to be a substitute for some over-the-counter pain medications.[22]
- Salmon: This is a very good source of protein, which is responsible for a patient's tissue growth and repair.[23] It is also rich in omega-3 fatty acids that serve as lubricants for the body's joints.[24]

Antiseptic Group

The second "anti-pain" food group is known to have antiseptic, antibacterial, or healing properties. Foods that belong to this group have been traditionally used to sterilize and cure wounds and further fight infection. Examples are as follows:

- Artichoke: Originating from Mediterranean locales, artichoke contains a healing substance called *cynarin* (also spelled *cynarine*) that helps lower blood cholesterol levels, enhances liver function, and aids in the treatment and prevention of painful gallstones in the gallbladder.[25]
- Banana: A widely grown tropical fruit, banana is the perfect food for people who are recovering from an illness and gradually regaining strength. It is also a known remedy for painful upset stomachs and ulcers.[26]
- Blackcurrant: Used in herbal medicine, blackcurrant is a widely used remedy for fever and diarrhea. It has anti-inflammatory and anti-infective properties that can treat sore, painful sore throats as well.[27]
- Blueberry: Containing *anthocyanidins* (healthy plant dyes), blueberries provide protection against excessive amounts of E. coli, one of the many bacteria found in the gut. When dried, it is used as a popular herbal medicine to cure digestive complaints, such as food poisoning.[28]
- Cabbage: Juice is extracted from raw cabbage to promote healing of gastric ulcers and other digestive issues in traditional medicine. The chemical compound responsible for this juicy "medication" is *s-methylmethionine (SMMS)*.[29]
- Honey: Traditionally used to treat burns and wounds, honey is a mild antiseptic that alleviates sore throat and common cold symptoms.[30] According to German academic research, a honey-based dressing called *medihoney* is an effective medication for diabetic patients with painful foot ulcers.[31] Its potency reduces inflammation, kills germs, speeds up healing, and even eliminates any foul odor smell of infected open wounds.
- Onion: A popular remedy to cleanse wounds during the war era, an onion has antiseptic properties that can heal insect bites, bee stings, burns, scurvy, and even athlete's foot. It also acts as a sterilizing agent in the mouth and the throat when consumed raw. Aside from antibacterial properties, it has antiviral capabilities that enable it to prevent a number of digestive diseases.[32]

- Wheatgrass: Wheatgrass can be used to treat ulcers of the digestive system, joint pain, and painful skin disorders. It also controls excessive bleeding of wounds and restores the blood pH level to optimal levels. Furthermore, it increases the metabolism and recovery rate of the body by boosting nutrient absorption.[33]

Laxative Group

The third group of pain-reduction foods is characterized by its laxative and diuretic properties. Examples of foods that belong to this group are as follows:

- Asparagus: A mild laxative, asparagus relieves a person from painful bowel movements and also ensures that the kidneys are functioning properly. It could also be used as a sedative in herbal medicine to cure *neuritis* (nerve inflammation).[34]
- Cape gooseberry: This has diuretic properties and powerful antioxidants that can dissolve kidney stones in the long run.[35]
- Dandelion: These leaves have natural diuretic properties used to purify the blood, cure digestive complaints, and treat painful kidney and liver disorders. It can also be used as a substitute for coffee when its roots are roasted and ground, which can improve symptoms of rheumatism, gout, and *dyspepsia* (indigestion).[36]
- Fig: The natural laxative property of fig syrup is a popular remedy for constipation. Traditionally, fig is used to treat catarrh, mouth ulcers, boils, tooth abscesses, and carbuncle.[37]
- Horseradish: Considered a strong diuretic, horseradish is used traditionally to cure urinary tract infection, kidney stones, cystitis, rheumatism, and gout. It is also a potent stimulant that is beneficial to the digestive system.[38]

It is of utmost importance that health professionals consider a wide variety of factors before prescribing and administering any of these short-term pain-relieving therapeutic diets. Every diet implementation needs a careful consideration of a number of aspects that could include the following: a patient's normal dietary intake, what foods the patient is able to eat, the patient's existing weight condition, and the ability of the patient to chew or swallow food.[39]

GENERAL DIETS THAT RELIEVE PAIN OVER TIME

Apart from the aforementioned specific therapeutic diets to relieve pain temporarily, there are general diets formulated for patients that will either help prevent the occurrence of pain, alleviate pain for a longer period of time, or completely eradicate pain in the long run. The composition of such therapeutic diets depends on the disorder causing the painful sensations and symptoms. Clinical studies have shown that patients of chronic pain disorders such as diabetes who go undergo their usual medical care combined with appropriate diet therapies, have reduced pain and increased quality of life.[40]

Diets without Food Additives

Dieticians may recommend avoiding diets with food additives that contribute to or even cause chronic pain. Information regarding food additives that need to be eliminated or lessened becomes increasingly useful, especially for pain conditions where the source is not readily apparent. Additionally, painful conditions such as migraines and arthritis are increasingly common and afflict a substantial number of individuals. Patients suffering from migraine headaches and arthritis are encouraged to stay away from natural and artificial sweeteners as well as high-fructose corn syrup. Salt and monosodium glutamate, a common flavor enhancer, are common culprits as well. In general, patients are encouraged to steer clear of synthetic types of preservatives. Ultimately, the diet approach in pain management advocates choosing fresh food over instant or ready-to-eat items, not just to help decrease pain, but to improve overall health.[41]

Bland Diet

A bland, non-spicy diet is a special kind of diet formulated for patients with either *gastric* (stomach-related) or *enteral* (intestine-related) peptic ulcer. It is comprised of high-protein foods such as milk and eggs to neutralize the acidity caused by gastric juices. The main goal of this treatment is to prevent the stimulation of gastric secretion by avoiding items that can aggravate ulcers (1) chemically, against excessive spices, strong coffee or tea, and carbonated or alcoholic drinks, or (2) mechanically, against sharp seeds, tough fruit skins, or foods that are too hot or too cold. For patients who have difficulty chewing or swallowing, a bland diet is often combined with a "soft" one that consists of foods that are almost in liquid form.[42]

Vegetarian Diet and Pain

According to scientists at Georgetown University School of Medicine, a low-fat, vegetarian diet tremendously reduces the intensity and duration of pain associated with dysmenorrhea and premenstrual symptoms. This diet mainly consists of grains, fruits, vegetables, and legumes that are low in fat but high in omega-3 fatty acids. This chemical composition makes the diet anti-inflammatory, thereby significantly reducing the intensity and duration of menstrual pains in women.[43]

Diets for Painful Esophagus

Based on a study conducted by a team of doctors at Children's Hospital of Philadelphia, symptoms of *eosinophilic esophagitis (EOE)* in children and even in adolescents can be treated by administering an elemental diet that reduces the symptoms within ten days. EOE is an infection of the esophagus, the tube through which food passes after swallowing. Common symptoms of EOE include nausea, epigastric pain, vomiting, regurgitation, and heartburn. The elemental diet here is comprised of a combination of amino acids, corn syrup solids, and triglyceride oils. This diet is taken together with water, a single fruit such as a grape or apple, and its equivalent pure fruit juice.[44]

Diets for Crohn's Disease

Crohn's disease is another painful chronic disorder characterized mainly by the inflammation of the small intestines that can be treated with another elemental diet. Potentially fatal inflammation can cause excruciating pain, diarrhea or constipation, loss of appetite, and even internal bleeding when neglected.[45] The diet devised by a group of medical researchers in London for patients suffering from Crohn's disease consisted of a feeding formula called Vivonex (common name is "medical food") that replaced the participant's entire diet with the exception of coffee and tea. This was administered for four weeks, after which normal food was slowly introduced to the diet again. Because of the chemical composition of elemental diet, the digestive enzymes are prevented from further aggravating the inflamed condition of the intestines, thus improving the overall condition of the pain patients. Moreover, it is an effective, nontoxic alternative to the conventional administration of pain-relieving drugs and surgery in hospitals.[46]

Herbal Diets

In Taiwan, a modified traditional herbal diet is found to reduce and eventually eradicate pain in terminal cancer patients. The herbal diet is made up of analgesic herbs (*peony root* and *licorice root*) and a Taiwanese tonic vegetable soup from lily bulbs, lotus flower seeds, and jujube fruit. Because of the inherent analgesic property of the herbs, the diet aids the person in his battle against pain. It is also much safer to administer the herbal diet to patients as compared to morphine, which could lead to addiction or even more problematic side effects.[47]

Fasting

Fasting involves partially or completely abstaining from food for a given duration of time. Since the word *diet* can also mean reducing food consumption, fasting will be considered a dieting practice for the purpose of this chapter. According to the University of Linkoping in Sweden, fasting can reduce pain and stiffness in patients with rheumatoid arthritis.[48] Their fasting course does not exactly imply "zero calories," but the diet must contain fruit and vegetable juices that would provide a daily energy supply of approximately 800 kilojoules (kJ). Purgation with castor oil and *water enema* (flushing out the digestive system) is also an important part of this fasting course. Overall, the fasting aims to provide the pain sufferer with adequate amounts of water and minerals.

Low-Cholesterol Diet

A low-cholesterol and low-fat diet is commonly prescribed to prevent cardiovascular diseases that are characterized by elevated blood cholesterol levels, which can result in chest pain. This diet is comprised of fiber-rich foods such as rice bran, oat bran, peas, lentils, barley, apples, oranges, pears, and prunes, which effectively reduce cholesterol levels. As for animal products, it is recommended to eat lean meat, skinless fish and poultry, and dairy products that are low in saturated fat.[49] This low-fat diet can be modified further to help prevent painful liver and gallbladder disease.[50]

Gluten-Free Diets

Based on clinical research in the United States regarding the symptoms of *celiac disease* (a painful inflammatory disorder of the gut), a gluten-free diet is advised for patients to speed up recovery from abdominal pain, diarrhea, and other gastrointestinal symptoms.[51] The research found that once a gluten-free diet is introduced, the patient will experience relief from abdominal pain within days after it is administered. The frequency of diarrhea will drop substantially until it is completely eradicated after sixth months of following the diet, and, other gastrointestinal symptoms such as nausea and vomiting will also be resolved.

ANALYSIS

Therapeutic diets can be helpful in preventing, alleviating, controlling, and further eliminating symptoms of painful medical disorders. However, one must understand that it is always a good practice to consult a health professional such as a physician or a registered dietician before self-administering any pain-relieving diet. An assessment of an individual's physical condition and dietary needs will have to be performed and further compared with existing dietary standards. The means of implementing the therapeutic diet, whether it will be given orally or via a *nasogastric tube* (a feeding tube that goes from the nasal cavity to the stomach), should also be taken into consideration for further research.

25

EXERCISES FOR PAIN RELIEF

Centuries ago when a person suffered from pain the primary prescription would have been bed rest or cessation of the activity thought to induce the pain. Following extensive research, professional caregivers found that a painful state of discomfort can be reduced to a certain extent with necessary and accurate exercise. With the help of exercise, pain patients' well-being can be increased, their health improved, and the suffering reduced. Appropriate exercise helps improve flexibility as well.

SIGNIFICANCE OF EXERCISE FOR THE PAIN PATIENT

Exercise has an important contribution to a person's physical state because it really puts strength and endurance to the test. Exercise also improves *cardiovascular* (heart and blood vessels) and *cardiorespiratory* (heart and lungs) capacities. These types of exercises are based on repetitive movements that accelerate the pulse and maintain its steadiness for the duration of the workout. Moreover, exercise reduces arterial pressure as well as the amount of fat deposited in the blood vessels. This prevents the formation of blood clots. Another benefit of exercise is the prevention of cancer. Research has discovered that men and women who work out thirty to sixty minutes a day have a 30–40 percent lesser risk of colon cancer. In the case of breast cancer, the percentage is 20–30. Although it is presumed that exercises for pain can lower the risk of disease and the development of other types of cancer, the studies are not 100 percent decisive.[1]

Exercise maintains and improves the health of muscles, bones, and joints. It prevents osteoporosis because it increases bone density. Workouts increase the body's immunity, provide a better muscle tone, and help in losing weight or keeping it constant. They also provide for better prevention of painful conditions such as diabetes. A study conducted by The National Diabetes Prevention Program revealed that patients who lost weight and walked for twenty minutes daily for three years have a 58 percent lower risk of confronting diabetes later on.[2]

BEST EXERCISES FOR PAIN PATIENTS

There is a temptation to avoid exercising when in pain. People experience all sorts of pain, ranging from backaches to headaches. For each type of pain, there is a set of exercises meant to reduce and improve the quality of the pain patient's life.

Exercise and Back Pain

Back pain usually appears after an everyday activity, and most of the time, recovery is unpredictable. While few people have a "diagnosable pain" (irritation of a nerve root), an increasing number of individuals experience back pain because of a sedentary lifestyle, weight problems, smoking, or incorrect working posture. These aren't the only causes of back pain that would otherwise be relieved with the help of proper exercise. Tuberculosis, postural defects, metabolic bone illnesses, and even inner organ illnesses can produce back pains. Studies report that 75–85 percent of adults have problems with their back and that they experience it at least once in their life.[3]

When back pain occurs, professional caregivers can advise simple back pain exercises. A strict control of intense physical activities is recommended, as well as control of weightlifting and carrying positions. In order to protect the body from back pain, there needs to be an understanding of how different exercise positions can cause damage. When lifting objects, a pain patient should never try to pull the object from the ground at an uncomfortable angle or turn his waist, which should be flexible while the object is put down. While lifting, the person's back can be placed against a wall, with the heels and shoulders touching the wall. The backbone should be straight and parallel to the wall.

A person with a healthy back should be active and strong. The position should be changed frequently; any heavy load that needs to be carried should be divided in two, and objects should be lifted with the legs—not with the back. A sturdy orthopedic bed is indicated for sleeping, and the back pain patient should also keep his or her weight under control. Ideal sports for this kind of pain are running and swimming.[4]

Exercises for Neck Pain

Neck pain is a common occurrence among humans. Two out of three people worldwide suffer from this kind of pain at least once in their lifetime.[5] In many cases, the exact cause of the pain is not known, and doctors call this *idiopathic* or nonspecific neck pain. Neck pains can also result from a sprain after the neck is bent in unusual angles, from poor posture, or after sitting stationary for too long. To control neck pain, it is recommended to consult with a physiotherapist, a manual therapist, or a medical practitioner. They will prescribe a range of motion exercises meant to be executed daily so as to put the neck through full movements. This will prevent stiffness and prepare the neck for daily physical demands.

The exercises presented will help a patient control the pain and regain mobility or allow more neck activity. Done slowly, for five times a day, the wanted result will be achieved. *Neck flexion* requires the head to be brought forward so the chin comes into contact with the chest and the face is staring down at the floor. This workout, when done with care, will properly stretch the muscles at the back of the cervical spine. These muscles tend to become tensed and they consequentially restrict the neck from natural movement.

Neck Extension

This exercise requires that the head angles back slowly until the pain patient's face is looking directly at the ceiling. If the movement is done forcefully, it can bring all the small joints into an extreme position and increase the pain. The neck should be eased back at the end of the exercise and relaxed for a few seconds. However, if dizziness occurs after this exercise, the patient should stop, since that could be an indication that the blood vessels in the neck are getting squeezed.

Rotation

This exercise suggests that the head be slowly turned around to one side until it cannot go any further. This motion should be repeated five times. The neck should be held at the end of the movement for a few seconds because the motive of this movement is to maintain or increase flexibility.

Side Flexion

Keeping the head straight facing forward, the ear should be tipped toward the same shoulder. Because this exercise is quite hard on the neck joints, slow movements are required. It is advisable not to twist from side to side too frequently while performing this exercise because that could aggravate the joints and muscles.

Neck Retraction

Also known as a "chicken tuck," this is a useful exercise as it controls the tendency of the pain patient's head to poke forward in a poor posture. The workout is based on the forward and backward movement of the pain patient's head, like a chicken. Experts recommended that a patient hold his neck at the extreme end of the backward posture for a few seconds.

Exercises for Shoulder Pain

Whenever neck pains appear, the discomfort usually involves the thoracic spine and the shoulder ring. It is advised to involve these areas in the exercises in order to loosen the muscles. Workouts proposed for this area of the body include shoulder shrugs. During this exercise, the shoulders should be lifted as high as possible and then lowered slightly farther than normal.

Pain Exercises with Shoulder Braces

Shoulder bracing is another solution to pain, requiring the shoulders to be brought to the front or trying to get them to meet at the middle. Sometimes the shoulder braces attempt to pull the shoulders back, as if bringing the shoulder blades together. A large, slow, repetitive movement is indicated when exercising with shoulder braces. The shoulder contains muscles, bones, nerves, arteries and veins, ligaments, and other supporting structures. Shoulder pain can have many causes, some being life-threatening, such as heart attacks and major traumas, while others are not so dangerous, such as strains and contusions.

Pendulum Exercises for Shoulder Pain

Exercises that provide relief from shoulder pain include pendulum exercises. While one hand holds a table, the other should move in free rotations forward and back as well as left and right.

Climbing Exercises for Shoulder Pain

Facing a wall with the arms straightened, fingers should be moved up the wall without bending the body. The second part of this exercise involves turning one side to the wall, placing the opposite hand on the wall and moving the fingers up as before.

Shoulder Elevation

Here, the patient stands with arms free at the sides. While lifting the shoulders, the patient inhales a deep breath. Bringing down the shoulders, the patient exhales. The same exercise can be done with one-kilogram weights held in each hand.

Stretching

In this exercise, the pain patient lies on his back, face turned to the side. The shoulders are raised without changing positions. While in the same pose, the hands are placed on top of the head. Another exercise requires this same position (still lying down) with the hands put next to the head.

Another type of exercise consists of sitting straight with the arms at chest level and pushing the hands against each other, counting to ten, and then releasing for five seconds. The same exercise can be done at the chin and forehead levels.

Room Exercises

The patient places both hands against the wall. While keeping the arms straightened, the person stretches as high as possible reaching up the wall. Then lying on his back, the patient puts his arms beside his body and, without bending the elbows, the patient raises his hands in the air. While the arms are perpendicular to the floor, they are rotated without raising the shoulders.

Exercises for Lower-Back Pain

A common health problem is lower-back pain. This type of issue is more frequent in elderly women, but due to lifestyles in the modern age, younger people suffer from it too.[6] Back pain is troublesome as it restricts the body from adequate movement. To better prevent the causes of lower-back pain, a general understanding is needed. When a person stands, the lower back is supporting the weight of the upper body. When bending, extending or rotating, the lower back is responsible for weight bearing, as muscles, tendons, ligaments and the spine are all involved in the process. Moreover, a critical function of the lumbar spine is to protect the soft tissues of the nervous system and spinal cord as well as nearby organs of the pelvis and abdomen.

Sources of this type of pain include excessive fat in the waist region. Also, surgeries performed around the stomach or backside area can weaken the muscles of the spinal cord. Because the bone nerves are shifted from their initial position, this induces lower-back pain. Pregnancy could also affect the area because nerves can deteriorate during labor, and even if the delivery is cesarean, they will still weaken. This usually results in heavy lower-back pain in female patients. In order to avoid this type of pain, it is recommended that the person consult with a physiotherapist who can prescribe the right exercises. It is advisable not to stand or sit in the same position for a very long period of time. Moreover, sleeping on a too-firm or too-soft pillow or bed can cause these problems. Losing weight around the waist and hip region can also prevent the pain. Yoga and a walk of two to three kilometers in the morning are also suggested.

Abdominal Exercises

The patient should lie supine on the floor and raise the head four to five finger lengths. This position should be held for three seconds and then the head lowered. The same movement should be done with (1) the hands holding each other across the chest, (2) hands touching the opposite shoulder, (3) hands on the forehead, or (4) hands interconnected at the back of the neck.

Mobilization and Rotation

On hands and knees the patient extends one arm at the front with the other bent at the elbow. The elbow is not on the floor at this point. This exercise involves switching the positions of the arms back and forth, and it is repeated several times. As far as rotation is concerned, the person sits in a chair and turns at the waist from one side to the other with the arms raised.

Stretching

Dorsal stretching: while lying on the back, one of the knees is held with one hand and pulled to the chest. The same is done with the other knee alternately. For hamstring stretching: with the back flat against the floor, one leg is held straight while the other is bent at the knee. The straight leg is lifted up slowly. The same movement is then repeated for the other leg. Stretching can be done just about anywhere, and it improves flexibility by moving body parts in a full range of motion. There are many programs for stretching, and as a result, some employers have developed schemes for workers who stand or sit for too long.[7]

Pelvic Tilt

While lying on the floor, the knees are bent and the feet are placed on the floor. The waist is lifted from the floor for ten seconds, then relaxed. It is advisable for the movements to be done slowly. These exercises, if performed correctly, will ease pain and improve mobility for the individual suffering from pain.

Exercises for Knee Pain

Overusing the knee or suddenly injuring it can result in immediate pain. Because the knee joint sustains the full weight of the body and the extra force when running or jumping, it is particularly predisposed to damage and pain. Pain patients who are overweight are more inclined to suffer from this type of injury. When knee pain occurs, there are certain exercises that can improve the health and mobility of the muscles, tendons, and ligaments.

Chairs

One exercise requires the patient to sit on a chair with the legs straight out, feet off the floor while the person supports himself with his arms. A rolled towel is put under the knees by an assistant, while the legs are pushed down by the helper at the knees. Basically, the idea is for the patient to resist these movements.

Lying on the Back

The person lies on his back and lifts a leg approximately fifteen centimeters from the ground. The patient should hold the position for a few seconds and then slowly put the leg down. This exercise can also be performed with one-kilogram weights tied to the feet. The person can also stand and lift one leg forward without bending the knee.

Weights

Experts recommend using different weights and instruments when exercising for lower-back pain. A good instrument is a heavy medicinal ball. While standing on relatively soft ground with some weights on her legs the patient tries to catch the ball from different directions while keeping the same position.

Another back exercise has the patient put a pillow under the knees, while bending them a little. The feet are crossed and then are pressed against each other for about seven to eight seconds. The same exercise is performed while the legs are hanging down from the bed. The legs will be bent in a 90 degree angle from the knees.

Cycling

Riding an exercise bike lightly will also help and improve the condition of the knees in pain. The pedal height must be set to where the knee becomes completely straight. The first training session can last five minutes. Then, the level of intensity and the time is slightly increased.

MORE PAIN EXERCISES

Pain is lessened and the quality of life is enhanced by exercising. Working out is for everyone, as it usually helps people to reduce the physical perception of pain and to overcome limited functionalities. The first step in working out is consulting with a physical therapist or personal trainer that can develop a set of exercises or recommend a specific activity.

Walking, Swimming, Yoga, and Tai Chi

Walking

One activity that will improve flexibility and mobility is walking. This is a low-impact exercise that is a good choice for pain patients with physical capability. The advantage of walking is that it can be done just about everywhere. It is easy to do and it can be practiced during all seasons outdoors if weather conditions allow it.

Swimming

Swimming is a great form of exercise for individuals who suffer from (1) osteoarthritis, (2) issues with the muscles, or (3) any joint disease that affects the body in an unhealthy way. What makes swimming so beneficial for human health is the fact that water exercises defy gravity, thus avoiding major impact to the joints.

Yoga

Another way to cope with pain is yoga. The movement and stretching combined with breathing routines can help and ease chronic pain. Because yoga requires certain postures and poses, experts at New York University recommend comfortable motions that are within a person's abilities.[8] The risk of injury develops from postures that involve the spine and joints. Moreover, it is advisable to avoid rigorous yoga at first.

Tai Chi

Pain can also be prevented by practicing *tai chi*. This is a martial art that originated from China, and much like yoga, it fosters mindfulness. Tai chi is recommended for the young as well as for the elderly. The National Health Interview Survey (NHIS) reports that incorporating tai chi in daily workouts reduces pain, stiffness and fatigue—all while building strength, endurance, and balance.[9]

Strength Training, Pilates, and Aerobics

Strength Training

To avoid pain, lightweight strength training is a solution. Usually, programs that involve this type of activity are helpful for people suffering from painful arthritis. This all works by strengthening the joints around the injury and relieving some of the stress off of the joint used in the exercise. A pain patient can begin by lifting small cans of soup at first. Pushups or sit-ups can help prepare the patient for more intense exercises requiring the use of five- to ten-pound weights.

Pilates

Pilates, developed by Joseph Pilates, has become one increasingly popular exercise for people in pain. This set of exercises helps with core strength building, and it is favorable for people with low-back pain as well as for patients who suffer from fibromyalgia.

Aerobics

Lastly, pain sufferers and their caregivers should understand that aerobics is a great form of exercise no matter the type of pain a person suffers from. This exercise helps with alleviating pain while also strengthening and toning one's physique. As an advantage, aerobics also helps the heart and activates the *endogenous* (internal or inborn) opioid mechanisms known to reduce pain.[10]

ANALYSIS

This chapter covered the relationship between exercise and pain. To prevent any strain, pain patients should try to protect their body from the dangers that can result from intense exercise. While some pains may result in surgical correction or specialized medical treatment, others can be solved with a proper set of exercises. In essence, not all types of pain require serious medical attention.

26

ADDRESSING THE MENTAL ASPECTS

To alleviate pain, one must pay attention to the source, but the ability to manage pain may still ultimately depend on the psychological state of the patient, which is why people express their pain differently from one another. The subtleties in how one deals with pain profoundly vary and involve genetic, psychological, and social variables. These variables can determine how one mentally perceives pain. Thus the mind has the power to alter a person's overall physiology, since pain centers reside in different areas of the brain.[1] In fact, chronic pain is now also considered to be a condition of the central nervous system, which may or may not originate from any physiological damage. According to studies that involve *neuroimaging*, the pain centers in the brain are made up of a pain perception system and a pain modulation system.[2]

More and more studies are giving credence to mental approaches to the management of pain versus the straightforward use of pharmacology. These mental approaches include, but are not limited to:

- hypnosis;
- visualization and imagery;
- mind-body therapies such as relaxation;
- music and art therapy;
- rhythmic breathing;
- cognitive-behavioral therapy; and
- meditation.

These approaches may come across as unorthodox, and some need additional evidence to validate study results, but the potential of these techniques cannot be underestimated. Ultimately, therapeutic intervention that reduces pain and provides long-term relief to a patient without the use of medications is always advantageous. This chapter will therefore challenge the conventional understanding of pain and its corresponding management.

MENTAL CONNECTION TO PAIN

Introduction to the Processes

To fully grasp the mental aspect of pain, one must be able to determine four processes involved in the experience and psychological mitigation of pain. The first process of mentally perceiving pain is *transduction*. This is a process by which a physical source of energy, in this case a pain stimulus, moves in the form of a neural impulse. A neural impulse is really an electrical charge that travels to the brain through a nerve fiber.

The second process is *transmission*, in which the stimulus of pain, in the form of a neural impulse, is conveyed to the brain (particularly the cerebral cortex), which enables the patient to mentally "get the message" that he's actually hurting.[3] Based on the process of transmission, the psychological experience of pain is generally created from the brain's interpretation of the painful stimulus. As they say, it's "all in one's head." Clearly, this is where the mental aspect of pain should be primarily understood, since this is where the psychological feature of pain originates.

The third process of psychologically recognizing pain is *perception*. This is the process by which the cerebral cortex of the brain assesses the location and intensity of the pain. This is when the person realizes what part of the body the pain is coming from. Moreover, the intensity of pain will then be measured, as the patient is now able to mentally quantify *how much* pain he's experiencing. The concept of pharmacology (chapter 28) applies to this third process. The action of certain drugs may affect the physiological function of the brain, thus altering one's overall perception of pain.

The fourth process is *modulation*, which refers to the psychological manner of dealing with pain. The approach to reducing, diminishing, or altering pain is considered in this process.[4] Due to the high subjectivity of pain perception, the treatment and remedy may prove to be a very challenging feat. In order to understand the nature of pain and how to ultimately relieve it, various mental issues that people experiencing pain might face will be explained in the following sections.

Terrible Two: Pain and Depression

Without a doubt, pain diminishes the sufferer's ability to perform tasks and to interact socially. This diminishing may lead to depression, seclusion, and feelings of low self-worth. This is especially true in cases where pain lingers and becomes chronic pain. Chronic pain isn't only a physical condition but also a mental one that needs to be treated, as it normally brings about emotional problems, sleep disturbances, irritability, and lack of concentration, which in turn can lead to fatigue, reduced physical activity, and even weight gain. Clearly, chronic pain and depression have a deep relationship. The relationship between the two can be illuminated by the fact that depression and chronic pain actually share the same neurotransmitters. In the second process of pain perception, which is transmission, neurotransmitters carry the message of pain to the brain. So, in the case of depression and chronic pain, the same neurotransmitters are employed to carry the signal to the brain. As a result, the depression can make the pain more unbearable.

Considering the relationship of pain and depression, while pain can result in depression, in certain cases, depression can also cause pain. A brain scan may show that the pain's psychological origin may very well be attributed to depression, since pain involves active brain activity that can be comparable to people experiencing depression.[5] Pain (especially chronic pain) affects one's behavior, thoughts, or mood resembling that of depression. Sufferers of chronic pain have a higher risk of developing depression and other psychiatric problems, and the occurrence of depression further intensifies pain.

Since pain and depression are considered inseparable, treatment protocols have been improved to aid both. Most physicians treat pain by initially taking a full medical history and performing physical examinations that will further assess the biological and psychological background of the pain sufferer. It is necessary to identify the correct cause of the ailment so proper treatment may be taken.

Substance Abuse

There have been numerous studies confirming that chronic pain sufferers have higher rates of substance abuse.[6] This creates a problem in treating chronic pain with drugs, especially in patients who have substance abuse disorders. If the treatment of chronic pain through strong painkillers or narcotics leads to substance abuse, it could worsen a pain patient's mental condition.

Anxiety

Anxiety disorders have also been frequently diagnosed with people having chronic pain. Anxiety disorders include phobias, panic disorder, and obsessive compulsive disorders. Anxiety gives the pain sufferer a very low mental tolerance for pain. An anxiety disorder can also be exacerbated through fear of possible side effects. This situation worsens the experience of the pain. [7]

Somatoform Disorder

Somatoform disorder is a mental disorder wherein there is chronic pain that cannot be explained by medicine, as there is no noticeable effect from any physical illness. This disorder is related to chronic pain. [8] While the entire biological function of somatoform disorder is still a mystery, there is a promising conjecture that a sufferer's amplified consciousness of the sensations of his body may engender a preconceived notion of pain, thus explaining the presence of pain without a known biological cause.

Personality Disorders

Chronic pain and personality disorders have also been shown to have a concrete relationship. Certain personality issues such as hysteria and hypochondriasis have been found to be more common in sufferers of chronic pain. Moreover, personality disorders are higher in individuals experiencing chronic pain. Those who are unable to cope with their condition tend to show a certain pathology of personality. They may show feelings of suspicion, exhibit poor interpersonal relationships, and be exploitative of others. [9]

DIFFERENCES IN PAIN TOLERANCE: A PSYCHOLOGICAL VIEWPOINT

There is no clear-cut way of knowing how much pain a person is experiencing. If pain is rated by a group of persons experiencing pain in the same region of the body, five being the most painful, one person's "three" may be another's "five." There is a possibility that some persons are psychologically more resistant to pain than others, able to withstand excruciating certain amount of pain and remain relatively unbothered by it. In some cases, an athlete might not feel intense pain from physical impacts and stress during the height of the game. Thus, the term "mind over matter" can be applied, since pain tolerance may vary regardless of the pain's source.

Pain endurance or conscious suppression of pain may be due to various factors such as mood, individual personality, and mind-set. Perception of pain during the pain process may be magnified by factors aside from the pain stimulus. If the person is already anxious or fearful, a hormone in the body called *prostaglandin* is stimulated, making pain more intense. Prostaglandin makes the neural fibers more likely to respond sensitively to pain. Moreover, stresses inhibit a certain type of hormone in the body called *endorphins*, which are considered to be the body's natural pain relievers. Therefore, different types of psychological factors will determine how well the body tolerates pain and how pain tolerance differs among people.[10]

Mental pain tolerance may vary according to gender. A study at the University of Washington in Seattle suggests that men have a higher tolerance of pain than women.[11] An explanation suggests that men are more conditioned to hold back and tolerate pain because of cultural notions of masculinity. Conversely, there is a cultural notion of women being the weaker gender. Moreover, it is more socially acceptable for women to express their pain as compared to men.[12] These circumstances imply that it is emotional factors that may bring about pain.

STAYING HAPPY AMID CHRONIC PAIN

While the opposite of chronic pain accompanied with depression or other mental disorders is happiness—it is likewise true that happiness is a tool for better mental health. Pain isn't only a physical condition but also a mental one, and happiness, therefore, can alter the austere mental state of the chronic pain sufferer.

To have a positive outlook in life and be in good emotional health is basically to have learned to better manage and cope with the stress of daily problems and physical and emotional suffering. This does *not* mean that one should neglect the realities of life; rather, it's a way of embracing life with an optimistic and encouraging standpoint. Pain patients and caregivers should have a clear and definite meaning of the term *happiness* and steer clear of its misconceptions to better understand its vital role in the relief of chronic pain. For the pain patient, being happy doesn't mean abandoning the realities of life while just pretending to be happy. It involves various science-based steps toward happiness.

One has to look at life with a realistic attitude and be able to accept that current situations can change at any moment. Furthermore, it is a common misunderstanding that in order to be happy, one has to disregard physical pains and refrain from speaking openly and honestly about one's long-term ailments. One of the many reasons why chronic pain sufferers succumb to depression is refusal to talk to others about their pain, believing that no one can actually understand what they are going through. Sometimes it helps to complain, and it always helps to find a supportive person or group with whom thoughts and feelings can be shared. Happiness does not mean being ignorant of the negative things one is experiencing. Misfortunes in life are normal and unavoidable. It is really how the pain patient *deals* with misfortunes that truly matters. A person who rationally acknowledges emotional traumas in life is better able to understand why people have negative feelings, and thus can improve mentally. Since the conception of pain is derived from the mind, in order to address pain it is logical to heal the mind through the introduction of positivity.

Another method for staying happy is avoidance of any form of illegally obtained pain drugs, as they compound the problem with drug dependence. Happiness is a natural pain reliever to a certain extent. Happiness, which can be expressed either by just smiling or maintaining positive thoughts, releases "happy hormones" such as serotonin and dopamine. These hormones are able to aid people in their struggle against chronic pain. This further alleviates the actual pain and the emotional trauma linked to it. [13]

Based on research from the University of Kentucky, happiness (1) improves one's mood, (2) boosts the immune system of the sufferer, (3) releases natural painkiller hormones that inhibit stress hormones, and (4) lowers the risk of heart failure and blood pressure. [14] These reasons alone are enough for staying happy, but a happy state of mind may even relieve the pain sufferer from further pain and depression.

HOW TO AVOID SPECIFIC MENTAL OUTCOMES OF PAIN

Facing the mental outcomes of pain is very challenging as the sufferer attempts to deal with the physical and emotional aspects of pain. Fortunately, the following can be practiced and observed in order to avoid mental distress that pain may bring.

Maintaining a Healthy and Well-Balanced Diet

As much as it involves mental anguish and distress, chronic pain is still considered a physical pain since it debilitates the body. Therefore, it is important to practice well-balanced nutrition so the patient will have the necessary nourishment to battle the physical aspects of chronic pain. Feeding one's body is as important as finding ways to alleviate pain. The individual suffering from pain must always maintain a healthy diet since the body and the mind are interrelated.

Exercise

Although exercises for pain were discussed extensively in chapter 25, this section explains the role of workouts as they pertain to the *mental aspects* of pain. Much like a well-balanced diet, staying fit is important for those suffering from chronic pain in order to avoid discomforts brought about by pain such as stiffness, joint and muscle pain, and even emotional lethargy. Exercise also builds strong muscles, which in turn promote the release of stress from the joints, and subsequently, the mind. With a proper routine depression can be alleviated as well as cognitive abilities improved. Specific activities for mental pain can be constituted as a complementary treatment for depression and anxiety. Researchers have shown that certain movements and exercises can help combat cognitive disorders such as Alzheimer's disease.[15] Moreover, the Duke University Medical Center published a study that demonstrated the benefits of exercises for a person's mental capabilities.[16]

Stress Management

Emotional and physical pain have a tendency to overlap. Persistent pain can thus lead to higher levels of stress, and therefore it is important to stay focused and find ways to "detoxify" the pain patient's mind. Listening to calming music, a walk in the park, or playing with a child may provide satisfactory stress management. It is also useful to occasionally self-converse. While it may seem silly, talking to oneself boosts self-motivation. A huge difference can be made by just creating the perception in one's head that the pain felt today is far less than that of yesterday.[17]

CHRONIC PAIN AND PSYCHONEUROIMMUNOLOGY

The oftentimes ambiguous relationship between chronic pain and mental health can be explained scientifically by way of *psychoneuroimmunology* (PNI), which is a study of how the psychological processes of the brain interact with various organs, particularly those of the immune and nervous systems. The brain and the immune system have the ability to communicate with each other through their common signalling pathways. The correlation between the nervous system and the immune system is already seen to be evident through the body's natural reaction to various stimuli such as cold or heat. In other words, a stimulus through the nervous system has a direct effect on the pain sufferer's immunity functions. There is also a very interdependent connection between the immune system and emotions, since both share the same neural pathways in the brain. Pain thus affects the emotional condition of the patient, while possibly causing severe mental suffering.[18]

Therefore psychosocial conditions can actually affect the health condition of the sufferer. This is considered to be the main idea behind PNI. According to PNI, the variety of body systems that are involved in pain management means that the treatment of chronic pain should be holistically treated so as to relieve all the systems that have been affected by it.[19]

ANALYSIS

The intricacy of the pain processes involved in the human body causes a ripple effect mentally. This presents a challenge since treatment needs to involve both the body and the psyche. Perhaps the best way to address the mental aspects of pain is to try to maintain a positive mind-set at all times, which will provide psychological and clinical benefits.

27

SURGERY AND OTHER
NONPHARMACOLOGICAL APPROACHES

Pains that do not respond to conservative management are targeted with more aggressive forms of treatment. This chapter will discuss the advanced therapies indicated for protracted pain, namely surgery, and other nonpharmacological approaches.

INTRODUCTION TO SURGERY FOR PAIN

It is a generalized rule that the last resort in any treatment is surgery. This rule also applies to severe pain, but it also depends on the disorder that caused the pain in the first place. Surgery will relieve the pain, but it can also damage receptors in that part of the body. Few people have tried surgery for the sole purpose of eliminating chronic pain. Like most clinical cases, surgery for pain also involves making the right choices. *Intrathecal surgery* is the insertion of a small tube in the spinal canal where the pain signals go to the brain. With this technique, the brain can no longer detect extreme pain in that part of the body. Other surgical options include *spinal cord stimulation*, and *radiofrequency ablation*. These will be discussed later in this chapter.

When Surgery is the Best Option

Surgery is carried out to achieve either of two purposes: (1) to repair an anatomical defect or to address another anomaly caused by an illness or injury, or (2) to interrupt the transmission of pain signals sent to the brain. The different surgical approaches to pain will be discussed here according to the different kinds of pain for which they are indicated.

When Surgery is Indicated for Back Pain

Pain in a person's back is almost always triggered by defects along the length of the spinal column. Those requiring surgical methods are commonly caused by *disk herniation* (protrusion of the vertebra) and *spinal stenosis* (narrowing of the spine).

Diskectomy is a procedure indicated for disk herniation. Disk herniation happens when a spinal disc protrudes from its normal alignment. An accident or habitual straining of the back, especially for elderly people, usually triggers disk herniation. The protruding disk pressing against the spinal nerves and the spinal cord causes a sudden shooting pain. Disk herniation is also commonly referred to as "slipped disk." Pain will originate from the *cervical* (neck) region to the arms or from the lumbar (lower back) region to the legs, depending on where the compression occurs. Diskectomy involves the surgical removal of the damaged disk to relieve the spine and allow the nerves to heal.[1] Diskectomy procedures have become less invasive and there are several ways of performing it today, such as *microdiskectomy, endoscopic diskectomy, laser diskectomy* and *nucleoplasty (or percutaneous diskectomy).*

Back pain can also arise from spinal stenosis, the abnormal narrowing of the spinal canal. This restriction of the spinal canal results in a neurological deficit. The symptoms include severe pain, numbness, and lessened motor control. Spinal stenosis can occur at several locations along the spine. When it occurs near the neck, it's called *cervical spinal stenosis.* This is very dangerous and painful because it implies the compression of the spinal cord.[2] Spinal stenosis taking place in the lower back is called *lumbar spinal stenosis.* This is the more common and less dangerous form of spinal stenosis. It involves narrowing of the spinal canal, thereby causing compression of the spinal nerve roots in the lower back. *Laminectomy* is a surgical procedure to treat back pains caused by spinal stenosis. It is performed to relieve the pressure on nerves and involves widening of the spinal canal by removing or cutting away thickened tissues and bone parts. This procedure has a high rate of success in pain palliation and improvement in quality of life.[3]

Spinal fusion surgery is commonly an adjunct surgery to the two previous types of surgical procedures mentioned. It may also be done as an exclusive procedure, especially when indicated to treat fractures and other spinal problems. The objective of this major surgical procedure is to allow new bone to grow between two or more vertebrae, hence fusing them together. Sometimes, immobilization of a vertebral area is the solution. In spinal fusion, the vertebrae are conjoined to inhibit motion in a particular region of the spine or to correct rare spinal curvatures. This can be done by using bone grafts or metal implants to fasten the vertebrae together until new bone develops.

Medical conditions necessitating the full movement of the spine do not benefit from spinal fusion surgery. *Arthroplasty* is an alternative to spinal fusion. It has the advantage of retaining motion of the spine and preventing the collapse in adjacent levels. Arthroplasty can either be *artificial disk replacement (ADR)* or *total disk replacement (TDR)*. Artificial disk replacement involves implanting cushion structures made of metal or polymer to replace the *invertebral space (space between the vertebrae)*. These surgical procedures are indicated for chronic and severe lumbar and cervical pains brought about by degenerative disk disease (see chapter 21). The surgery is performed to replace degraded invertebral disks in the spinal column with artificial ones. This procedure also helps to preserve the disks below and above the replaced part.

Vertebroplasty, also called *percutaneous vertebroplasty*, is a spine surgery done to strengthen and stabilize a collapsed or fractured vertebra. Specialized cement is simply injected into the damaged vertebra to form a support structure. The bone cement used in this procedure is *polymethylmethacrylate*. *Kyphoplasty*, or *percutaneous kyphoplasty*, is a similar procedure. The procedure is usually recommended for pain caused by *osteoporotic spinal fracture* (when the vertebra fractures due to holes in bones).[4]

When Surgery Is Indicated for Pelvic Pain

The etiology of pelvic pain is not all that clear. It is therefore necessary to evaluate pains identified in the pelvic region very thoroughly before considering surgery. Pelvic pain could be associated with other problems such as reproductive and genital disorders, bladder or bowel dysfunction, or musculoskeletal or neurological conditions.

Chronic vulvodynia and *vestibulitis* are treated by the surgical removal of vulvar or vestibular tissues. Vulvodynia and vestibulitis are women's diseases characterized by inflammation and pain in the vulvar region that radiates to the whole pelvic area. A narrowing cervix (not the neck), called stenotic cervix, usually causes bleeding and pelvic pain. Cervical dilation is performed to treat a stenotic cervix. The presence of a *myoma*, sometimes incorrectly called fibroids or polyps in the uterine cavity, usually cause pain in the pelvic region. Surgical options include *myomectomy* or *myolysis*. The procedures can be done by several methods. *Hysteroscopic resection* uses an instrument called a *resectoscope* that makes the incision-free vaginal procedure possible.

Laparoscopy for pelvic pain is a method that may involve small incisions through the abdomen. Laparotomy is the method used for myomectomy that will require larger incisions in the abdomen. The size and location of the painful region determine which of these methods will be used. Pain patients and their caregivers should understand that laparotomy is also the procedure commonly performed when endometriosis or scar tissues cannot be removed by laparoscopy. When it is necessary to remove an ovarian cancer and it becomes complicated because of adhesions, laparotomy is again preferred.

Recurrent pelvic pain is sometimes caused by dense *periovarian adhesions* that trap fluid from ruptured cysts. Surgery is performed to remove the adhesion. *Adhesiolysis*, or surgical removal of adhesions, is conducted for *peritubular* (surrounding the fallopian tube) and *periovarian* (surrounding the ovary) adhesions. Adhesions can also occur in the intestines and are initially felt as pain. Enterolysis is the standard surgical separation of intestinal adhesions, and it is also performed to remove small bowel obstructions.

Recurrent abdominal and pelvic pain necessitating surgery can also be caused by a condition called a *hydrosalpinx*. This occurs when fluids fill the fallopian tube and it gets infected. *Salpingectomy* or *neosalpingectomy* is the surgical removal of the painful fallopian tube. This is also commonly performed for tubal pregnancies. Endometriosis, a painful condition when cells from the uterine walls attach to surfaces other than the uterus, has been the usual culprit in cases of bleeding and pelvic pains. Endometriosis may be found in the walls of the bladder, the bowel, and other internal surfaces. It is usually responsible for the unmanageable pain experienced by some women in their reproductive age. The pain is usually associated with dysmenorrhea which is a common condition for ovulating women. Those that cannot be treated by the common pain relievers are evaluated for underlying conditions. Removal of endometriosis is done by surgical resection.

Uterosacral nerve vaporization may also be done by interrupting nerves in the uterosacral ligaments. Relief from pain through this procedure is achieved from (1) the treatment of endometriosis, if that was indeed the principal cause of the pain, and (2) severing the nerve fibers that are transmitting pain messages to the brain. *Presacral neurotomy* can also be performed to remove the nerves responsible for sending pain messages from the uterus to the brain. This procedure also treats pain that originates from the bladder.

Hysterectomy is performed if (1) resection of endometriosis and (2) presacral neurectomy fail to stop the disabling pain. A possible condition called *adenomyosis*, also called *internal endometriosis*, may require more than just resectioning and *neurectomy* or cutting through the nerves. Adenomyosis, when glands are found connected to muscle, is characterized by bleeding and extreme uterine pain. Hysterectomy will treat this condition by surgical removal of the uterus.

Infection of the appendix, called *appendicitis*, initially results in pain felt around the navel. The pain increases and becomes more concentrated in the lower right quadrant of the abdomen. If confirmed, appendicitis is treated with a procedure called *appendectomy* or removal of the appendix.

Uterine suspension, a surgical procedure involving suspension of the uterus in the pelvis, is usually the only treatment for numerous uterine conditions displaying signs of pain. It is indicated for the following:

- *Pelvic congestion* (varicose veins occurring in the abdomen);
- *Uterine prolapse* (when the uterus slides into the vagina);
- *Collision dyspareunia* (painful sexual intercourse);
- *Severe dysmenorrhea* (irregular menstrual cycles); and
- *Endometriosis in the anterior or posterior cul-de-sacs* (closed cavities).

A hernia is the protrusion of a reproductive organ through a cavity near the pelvic region. It is called an inguinal hernia when the bulge involves the groin up to the scrotum. Femoral hernia is common in women and the bulge appears just below the groin. Hiatal hernia occurs when the upper stomach pushes into the chest. It is called an *incisional hernia* when it pushes to a scar in the abdomen, and *umbilical hernia* when it bulges around the navel. Hernia can cause severe pain and discomfort. Surgery is the only treatment for a painful hernia.

Sacral nerve root stimulation, also referred to as *sacral neuromodulation*, is a low-invasive procedure involving the implantation of a programmable pulsar in the buttocks. It is attached to a lead wire with an electrode tip that delivers low-amplitude electrical current to the sacral nerve where it is secured. Studies show that sacral nerve stimulation can benefit patients suffering from intractable pelvic pain.[5]

When Surgery Is Indicated for Joint Pain

Joint pains can come from injuries, allergies, inflammations and infections. The following are some of the surgeries performed:

- *Arthroscopy* is a minor surgical procedure that involves the examination and sometimes the treatment of a damaged joint with the use of an endoscope.
- *Osteotomy* is the cutting and repositioning of bones in osteoarthritic joints to shift the weight away from damaged cartilage.
- *Arthrodesis*, also known as joint fusion, is the surgical joining of joints with the purpose of relieving pain by immobilizing the joints.
- *Resection arthroplasty*, also known as *Girdlestone resection arthroplasty*, is an alternative to hip replacement surgery for patients with severe hip arthritis. Surgery is performed to remove the bone around the hip joint. The joint space is then filled with scar tissue.
- *Radiofrequency ablation* is a procedure that is quite successful for treating pain coming from disorders of the sacroiliac joint. The procedure involves the use of a radiofrequency probe to "burn" nerves that allow pain to be sensed from the joint.

Jaw Joint

There are various surgical options for painful disorders of the jaw joint, also referred to as *temporomandibular joint* (TMJ) disorder. TMJ disorder causes, among many other symptoms, lifelong pain that adversely affects a person's quality of life. An individual suffering from TMJ disorder has several surgical options. A simple *arthrocentesis* is the least invasive because it involves joint irrigation, but the pain may still warrant minor surgery later on. *Articular eminence recontouring* is the reshaping of the socket of the TMJ. Replacement surgery is the most extreme option because it involves the removal and replacement of the joint.

When Surgery Is Indicated for Limb Pain

Surgery for carpal tunnel syndrome, either open or endoscopic, is performed to release the pressure on a strained nerve in the wrist. This involves severing the ligament that puts pressure over the median nerve. Carpal tunnel syndrome is detectable because of intense and persistent pain in the arm that stems from the wrist.

Pain, numbness, and tingling sensations along the legs can often be traced to a condition called *sciatica*. The affected nerves exiting through the *foramen* (opening) are compressed, and this results in the symptoms. *Foraminotomy* is the surgical procedure employed to make a lesion in the tissues of the foramen. This is done to decompress the sciatic nerve. Sciatica can also be relieved with the previously discussed percutaneous endoscopic diskectomy. Another procedure is *laminectomy*, which is the surgical removal of *the lamina*, (linings of thin bones), which are supposed to protect the sciatic nerve. The purpose of the procedure is to decompress the nerve root or the spinal cord and relieve pain from sciatica.

Tendonitis surgery, either open or endoscopic, is performed to treat tendonitis. When there is pain in moving or pulling a muscle, one of the reasons could be inflamed or impaired tendons. This occurs when the band (tendon) that connects a muscle to the bone is torn, ruptured, or irritated by a bone spur. The surgery repairs tendons and excises bone spurs. *Hallus valgus* or *bunion* surgery is usually performed by a podiatric surgeon to solve painful foot problems caused by bunions. A bunion is a bony protuberance that develops under the big toe. This will cause pain and difficulty in walking. The surgery is carried out to (1) remove the bony enlargement, (2) realign the bone with the other *metatarsals (bones behind the toes)*, and (3) correct misaligned cartilages and other deformities of the bones.

When Surgery Is Indicated for Abdominal Pain and the Like

Severe abdominal pain (a strong "stomach ache") is usually a symptom of serious ailments such as gastrointestinal, renal and urologic, gynecologic or obstetric, and glandular disorders. Surgery is commonly resorted to after determining the cause of the symptom and after exhausting all preliminary procedures. *Neurolysis* is another option used to destroy sympathetic nerve tissues responsible for the control of most of the body's internal organs.

Surgery, either *open repair* or *endovascular stent grafting*, is generally recommended for patients with abdominal aortic aneurysm (AAA). Abdominal aortic aneurysm is the enlargement of the aorta that supplies blood to the abdomen. The pain is severe and persistent, spreading from the abdomen to the groin and legs.

Thoracoscopic splanchnicectomy is indicated for upper abdominal pain syndromes that are characteristics of many conditions such as, chronic pancreatitis, *supramesocolic (above the mid-colon) malignant neoplasms*, and *unresectable pancreatic cancer*. For these conditions, surgical procedures can be done as solutions to pain. In this precise surgical procedure, either the nerve roots or only the splanchnic nerve are lesioned or "denerved" to cease the perception of pain in the area in question.

The painful passing of human waste is not an uncommon condition. The usual cause of the pain is a chronic anal fissure due to pressure on the internal anal sphincter. *Lateral internal sphincterotomy* is the surgery recommended for chronic anal fissures. This procedure can be carried out through open or subcutaneous techniques to remove the resting pressure in the sphincter. It is indicated for patients with chronic anal fissure when other medical therapies have failed.[6]

A *celiac plexus neurolysis* is performed to destroy the sympathetic nerves controlling the organs in the abdomen. This operation is indicated for individuals with severe chronic abdominal pain from cancer or chronic pancreatitis. Long-term pain relief is expected until the destroyed nerve regenerates. Neurolysis is also performed for the lumbar plexus nerve, the superior hypogastric plexus nerve, the ganglion impar nerve, and the stellate nerve.

Surgery for Musculoskeletal Pain

Pain of the muscle and/or bones can come from a fall, fracture, sprain, direct blow or trauma, degeneration due to age, or defective posture. The pain will sometimes be perceived as a pain throughout the entire body. Fibromyalgia is widespread pain in the muscles. A decompression operation on either the base of the brain or neck spine (cervical spine) is indicated for fibromyalgia as a last resort for debilitating pain. This operation is also an option for cervical spinal stenosis. Paget's disease of the bone is a chronic disorder that may cause much suffering to afflicted patients. This disorder results in enlarged, misshapen bones that cause pain and fracture to weight-bearing joints. To alleviate the pain, surgery is often resorted to by cutting and realigning "Pagetic" bones of the hip or knee. Osteotomy can also be performed to remove damaged wedges of bones in Paget's disease. However, if a hip or knee has already been badly damaged, a surgery to repair the bones or replace the affected joints may be indicated.

Pain in *spastic cerebral palsy* is usually felt in the bones, joints, and in the stiff muscles. *Rhizotomy* is the surgical sectioning of nerves in the spinal cord to treat pain brought about by this condition. The procedure will interrupt the transmission of sensation by selectively destroying damaged nerves and relieve pain by shutting off the pain signals sent to the brain. Generally, more than one nerve needs to be sectioned to achieve the desired result. Variants of simple rhizotomy include *selective dorsal rhizotomy* (SDR) for spastic cerebral palsy. Problematic nerves are isolated during the procedure and severed with tiny electrical pulses. This fixes spasticity issues permanently. The unaffected nerves and nerve routes remain intact and are able to carry the desired messages to the brain.

Surgery for Painful Sports-Related Injuries

Sports injury surgeries are performed as a last option for sports-related accidents that mostly cause chronic and excruciating pain. There are several surgical interventions that could eventually become necessary because other options have failed or have become unfeasible. Knee and shoulder surgeries vary as to the level of invasiveness and procedure required, depending on damage to the knee or arm. Knee arthroscopy is a minor surgery to treat many conditions within the joint. Meniscus tear surgery involves removal of a torn meniscus. Meniscus repair involves suture of the damaged meniscus. Anterior cruciate ligament (ACL) reconstruction is a major knee surgery and it is the only pain relief option for a torn ACL. Lateral release is an arthroscopic surgery to treat *patellofemoral (knee and femur) pain syndrome*, which is caused by softened cartilage under the knee cap.

Labral repair is an open surgery to correct a torn *labrum* (cartilage) of the shoulder. Overhead arm movements of swimmers and throwers often result in *shoulder impingement syndrome* or *painful arc syndrome*. This is treated by performing an arthroscopic procedure called *subacromial decompression*. Rotator cuff surgery can be performed, either open or arthroscopic, to repair torn rotator cuffs. *Superior labrum and posterior* (SLAP) repair is performed when pain is unabated despite other treatment carried out for SLAP tear. This happens when the cartilage ring surrounding a shoulder joint is torn.

Surgery for Cancer Pains

Pain in cancer is mostly caused by a tumor that imposes nerve pressure or assaults bone. Bone metastasis is usually associated with tormenting pain. Cancer pain palliation is enormously important in improving the quality of life—if not in lengthening it—for a metastasized cancer patient.[7] Surgical and nonpharmacological therapies may include radiotherapy, intrathecal neurolysis, sympathetic nervous system blockade, nerve blocks, vertebroplasty and other more invasive surgical procedures. External beam radiation therapy (EBRT) is a pain relief regimen. A study on the efficacy of EBRT in relieving pain and improving the quality of life of patients with bone metastasis confirmed that EBRT has the ability to relieve bone pain.[8]

Cordotomy (or chordotomy) is the surgical interruption of pain pathways in the spinal cord. It is accomplished by cutting bundles of nerves and is presently indicated for pain experienced by patients with asbestos-related cancers, such as pleural and peritoneal mesothelioma. Anterolateral cordotomy is effective for unilateral somatic pain. Bilateral cordotomy is recommended for visceral or bilateral pain. Cordotomy is generally done percutaneously, or by needle puncture with fluoroscopic guidance. Percutaneous cordotomy is always the first option for patients where it is indicated because of its relative safety. However, open cordotomy may still be resorted to when percutaneous cordotomy is not feasible or has failed as a first option.

Percutaneous cementoplasty is used to strengthen bone by infusing cement into diseased bones in bone cancer. This is a similar procedure to kyphoplasty and vertebroplasty of the spine. Thalamotomy is a highly invasive procedure and is done only after extensive examination of a particular case of intractable chronic pain because of the possible complications and risks. The affected part of the thalamus is surgically ablated or destroyed either by liquid nitrogen, which kills the cells, or by a heated electrode that burns the cells.[9]

Spinal cord stimulation is the standard care indicated for these types of patients to minimize dependence to pharmacological medications. A tiny programmable device is embedded under the skin. This device has a generator and electrical leads that produce electrical currents to the spinal cord. The electrical nerve stimulation causes a tingling sensation and blocks the brain's ability to perceive pain.[10] The device is placed nearest the location of the pain. Moreover, this technology is gaining wide attention due to the possibility of adjusting the intensity of nerve stimulation, and it provides relief to different types of pain. It is battery-powered and the patient can be taught to use the device without assistance.

Low-dose radiotherapy is one of the methods used in treating bone pain. The periosteal layer of bone tissues is highly pain sensitive, which causes severe and debilitating pain in many conditions. Some of these disorders include osteoarthritis, fractures, osteomalacia, osteonecrosis, and bone cancer.[11]

PREPARATION AND RECOVERY

Preparing for Pain-Related Surgery

A person who goes for surgery, except for those who constitute emergency cases, should have decided to go under the knife only after giving it very careful thought. Even then, it is normal for anxiety to build up as the day of the surgery approaches. Anxieties come from fears and uncertainties. A well-informed patient is less likely to be fretful about the procedure. A patient needs to have all his questions answered and his doubts cleared away. Emotional and mental preparation for the patient is crucial when it comes to surgery for pain. This is something that the pain patient himself must actively take part in. His usual concern will be the competence of the surgical team who will perform the procedure, and he must therefore inquire about the surgeon, the anesthesiologist, and the other professionals who comprise the whole team. He may inquire as to their experience, their fields of specialization, and similar cases they have handled previously. Assuring information on this will lessen the pain patient's uneasiness.

During pre-surgery consultations and counseling, the patient may ask questions regarding the procedure, such as how long the procedure will be and whether he will be half awake during the procedure. The patient may also like to know what to expect right after the surgery, what precautions to observe, the length of the recovery period, what aftercare is required, and locations of nearby recovery facilities. Any health issues bothering the patient should be inquired about as well; for example, high blood pressure, allergies, alcohol and smoking problems, medicines currently being taken, and addictions—all of these are issues relevant for the doctor. Personal concerns such as the effects of the surgery on appearance or on sexual capabilities also need to be addressed.

Preparations should be made for the surgery well in advance of the day. Lack of preparedness will cause increased nervousness and make the surgery a more stressful event. The pain sufferer can ask a friend or family member to be there during and after the surgery when he or she will most likely be drowsy for several hours. Arrangements can be made for post-hospital necessities. A friend can be requested to walk the dog or do the shopping for a week or two if need be. Preparing for these small details, with all the things to be done before, during, and after the procedure clear and planned for, puts the mind in a more optimistic and calmer mode.

Recovery Phase

For some *percutaneous* (through the skin) and less invasive procedures, the pain patient simply gets up and goes home a day or two after the surgery. Highly invasive procedures, however, will require longer after-care and recovery. Right after the surgery, the patient will still be sedated. Anesthesia can wear off several hours later. Most surgeries will require that patients begin sitting and walking as soon as they are able. Vital signs are closely observed. Dressing of wounds and changing of bandages will be required regularly or upon the surgeon's orders, and the patient might be asked to do a cough-and-deep-breath exercise to expand the lungs. Food intake usually begins with a diet of clear liquid before it returns to the regular routine.

The home must be prepared ahead of the surgical patient's return for medical and personal necessities. A bed with specified height or design may be required, or a breathing apparatus and other equipment may need to be provided. The patient must take things in stride. It is important to adjust physical activities accordingly. Physical therapy serves as a great adjunct to recovery management, but the doctor must be consulted as to the extent of activities the pain sufferer can continue doing.

OTHER NONPHARMACOLOGICAL METHODS

Headaches are often just "tension" aches involving the neck, scalp, and the general head area. However, pounding headaches and facial pains are characteristic of serious migraines and inflamed sinuses. Even worse: there are "cluster headaches," which cause a sharp kind of pain. Headaches can also be symptoms of serious problems such as meningitis, encephalitis, or brain tumor. In deep brain stimulation (DBS), the hypothalamus is electrically stimulated to relieve chronic cluster headaches in pain clients who are unresponsive to drug therapy. A small generator is implanted under the collarbone. This generator provides electrical pulses to tiny wires attached to the hypothalamus. Pain relief in this manner has been successful for some patients, but there are always risks attached to DBS, such as fatal cerebral hemorrhage. [12]

Vagus nerve stimulation (VNS) is another treatment for cluster headache and chronic migraine. The vagus nerve extends between the brain and abdomen. The procedure involves the implantation of a small generator under the skin on the left side of the chest. A tiny wire runs from the generator to the vagus nerve to continually send mild electrical pulses to stimulate the nerve.

Occipital nerve stimulation (ONS) is an alternative to DBS and is considered to be less invasive and less risky. It involves the use of an electrical impulse to the nerves at the back of the head to treat intractable migraine.

A disease that causes intense facial pain is *trigeminal neuralgia*, also known as *prosopalgia* or "suicide disease." The pain emanates from compression of the trigeminal nerve. *Microvascular decompression* is a surgical procedure for repositioning or eliminating facial blood vessels that are in contact with the trigeminal root. Gamma knife radiosurgery uses radiation directly to the trigeminal nerve root. Pain is relieved gradually in people suffering from this condition. Microvascular decompression is the preferred procedure among many formal caregivers because of its noninvasive nature.

Support Groups as Nonpharmacological Approaches to Pain

It takes a while to cure pain because most pains are deep seated. In fact, pain *management* is a more correct term than pain *cure*. As the body undergoes medical procedures for pain, the mind and the psyche must also undergo processes of wellness. One way to facilitate this process is by sharing information regarding the condition. Learning about any feared thing removes much of its mystery and makes it less frightening. A support group can bring in people with similar experiences and present an assurance that the pain is not so uncommon. If others have lived with or survived it, then it is perceived as more manageable. Exercise and recreational activities, if not contraindicated for current medical treatment and conditions, can also be done. The semblance of normalcy conveyed by these activities can often make the pain bearable. Other useful adjuncts to the core treatment of pain that can be provided by support groups are laughter, games, and relaxation therapies.

The primary support group of a person suffering from pain usually includes family, friends, care providers, and medical professionals. A support network will help the patient communicate and clarify feelings of alienation, helplessness, and despair. The ability to articulate and address all these issues assures a better healing environment and quality of life, as there is comfort in knowing that there are people willing to listen and understand. While people should not be intimidated into thinking that professional psychological help is essential simply because they are in pain, more often than not, a comprehensive approach that includes the use of support groups is for the better.

ANALYSIS

Surgery for pain must be performed only after other measures to counter persistent pain have truly been exhausted. The medical history of every patient suffering from debilitating pain must be carefully evaluated and understood before an invasive procedure—or any other non-pharmacological approach for that matter—is indicated.

28

PHARMACOLOGICAL APPROACHES

Pharmacological action, or *pharmacotherapy*, is an interdisciplinary approach of the professional caregivers assigned to the pain patient. Although they are not aimed at eradicating the cause of the pain entirely, pain medications act toward alleviating pain symptoms and reducing the pain experience temporarily.[1]

PRELIMINARY EXPLANATIONS

The pharmacological approach focuses on the role of drugs and medication in the management of pain. These medicines include but are not limited to acetaminophen and opioids. The pain management specialist needs to be aware of all pain medications prescribed to a patient and be able to evaluate the patient's response to these drugs within a given time frame. Administration of these drugs should be under the guidance of pharmacological principles that outline proper usage and inform of side effects to be on the watch for. These principles act to ensure that patients are given proper education about the medications they are consuming. Institutions and organizations offering pain management are governed by their own set of pharmacological principles. Guidelines need to be in place especially because of the number of drugs known to be addictive and, therefore, prone to abuse.[2] If managed properly, pharmacological interventions can alleviate most pains and restore quality of life and normal levels of functioning. However, it must be noted that although pain medication can be helpful and provide relief, it is not *the only* available option and solution.

In 1986, the World Health Organization (WHO) formulated a three-step ladder in prescribing analgesics. Although formulated for use in cancer pain, it was adapted by health systems and became a standard for pain management for the next three decades. The three-step ladder categorizes analgesics by pain severity. For mild pain, it recommends the use of non-opioids. Weak opioids are given to moderate pain and strong opioids for severe pain. This is with or without adjuvant drugs.[3] Special considerations were made for children and geriatric patients. Presently, research is aimed toward evaluating the efficacy of the pain ladder. Although the WHO "pain ladder" globally remains a basis for prescribing analgesics, different approaches and innovations are being formulated in treating pain.[4]

Pharmacological therapy for pain is often based on individual need. It is a collaborative approach that necessitates effective communication and close management. In basic home-care settings, pharmacological therapy can be somewhat managed by the family. In cases of palliative home care, the home-care nurse evaluates the efficacy of the pharmacotherapy and relates this with the health team. In fully functional individuals, over-the-counter (OTC) analgesics are recommended for use. However, since pain relievers may cause adverse effects and addiction, close supervision is required in persons with constant use of analgesics.

Right Dose

The right dose of analgesics is needed to achieve a certain level of pain relief and maintain the serum level of the drug at the therapeutic level. In the hospital setting, this is routinely monitored by the pain patient's health team and evaluated. The dose is modified to satisfy specific requirements and to prevent side effects. The possibility of a drug addiction is also taken into consideration. Since there is minimal opportunity for continuous monitoring in the outpatient setting, health care workers often prescribe analgesics with a lower dosage because of fear of unintentionally promoting drug addiction. Side effects may still appear even with a relatively small dose of painkillers. The lower dosage leads to only minor pain relief or no relief at all, thus leading to increased drug consumption.

Frequency of Use

The standard practice in the past was to administer analgesics only when there were complaints of pain. This often led to unrelieved pain because patients in the hospital were unaware that they needed to ask for pain medications. Some individuals, even those in the outpatient environment, wait for the pain to become intolerable before seeking help. WHO included in its guidelines the administration of analgesics around the clock, rather than *pre re nata* (PRN), or "as needed." This is done to maintain the effect of the drug at its therapeutic level. Since the serum level of the painkiller gradually decreases, its therapeutic level decreases as well. Analgesics are administered at intervals before the pain becomes severe. This proves to be a better pain control method since only smaller doses are required at this stage.

Time Intervals

The time interval between dosages is individualized as well. Metabolism rate and absorption time of medications is often different from one person to another. A certain schedule may be effective in one pain patient, but not in another. This may also depend on the level of pain that the client is experiencing. To determine the proper time interval between administrations of the drug, health care workers often assess the magnitude of pain at every dosage, in order to avoid possibly sedating someone who is *not* experiencing pain.

Combined Usage of Analgesics

The combined approach refers to the use of more than one analgesic agent at a time. Sometimes, when a single analgesic is used, the drug is given more frequently in higher doses to achieve its optimum effect. This may lead to adverse consequences. Three different categories of analgesics are often used in a combined approach: opioids, local anesthetics and NSAIDs or nonsteroidal anti-inflammatory drugs. Since these agents work on different mechanisms, maximum relief of pain can be achieved while potential toxic effects of a single drug are minimized. Although research about drug efficacy of pain relievers is often extensive, fewer studies have been carried out for the combined therapy versions.[5]

Adjuvant medications are usually the drugs that have medical indications other than basic analgesia. These are given along with the analgesics in the pain ladder. They are usually administered to provide better pain moderation while promoting lesser opioid requirement.[6] A few examples of these are antidepressants and anticonvulsants, which are used either to modulate side effects or to enhance pain relief offered by opioids.

Patient-Controlled Analgesia

Nowadays, a new approach to pain is implemented by hospitals. Patient-controlled analgesia or PCA is a pain-relief method that allows the patient to administer his or her own pain medications. An intravenous, subcutaneous, or epidural catheter is inserted and is connected to a PCA pump. The PCA pump is electronically controlled by a timing device. A patient can self-administer a preset amount of medication in episodes of pain through a push of a button. An extra dose may also be administered, but the pump does not allow administration after multiple pushes in rapid succession. The timer can be programmed to disallow administration until a certain amount of time or until the effect of the first dose has exerted its optimum effect. It can also be programmed to deliver constant background infusions and have the patient administer an extra amount when needed.

Pharmaceutical Industry Advertising

In order to sell pain-related products, most pharmaceutical companies come up with different techniques for advertisement. One strategy is *direct-to-consumer pharmaceutical advertising* (DTCPA).[7] Usually, it makes use of popular mass media such as newspapers, television commercials, billboards, and the Internet, among other forms of mass media. These are reviewed by governing agencies before being shown to the public. Although certain requirements and limits must be met before a DTCPA is approved, there have been recent difficulties in implementing these regulations.[8] A few DTCPA campaigns were found to omit important information while overemphasizing drug benefits. Some pain drugs are sold for a higher price but do not offer any significant benefits with other medicines. Health care professionals, however, report a few benefits from DTCPA. It is regarded as a way for empowering patients and even increasing their compliance toward treatment. Pain patients are often prompted to seek medical advice due to DCTPA, and information about illnesses is often provided thereof. This whole process can prevent under-diagnosis and under-treatment of various medical conditions.[9]

Another tactic utilized by pharmaceutical companies involves sending out representatives to sell or persuade physicians to prescribe their drug. Medications for pain patients are quite expensive, and there are claims by pharmaceutical companies that these drugs are more expensive because of the extensive research done on them. A few critics, however, claim that these drug representatives usually have neither medical nor scientific education. This implies that exaggeration, misleading information, and incomplete information may be provided to unsuspecting caregivers.[10]

PSYCHOACTIVE APPROACHES

Psychoactive drugs are chemical substances known to cross the blood-brain barrier and directly act on the central nervous system, resulting in alterations in perception, mood, consciousness, pain, cognition, and behavior.[11] Each drug has a specific action on one or more neurotransmitters or neuroreceptors in the brain. Many psychoactive drugs are abused due to the subjective changes in consciousness and mood that one perceives as pleasant or advantageous. Many of these drugs cause dependence, making it difficult for the pain patient to break free of the cycle of abuse. Psychoactive drugs can be classified into three categories, stimulants, depressives, and hallucinogens. Continual abuse of these drugs may lead to permanent damage to the nervous system.

Stimulants

Stimulants are psychoactive drugs that temporarily improve either the mental or the physical functions of a person or both.[12] Some of these effects may include enhanced alertness, wakefulness, and locomotion, among others. They may also improve mood, relieve anxiety and induce feelings of euphoria. These effects are induced by temporarily enhancing the effects of the central and peripheral nervous systems. As the effects of these drugs are fleeting, an individual will eventually sleep when the effects wear off, since they leave the person exhausted. As a person abuses such substances, tolerance to their effects grows higher while the negative effects intensify. Some of these substances include amphetamines, MDMAs, cocaine, caffeine, and nicotine, with the last two substances being the most abused of stimulants.[13]

Depressants

As opposed to stimulants, depressants contribute to temporary feelings of relaxation, sedation, muscle relaxation, and pain relief. They are often abused because of these effects. High doses of depressants can result in cognitive and memory impairment, dissociation, lowered heart rate, respiratory depression, and even death. Pain sufferers and their caregivers should know that substances associated with this classification include[14]

- barbiturates;
- benziodiazepines;
- cannabis;
- opioids; and
- alcohol.

Hallucinogens

Hallucinogens can lead to subjective changes in thought, perception, emotion, and consciousness.[15] They are divided into three broad categories: (1) psychedelics, (2) dissociatives, and (3) deliriants. Unlike other psychoactive drugs, hallucinogens not only amplify familiar states but also induce experiences that are entirely different from those of ordinary consciousness. Such experiences can be likened to meditation, trance, daydreams, or insanity. Abuse of these types of drugs may lead to several mental conditions such as Parkinson's disease, Alzheimer's disease, senility, and schizophrenia. Among the commonly abused are the Colorado River toad (a toad that is tongue-licked for "getting high"), LSD, psilocybin mushrooms, mandrake, salvia, and cannabis.[16]

PAIN-RELIEVING PHARMACOLOGICAL AGENTS

Acetaminophen

Acetaminophen, sometimes called *paracetamol*, is the most commonly used over-the-counter analgesic. Its primary effect is in the spinal cord and cerebral cortex. It also inhibits the synthesis of prostaglandin and COX-2 dependent pathways of the pain patient.[17] It is used in relief of mild to moderate pain and in cases of osteoarthritis. It is also the most common remedy for muscle aches, headaches, sore throats, menstrual cramps, and backaches. Because of its *antipyretic* (anti-fever) effect, it is also commonly used for the reduction of fever in those who also happen to suffer from pain. Side effects of acetaminophen are usually itching, swelling, rashes and in worst cases, difficulty in breathing. Intake of acetaminophen must be controlled because of its potential to cause liver damage.

Nonsteroidal Anti-Inflammatory Drugs

Nonsteroidal anti-inflammatory drugs (NSAIDs) modulate pain by inhibiting an enzyme called *cyclooxygenase* (COX). Common generic NSAIDs available for market are

- salicylates (aspirin, diflunisal, and salsalate);
- pyrazoles (phenylbutazone), celecoxib, and meloxicam;
- naphthlyalkanones (nabumetone);
- acetic acids (indomethacin, tolmetin, diclofenac, and ketorolac);
- proprionic acids (ibuprofen, naproxen, fenoprofen, ketoprofen, and oxaprozin);
- fenamates (mefenamic acid and meclofenamic acid); and
- oxicams (piroxicam).

Since NSAIDs inhibit both types of COX, they may cause gastrointestinal toxicity. COX-1 is an enzyme that maintains normal physiologic function. It increases gastric mucosal blood flow, promotes mucosal integrity and prevents ischemia. Hence, too much inhibition of COX-1 can lead to gastric ulceration and bleeding. COX-2, the second type of COX, facilitates prostaglandin formation that in turn results in symptoms of pain, inflammation, and fever. Inhibition of COX-2 leads to relief of mild to moderate pain. COX-2 inhibitors, in combination with opioid medications, provides better pain relief than with opioid alone. All NSAIDs have been found to cause kidney toxicity.

Aspirin is the most frequently purchased over-the-counter NSAID.[18] This drug was found to suppress production of prostaglandins and thromboxanes. It is commonly used as a preventative drug for heart attack and stroke, but is has been known to cause anaphylactic reactions or even death when combined with other medications or when used in patients with specific disorders such as *urticaria* (hives) and asthma.[19] Aspirin is harmful when used as a prophylactic since it can cause stomach bleeding and even kidney failure.[20]

Topical NSAIDS are most often in gel, spray, or cream form. The most common types of topical NSAIDS are salicylate and diclofenac. Topical salicylate is useful for acute and chronic pain. Topical diclofenac is commonly applied for sports-related pain and osteoarthritis. COX-2 inhibitors are now being developed to control the effects of NSAIDs to COX-1. COX-2 inhibitors are formulated to provide pain relief without causing inhibition of COX-1, and the former is now used in cases of osteoarthritis and rheumatoid arthritis. COX-2 improves analgesic efficacy with decreased incidence of side effects, but it is contraindicated in patients with ischemic heart disease or who are at risk for coronary artery diseases. These pain drugs have been found to increase the risk for NSAID-induced bronchoconstriction as well as *myocardial infarction* (heart attack).

Tramadol

Tramadol mainly directs its action to the central nervous system. It has both opioid and non-opioid effects. It is an "opioid agonist" and inhibitor of the reuptake of norepinephrine and serotonin. It does not suppress prostaglandin synthesis and so it causes fewer gastrointestinal and cardiac side effects than NSAIDs. It is most commonly used in malignant pain, osteoarthritic pain, low back pain, fibromyalgia, and diabetic neuropathy. Usually, it is also used as anesthesia for surgical and dental procedures. Nausea, vomiting, lethargy, dizziness, and constipation may occur with use of tramadol. Adverse effects include seizures and serotonin syndrome. Seizures are most commonly seen in patients who use tramadol together with antidepressants, neuroleptics, and other opioids. Serotonin syndrome is an increase in the serotonin levels in the central nervous system. This can cause abrupt changes in the mental status of the patient.

Opioids

Opioids continue to be one of the key agents in the treatment of pain. It is a *broad-spectrum analgesic*, which provides the most reliable and effective way for achieving rapid pain relief. Opioids (1) act mainly on *mu receptors*, (2) activate pain-inhibitory neurons, and (3) impede pain transmission. They are most often used in chronic pain conditions along with other analgesics or adjuvant drugs to reduce the total opioid amount.

Due to possibilities of drug abuse and dependence, strong opioids are used only when first-line medications fail to provide basic pain relief. Before prescribing, the physician weighs the benefits with the possible effects that may arise from opioid use. Moreover, constant monitoring and evaluation of efficacy is done throughout the course of treatment. Administration of opiates can be done through different routes. The intravenous route is the most rapid acting. Spinal infusion of opioids can cause regional analgesia even with just the use of a relatively low dose. Since the goal in treatment is to improve quality of life, the route with the least discomfort is most often used.

A patient taking strong opioids should be monitored closely for adverse effects. The opioids should be stored safely and kept away from unauthorized persons. Careful observation is also a part of the process, as it is the main criterion for successful treatment. Any miscalculations in the administration of the drug will be detected promptly if the individual suffering from pain is carefully observed. The ability of the patient to "retire" from the drug is also important, as there could be significant withdrawal symptoms when strong opioid medications are stopped abruptly. Once an individual absorbs the drug, the body adapts to it. The result is an addiction that is difficult to fight off. To avoid these problems, strong opioid doses should be lessened slightly over time until the body is no longer physiologically attached to it.

Opioid drugs can be very dangerous if consumed improperly, and therefore the right dose has to be established to lessen the risks. Opioid drugs for pain should be consumed on schedule and not just "on demand." In other words, the pain patient should not consume opioids every time he or she experiences pain. This is also done to avoid overdosing. The WHO has set a time frame regarding intake of narcotic drugs, which is an interval of three to six hours, concluding that pharmacological approaches are 80–90 percent effective and less expensive when the person administers the right drug and the right dosage at the right time.[21]

Patients and caregivers should also understand that some opioid drugs are illegal. One example is heroin. This drug is very addictive and can result in death. The dangerous aspect of this drug is that it goes directly into the bloodstream and travels up to the brain. The affected opioid receptors in the brain are normally responsible for breathing, blood pressure, and arousal. Heroin can suppress respiration, which can result in serious difficulty in breathing. All opioids may cause nausea, vomiting, and sedation, but the most serious side effect of opioids is *respiratory depression* (difficult, shallow breathing), or *hypoventilation* (low ventilation). Opioid rotation, which is the practice of changing from one opioid to another, may be done to lessen side effects. This takes into account the principle that each individual reacts differently to drugs from a pharmacological standpoint.

Anesthetics

Local anesthetic agents are applied directly to the site to block nerve conductions. They inhibit the opening of sodium channels to prevent transmission of nerve impulses.[22] They can be given through patches, sprays, or intravenous injections. Topical agents such as lidocaine patches act solely in the peripheral tissues and nerves. *Lidocaine* has been proven to block activities in the neuronal sodium channels, believed to cause several types of pain. Lidocaine patches produce analgesia by delivering lidocaine to local tissues without causing sensory deficits. It is beneficial in diabetic neuropathy, HIV-associated neuropathy, low back pain, osteoarthritis, and other peripheral neuropathic pain. Due to significantly low systemic levels, side effects are usually mild and resolve without need of further intervention.

Eutectic mixture of local anesthetic (EMLA) cream is a topical anesthetic used only on normal, intact skin. The cream induces anesthesia by blocking sodium channels of sensory nerves. This is often used postoperatively or post-surgically. It is also the anesthetic most often used on genital mucous membranes for superficial minor surgeries. Adverse effects may include itching, rashes, edema, and pallor, among others.

Intramuscular (IM) injections of specific anesthetic agents have also proved to be effective in producing regional painkilling effects. Intravenous regional anesthesia is often administered through an epidural catheter and is used in surgeries or in labor and delivery. It is delivered directly to the nerve roots, which provides better analgesia. Intravenous regional anesthesia injections produce better postoperative outcomes such as early ambulation, fewer complications, and shorter hospital stays. Spinal anesthesia may cause delayed or prolonged sensory and motor deficits, since it affects nerve roots directly.

Local anesthetic agents induce toxicity when there is an excessive amount present at a site. This is often due to constant application of the agent on the same site without allowing the serum levels of the anesthetic molecules to be fully consumed. Toxicity from local anesthetic agents can cause systemic and localized side effects. It may affect potentially hazardous sites such as the brain and heart. Lidocaine and other local analgesics may cause slow heart rate and hypotension. *Bupivacaine*, a local anesthetic most commonly used in chronic pains, has been known to produce arrhythmias and cardiac collapse. When injected into skeletal muscles, local anesthetic agents may cause reversible histologic damage depending on the agent used.

Antidepressants and Anticonvulsants

Dose-related biological activities of antidepressants appear to include pain relief. Research often attributes this to the blockage of the hormones norepinephrine and serotonin, which in turn enhances the stimulation of inhibitory neurons.[23] Antidepressants also potentiate the effects of analgesic agents. Antidepressant medications have been found to cause orthostatic hypotension, cardiac conduction delay, memory impairment, and urinary retention.

Anticonvulsant (anti-seizure) drugs have been found to have an effect on multiple biochemical and pathophysiologic processes involved in maintenance of pain.[24] These drugs are largely beneficial for relieving lancinating pains. A few of these drugs are used for headaches and fibromyalgia. The most common side effects connected with the use of anticonvulsant drugs are mental clouding and lethargy.

Miscellaneous Pain-Relieving Drugs

Some drugs have analgesic effects when used in specific conditions. Studies on *phenothiazines* found it to be effective in postoperative pain. *Benzodiazepines* are helpful in the treatment of acute pain. Antihistamines, normally prescribed for allergies and colds, are useful for headache, low back pain and cancer pain. Corticosteroids are beneficial in advanced cancer pain, whereas muscle relaxants can decrease back pain. However, the use of these drugs as strong analgesic agents is yet to be established. Most often, these are used as adjuncts to opioids and other analgesic agents.

SPECIAL CONSIDERATIONS

The rate of metabolism and absorption is relatively different in a child, an adult and an older person. Certain modifications in the analgesic therapy are made to provide efficient pain relief without compromising the safety of the pain patient. There are a relatively small number of medications proven safe and effective for pediatric use. By modifying the WHO pain ladder, a two-step strategy is formulated for children. The WHO recommends paracetamol and ibuprofen as first options for mild to moderate pain. For children below three months of age, paracetamol is the medication of choice.[25]

Opioids are considered for relief of moderate to severe pain. Use of strong opioids proves to have better benefits rather than intermediate opioids. Tramadol and other strong opioids are currently being studied for possible use as an alternative to morphine. Medications should be given at regular intervals for persisting pain. The least painful, simplest and most effective route of administration would be the oral route. Other routes such as *intravenous* (IV), rectal, or subcutaneous should be based on clinical judgment *and* on the condition of the child. The intramuscular route is avoided if possible since it is painful to the child. In choosing the right dosage for a pediatric patient, it is most appropriate to use the weight and age as a basis. The nutritional state of the child must also be taken into great consideration. Overdosing of pain medications must be avoided at all cost, and it is important to keep in mind that even acetaminophen toxicity is a common cause of drug-associated death in children and adolescents.[26] Side effects must be constantly monitored since it may lead to occurrence of drastic effects.

Geriatric patients may have altered drug sensitivity, as the gastrointestinal "transit time" for drugs consumed by the elderly is less than that of younger adults. This means that drug absorption is affected. The changes in body composition such as decrease in total body water and lean body mass and the relative increase in adipose tissues may affect drug distribution. Hepatic and renal blood flow may also be altered in aging pain patients, which directly affects metabolism and elimination of the drug. These physiologic changes mean that pharmacological treatment should be initiated at a lower dose. Sudden escalations of the drug should be avoided. Treatment is given at regular time intervals, but considering that the pharmacokinetics of the drug have already been altered, PRN administration may also be considered.[27] The occurrence of side effects may be heightened due to decreased metabolism of the drug, which essentially means a prolonged *half-life* (the time it takes for half of a drug to disintegrate) of the drug. Reduction of dosage may be done along with change of routes and opioid rotation. Monitoring is emphasized.

RESPONSIBLE PHARMACOLOGICAL PAIN APPROACHES

Due to abundant options in pharmacological approaches to pain, it is strongly recommended that medical consultation be done before deciding to take medications. Not all OTC pain drugs are safe for use. Indications, mechanism of actions, side effects and recommended dosage should be on the label and should be accessible to the public. It is best to check this or consult a medical professional when in doubt regarding a drug. Moreover, analgesics and other drugs must be used cautiously in patients with renal and hepatic problems. Problems in metabolism and elimination of the drug may ensue and cause toxicity from the drug. This may also cause drug addiction due to the prolonged sedative effects of the drug. Constant use of analgesics in renal and hepatic patients may cause complete failure of the liver and kidney as well as heart problems.

From a general standpoint, product safety evaluations must be done before choosing pharmacological substances based on DTCPA, or sales pitches from pharmaceutical representatives. A few drugs have been introduced to the market even before full safety profiles were completed.[28] This means that side effects and adverse effects of the drug had not been determined before distribution. In these cases, patient awareness and prescriber education must be emphasized. The expiration date of most drugs should be clearly indicated on the packaging, as usage of expired medical products is perilous. An expired drug does not guarantee safety and efficacy, due to the possible change in the chemical composition of the drug over time.[29] The drug must be disposed of properly before it causes untoward effects.

As far as side effects are concerned, research is geared toward predicting positive drug reactions in organs and occurrence of side effects in order to provide better treatment plans or prepare for potential emergencies. New tools, standards, and approaches are currently being evaluated to enhance the assessment of the efficacy, safety, and quality of pharmacological drugs.[30] These side effects should not be ignored. Anaphylactic reactions to a drug can lead to serious brain damage or death. If side effects that are not indicated in the label of the drug are felt, immediate withdrawal from the drug and medical consultation should be done. Since pain drugs are metabolized in the liver, over dosage or improper use of drugs may cause hepatic failure.

Proper monitoring and control of taking analgesics must be done extensively on a person receiving treatment. Opioids may often lead to misuse, abuse, and in worst cases, death. In 2009, more than 15,500 people in the United States died after overdosing from pain relievers.[31] Addiction to opioids usually occurs because of the compulsion to take the medication to experience its psychic and sedative effects. While collaborative approaches of the family and caregiving team have always been recommended, certain protocols are now being developed toward safe prescription and usage of opioids. Prescriber and patient education is emphasized to address related public health issues.

ANALYSIS

Pharmacological approaches to pain are intended to reduce the intensity of perceived pain through different physiological mechanisms. Numerous analgesics are available in the market but none are proven to produce exclusively healthy results in all cases. The labeled indications and side effects must be taken into great consideration by pain patients and their caregivers prior to consumption.[32]

V

Wrap-Up

29

SECOND OPINIONS

A second medical opinion is a consultation with a health care provider concerning a health issue that was previously checked by another doctor. There is nothing wrong with having another physician look into a patient's medical condition; in fact, a second opinion is even advocated by doctors when prescribing pain regulators.[1] The patient's reasons for seeking a second opinion vary from case to case. Some consult multiple caregivers to rule out the risk of mistreatment. Others just want to get another expert's take on their condition.[2] Whatever the reason is for getting a second opinion, the pain sufferer is entitled to a clearer understanding of what they are going through and what to do about it. Since a "second opinion" in general can pertain to the contribution of ideas from just about anyone, this chapter discusses the involvement of both doctors and family members in the pain patient's comprehensive approach to their suffering.

SECOND OPINIONS FROM THE DOCTOR'S OFFICE AND FROM HOME

Doctor's Office

Pain is a clear indication that the body is in need of medical attention. Ideally, doctor-patient relations are grounded on the circumstance of the patient needing a solid opinion. This calls for both the doctor and the patient's willingness to listen to each other. The doctor, having the expertise to address the pain the client is experiencing, suggests treatments and prescribes medicines. The means that the physician uses to treat the patient is heavily dependent on the information disclosed to him.

A physician at the University of Sydney, concerned that pain patients' reluctance to openly speak to their doctors aggravates their illness, says their hesitation is attributed to their lack of understanding of the methods that their doctors apply to ease their physical pain. Furthermore, doctors need to get patients to talk about their suffering. Specialists have devised two methods to maximize doctor-patient relations: proactively ask about the pain, and comfort the patient accordingly.[3]

Individuals suffering from pain are urged to be as upfront as possible when discussing their condition with their physician. The earlier the discovery of the cause of the patient's pain, the higher the chances of healing—or at least mitigating—damage to health. Only when patients are completely honest with their doctor will they be able to get the full benefit of the services they are paying for.

Involvement When Getting a Second Opinion

The decision to get a second opinion does not have to be entirely up to either the patient or the doctor. There are cases when professional caregivers, especially when treating patients whose pain is caused by a terminal disease, initiate the review of their patient's case by a fellow physician. In situations where the patient doesn't need immediate medical attention, a doctor might forget to voluntarily ask their patient to go and get a second opinion. This is when the *patient* has to bring up the topic. Getting a second opinion is a common medical practice, so patients do not have to worry about their doctor being offended should they ask for another consultation with a different doctor.

The doctor's responsibility to the patients doesn't end with a second opinion. On the contrary, the first physician's involvement is crucial for updating and conferring with the second doctor. Medical records are also needed for reference and a more informed diagnosis by the second doctor.[4]

At Home

There is stress where pain is present. While a person in pain can make life difficult for everyone at home because of the need for special attention, it is important for family members to understand how their support, or lack of it, can affect a suffering loved one. According to the American Chronic Pain Association's family manual, pain patients need to be kept involved with family life by talking about the situation and even giving the patient some simple chores to make him or her feel useful. Individuals suffering from pain must not isolate themselves, nor should family members give up on living a normal life.[5]

Family members' involvement in the course of getting a second opinion is an essential part of the support they offer. Pain sufferers basically go through all the same tests over again, so they'll be relying on their family to get them through another round of assessment. Some of the patients, whom the Health Experience Research Group (HERG) interviewed, testified on how pain actually brought their family together.[6] In other cases, a family member of someone battling with pain may have the tendency to be overprotective. This can lead to the patient becoming uncomfortable with the extra attention and prefer to suffer through it alone. Often family members get frustrated if medications fail to work or feel guilty when they can't identify with the patient's feelings.[7] These are common responses to situations of ill health. The main thing is to allow the family to support the patient, including when a second opinion on how to proceed is necessary.

The family's involvement in the patient's medical endeavor goes beyond looking after their needs at home. In order to fulfill their duty as caregivers, they must understand the patient's sickness from a medical practitioner's perspective. This can only be achieved when the family member goes all the way in their support. What this basically means is that relatives can immerse themselves in the process of medication. This can entail: accompanying the patient to the doctor's office and helping the patient to decide whether to seek a second medical opinion or to begin certain treatments.

Getting at least one adult family member to thoroughly understand a pain patient's condition is very crucial when a second opinion is proactively recommended by the attending physician. At times when the sick individual is indisposed, a family member must be around for the doctor to explain the situation the patient is in. It is important to note, however, that unless the subject is totally incapable of deciding for himself or herself, the decision to seek a second opinion must be authorized by the one who needs medical attention.[8] A holistic understanding of a loved one's condition will ensure that their needs are met at home in spite of living away from a professional's watch.

BENEFITS AND DRAWBACKS OF GETTING A SECOND OPINION

Benefits

Anyone who suffers from serious pain should not think twice about having their case checked by another physician, no matter how tedious the overall process may seem. Undergoing duplicate cycles of testing can be challenging, and sometimes, people are so stressed by their pain that they refuse to even bother getting a second opinion. The true advantage of seeking a second opinion is "peace of mind." Affirmation of whatever the first physician said about the patient's cause of pain will determine the next step toward healing. The earlier this is done, the better. Not knowing enough about what to expect when undergoing treatments can cause anxiety. The more patients understand their condition, the more assured they will be that all their treatments are substantially backed by diagnostic data. There is always room for error, even in medical readings. One way of lessening this kind of risk is by going through another round of consultation.

Fortunately, seeking a second opinion has never been more convenient than in this age of modern technology. Should patients with a rare condition fail to find a doctor in their area to better evaluate their medical case, online consultation through the Internet should be considered.[9] This attests to the urgency of getting a second opinion. Patients can be checked online without leaving the comforts of their home. With this kind of advancement in patient care, there should be no reason for a patient not to entertain the prospect of getting another doctor's opinion.

With a second opinion, the pain patient can be more confident that they are getting the most up-to-date treatments and prescriptions. This is a great source of comfort for patients and their family members who are unsure of the next step to take. Just as with any other big decision in life, cross-referencing pain-related information leads to a better-educated conclusion.

Patients who seek a second medical opinion also have a more extensive choice of treatment plans.[10] If a treatment modality does not work, the second opinion may lead to a better option. The medical expense involved in getting a second opinion can discourage patients from understanding the real value of such opinions. But patients and their family members need to bear in mind the costs that limited consultations can entail if ultimately unnecessary medications or treatments are used.

Drawbacks

Waiting for the results of another round of tests to accommodate a second opinion can be detrimental for some who need immediate treatments. The delay is caused when health care professionals have to carefully deliberate on the patient's treatment plan. If time is an important consideration in the sick person's case, then it may be better to act expediently to avoid further harm.[11] In some cases, doctors give varied recommendations on what to do after a diagnosis is made. This can lead to confusion, as decisions are partially left with the patient. Pain sufferers may feel overwhelmed when faced with several choices. Unless the doctor agrees on which treatment will work best, patients are most likely the ones to decide on the approach.[12]

When treatments fail to work despite the concerted efforts of physicians, patients may feel hopeless. There is, of course, no guarantee that a second opinion will remedy their existing pain. Having to face that reality can shatter hopes of ever recovering from the pain they are experiencing.

WHAT TO REMEMBER WHEN GETTING A SECOND OPINION

Before Getting a Second Opinion

While a second opinion is more likely to be sought than not, it is still pertinent for the patient to use their own resources, if time permits, to gather as much information about their painful condition as they can. If the reason for getting a second opinion is mainly to address some questions about the nature of the sickness as diagnosed or the methods the doctor used to arrive at a conclusion, then it is practical to ask the same doctor. Patients should never hesitate to clarify their medical issues with their doctor.

Taking time to check what other sufferers do to counter pain may also help to inform the patient. While it is true that physical pain must be brought to the attention of a professional, it won't hurt to first ask others with a similar experience or condition, for example on online forums. First-hand information can be as valuable, though not as determinative, as a doctor's opinion. When patients take the initiative to do their own research, communication with their professional caregiver is much easier. Having questions prepared before an appointment with a doctor can make the time spent discussing the cause of pain more productive and efficient. The patient's insurance coverage should also be deliberated prior to getting a second opinion to make sure their coverage allows them to go through the process without having to spend too much.

What to Ask When Getting a Second Opinion

Drafting questions before seeing the doctor is a key factor in understanding pain. Patients may feel hesitant to ask their doctors questions, for fear of causing irritation or embarrassing themselves. But in reality, questions are clues to how willing the patient is to cooperate. In fact, since the patient going to a doctor for a second opinion already has a preconceived idea of their condition, it can be expected that he or she will ask in-depth questions based on the first opinion.

Questions may range from simple clarifications to more technical ones. As they feel more comfortable and get more exposed to equipment and treatment options, patients should have greater confidence to ask questions. First, pain patients need to confirm the accuracy of the previous doctor's findings. There are instances when a second opinion leads to a totally different diagnosis. This brings about the need of the patient to seek a *third* opinion in order to get rid of any doubts. Upon confirmation of the diagnosis, the patient can then ask about the next step: getting treatments. There are a variety of things to consider about treatments. Additional opinions can provide for more options to fall back on in case the first, second, or third recommendations do not work. Each treatment will have its own side effects and benefits. No matter how effective a particular approach seems to be, when the patient is at risk of worsening, reconsiderations are advised. [13]

After getting a second opinion, the pain sufferer can then compare both doctors' findings and start weighing options. If, in spite of all these preparations, questions still remain unanswered, perhaps a third opinion might just be the one that the pain sufferer needed all along. Only when the patient feels comfortable and confident of what to do will he or she become conditioned for the next step to recovery.

ANALYSIS

Pain patients and caregivers should understand that a second opinion has its own risks and pitfalls. Despite its disadvantages, a second opinion can better inform and further empower the one who is in pain. Since it provides more opportunity for patients to understand their condition, it will enable them to keep a positive attitude all throughout their difficult situation.

30

CONCLUSION

By now, the reader should understand that there are five common factors in assessing pain. First is the precipitating factor—that is, what is causing the pain, such as a fracture, laceration, or specific disease. Second is the quality of pain, which only the person feeling it can describe, whether it is "crushing," "burning," "stabbing," or any other sort of descriptor the patient can find to relate the experience. Third is the location and possible subsequent spread of the pain to other areas of the body. Fourth is the severity of pain. The most effective way to determine the severity of pain is by rating it, for example by using a pain scale where 0 is the absence of pain; 1–3 is mild; 4–6 is moderate; and 7–10 is severe pain. The fifth and last factor is time. Sometimes pains are persistent and aggravating; sometimes they are intermittent or recurrent, depending on the cause. By observing the timing of pain medical personnel may also be able to identify the cause or severity. This concluding chapter explains how the pain patient can (1) try to prevent pain from happening in the first place or from getting worse, (2) remain hopeful, and (3) attempt to stay motivated at all times.

SIGNIFICANCE OF PREVENTING PAIN

As with all medical problems, if possible, prevention is best when it comes to addressing pain. Regular checkups, daily exercise, and a well-balanced diet are very advisable, but some people only do these things after a serious illness strikes. These lifestyle factors are the key to a healthy life, as well as at the forefront of prevention strategies.

HOPE DESPITE THE DESTRUCTIVE NATURE OF PAIN

There are many different interventions that an individual suffering from pain can employ, so there is no reason to lose hope. In fact, pain is only indicative of a physiological disorder that must be addressed, so in a sense pain is the first step on the road back to health. Pain might be mild and inconsequential or derive from a severe disorder such as cancer. For some individuals it becomes chronic and thereby has a holistic effect on their life. Such a person must find the inner strength not to lose hope as well as seek the emotional support needed to get through the ordeal. The patient cannot overcome chronic pain without this encouragement and support.

Pain also intensifies if the person loses hope and the will to continue fighting against it. For this reason specialized caregivers encourage the patient's family to be involved and present in therapy when possible. That said, it is essential that caregivers understand two major pathways to hope for the pain patient. The first is noninvasive, and the second is invasive.

Noninvasive Strategies for Finding Hope

When it comes to finding hope, noninvasive pain intervention must be regarded as the "first aid" of pain. Diversion techniques such as meditation or systematic relaxation can be used to help the pain sufferer to relax and focus more on other things than the pain itself.[1] Relaxation will help the person to calm down and gather strength while disallowing the pain to affect him or her holistically. As a result, the pain patient will gain hope in the struggle against pain. Acupressure is another possibility. This can be done by massaging pressure points that can alleviate pain. The person experiencing pain must go to a doctor to seek advice about noninvasive techniques and to determine whether acupressure is possible for his or her condition. When the pain is at its peak, the professional caregiver might want to consider recommending *invasive* pain strategies, albeit with caution.

Invasive Strategies for "Finding Hope"

These interventions are best for pain that is most severe or is chronic in nature. The first invasive intervention is taking medications prescribed by a doctor. The patient should always get follow-up assessments to note improvements or deterioration in health as a result of medication.[2] Drugs also depend on the cause of pain. In some cases anesthesia is the appropriate invasive intervention.[3] If the patient cannot withstand the pain, local anesthesia under the advice and supervision of a doctor is used. Anesthesia is only available in hospitals, so, when taking such a drug, close observation by a nurse or physician is very important. It is not really advisable to use anesthesia as the sole treatment for pain. The last solution is surgery. Almost all pain can be cured by surgery, and therefore the person suffering from pain must never lose hope. There are hundreds of solutions in dealing with pain. As long as people follow the prescription of their doctors and there is eagerness to fight pain, hopelessness need not be a lasting concern.

FINDING MOTIVATION AND LEARNING TO STICK WITH IT

The most obvious results of pain are seen physically, but mental functioning is also affected. Sometimes, the pain patient can no longer think properly. For example, a student with a toothache takes an exam and gets a low score simply because of the pain. Obviously, pain can affect the sufferer's performance in any activity; therefore, it is important for anyone with pain to find motivation to get past it.

Steps to Getting Motivated

A major step here is the willingness of the pain patient to change his or her lifestyle in order to become healthier, and this cannot be done without self-confidence. People who believe in themselves can withstand any physical misfortunes. The individual suffering from pain must believe in the path chosen for recovery and trust themselves to follow it. The achievement of motivational goals is easier when there is self-trust. Another point to remember is that a patient must be goal-oriented to *stay* motivated. Goals can be achieved only if the individual takes the first step and stays on track until the last step, which is why discipline is equally essential for getting motivated to fight pain. Simply put, pain sufferers need self-control to stay motivated, because their body will be affected physically if they give in to pain psychologically.

Motivation *itself* is a great technique for handling chronic pain. Family members can enhance pain management efforts through their support and help the sufferer gain more motivation. Doctors usually encourage family and relatives to make hospital visits. Moreover, there are counselors to whom people can go for motivation. People might seek spiritual or psychological advice, and some experts also provide routine activities to help patients relax and be more in control of their pain, once again increasing the chances of lasting motivation.

IMPORTANCE OF SEEING A DOCTOR

Some people prefer to buy OTC drugs instead of seeking a doctor first. Their hope is to save time and money, or they simply perceive the pain as a minor problem. This is acceptable as long as they don't intend to manage their long-term pain entirely by themselves. Taking matters into one's own hands can be dangerous because stark pain usually occurs in the late stage of disease. For example, if a person with cancer experiences extreme pain, then he is probably in the late stage of illness. It is also possible that a specific organ does not have enough oxygenation and blood supply, so other organs automatically send signals to the brain to respond in the form of pain. This physiological mechanism can be lessened to a certain extent, and hence it is vital to see a doctor first rather than take inappropriate action.

Palliative care is primarily given to a terminally ill person who is experiencing pain. Seeing a doctor can help to ascertain whether the pain patient needs such care. The objective here is to provide comfort during the potentially permanent remediation of pain. For example: a doctor orders an opioid drug for a cancer patient in pain, not necessarily to treat the cancer, but to provide relief amid fear and unease. The safest and the most effective way to know "right versus wrong" in the effort to reduce pain is often consultation with a formal caregiver.

Dealing with severe, lagging pain without the necessary consultation is hazardous. The dangers include drug tolerance. If drugs are taken continuously without limitation, the pain sufferer's body may adapt by producing antibodies and drug tolerance. As a result, stronger drugs will be needed to fight off the physiological resistance, leading to overdose. Some painkillers are extremely addictive. For example, *morphine sulfate* can be addictive to the point where additional health issues surface. Some take morphine sulfate because they have no other alternative for their severe pain, but unfortunately, their desire to end suffering supersedes the realization that their health is in more danger if they consume the drugs without control.

ANALYSIS

In general, pain is a simple problem that everyone has to endure at some point in life, so it is essential to know how to treat pain appropriately and with the right kind of help. There is often no immediate or fast "cure" to pain, but with the assistance of a physician, pain can be overcome in a stepwise manner. The most effective step is consulting a doctor, since it is always better to be assured than to take unnecessary risks.

Appendix A

PAIN RELATED LINKS

www.aapainmanage.org
www.abpm.org
www.action-on-pain.co.uk
www.americanheadachesociety.org
www.americanpainsociety.org
www.ampainsoc.org/pub/journal
www.apsoc.org.au
www.asipp.org
www.aspmn.org
www.asra.com
www.blackwellpublishing.com/journal.asp?ref=1526-2375&site=1
www.britishpainsociety.org
www.canadianpainsociety.ca/en/index.html
www.chernydatabase.org
www.chronicpainanonymous.org
www.douleurchronique.org/index_aqdc.asp?node=2&lang=en
www.efic.org
www.emergingsolutionsinpain.com
www.epapain.org
www.geriatricpain.org
www.iasp-pain.org/AM/Template.cfm?Section=Home
www.informaworld.com/smpp/title~content=t792304028~db=all
www.instituteforchronicpain.org
www.inthefaceofpain.com
www.istop.org
www.journals.elsevierhealth.com/periodicals/jps
www.lww.com/product/?0882-5646

www.masp.org.my
www.massgeneral.org/painrelief
www.medicine.ox.ac.uk/bandolier/booth/painpag/index2.html
www.medscape.com/viewpublication/947_index
www.michigan.gov/painmanagement
www.pain.com
www.pain.org.sg
www.painaction.com
www.painandhealth.org
www.painandthelaw.org
www.painassociation.com
www.painclinician.com
www.painconsortium.nih.gov
www.painedu.org
www.paineducators.org
www.painfoundation.org
www.painjournalonline.com
www.painknowledge.org
www.painmanagement.org.au
www.painmed.org
www.painpolicy.wisc.edu
www.painreliefnetwork.org
www.pain-topics.org
www.patient.co.uk/support/Pain-Association-Scotland.htm
www.sciencedirect.com/science/journal/03043959
www.sppm.org
www.stoppain.org
www.theacpa.org
www.trc.wisc.edu
www.uspainfoundation.org
www.webmd.com/diseases_and_conditions/pain.htm

Appendix B

RESEARCH AND TRAINING

Alan Edwards Center for
Research on Pain
McGill University
Suite 3100, Genome Building
740 Dr. Penfield Avenue
Montreal, QB H3A 0G1
(514) 398-8975
Fax: (514) 398-8121
cynthia.macdonald@mcgill.ca
www.painresearchcenter.mcgill.ca

The Alan Edwards Pain
Management Pain Unit of the
McGill University Health Centre
McGill University Health Centre
Montreal General Hospital
1650, Cedar Avenue, Room E19-128
Montreal, Quebec H3A 0G1
(514) 934-8222
Fax: (514) 934-8096
www.painresearchcenter.mcgill.ca

American Academy of Pain
Medicine
4700 W. Lake Avenue
Glenview, IL 60025

(847) 375-4731
Fax: (847) 375-6477
www.painmed.org

Atkinson Pain Research
Laboratory
Barrow Neurological Institute
350 W. Thomas Road
Phoenix, AZ 85013
(602) 406-3000
www.thebarrow.org

The British Pain Society
Third Floor, Churchill House
35 Red Lion Square,
London WC1R 4SG
020 7269 7840
Fax: 020 7831 0859
www.britishpainsociety.org

Canadian Institute for the Relief
of Pain and Disability
#204-916 W. Broadway
Vancouver, BC V5Z 1K7
(800) 872-3105
Fax: (604) 684-6247
www.cirpd.org

Cancer Pain Research Lab
Norman Bethune College
Room 367
Toronto, ON M3J 1P3
(416) 340-4800
lucia.gagliese@uhn.ca
www.cancerpain.lab.yorku.ca

Center for Health and Healing
Oregon University
3303 SW Bond Avenue, 4th Floor
Portland, OR 97239
(503) 494-7246
Fax: (503) 346-6961
www.ohsu.edu

Center for Neuroscience and Pain
Research
University of Texas
MD Anderson Cancer Center
1515 Holcombe Boulevard,
Box 110
Houston, TX 77030
(713) 563-5838
Fax: (713) 794-4590
hlpan@mdanderson.org
www.mdanderson.org

Center for Pain Research
National University of Ireland
Galway, University Road
Galway, Ireland.
+353 (0)91 493266 / 5280
www.nuigalway.ie

Center for Pain Research
Faculty of Health and
Social Sciences
Leeds Metropolitan University
Civic Quarter, Calverley Street
Leeds, LS1 3HE
m.johnson@leedsmet.ac.uk

www.leedsmet.ac.uk

Center for Pain Research
University of Bath
1 West Level 3
Bath, BA2 7AY, UK
+44 (0) 1225 383054
l.austin@bath.ac.uk
www.bath.ac.uk

Center for Pain Research
University of Minnesota
308 Harvard Street SE
Minneapolis, MN 55455
(612) 625-2945
carfair@ahc.umn.edu
www.pain.med.umn.edu

Center for Pediatric Pain
Research
IWK Health Centre
5980 University Avenue
P.O. Box 9700
Halifax, NS B3K 6R8
(902) 470-8895
Fax: (902) 470-7255
www.pediatric-pain.ca

Center for the Study and
Treatment of Pain
317 East 34th Street, 9th Floor,
Suite 902
New York, NY 10016
(212) 201-1004
www.pain-medicine.med.nyu.edu

Center for Pediatric Pain
Research
IWK Health Center
P.O. Box 9700
Halifax, NS B3K 6R8
(902) 470-8895
Fax: (902) 470-7255

marsha.campbellyeo@iwk
.nshealth.ca
www.pediatric-pain.ca

Center for the Study of Pain
University of Toronto
155 College Str., Suite 300
Toronto, ON M5T 1P8
(416) 946-8270
nancy.mitchell@utoronto.ca
www.utoronto.ca

Center for Translational Pain
Research
Massachusetts General Hospital
101 Merrimac Street
Boston, MA 02110
(617) 726-3744
MSHpainresearch@partners.org.
www2.massgeneral.org/
painresearch/

Comprehensive Center for Pain
Research
University of Florida
1395 Center Drive
Gainesville, FL 32610
(352) 392-3032
Fax: (352) 392-3031
ryezierski@dental.ufl.edu
www.painresearch.ufl.edu

Chronic Pain and Fatigue
Research Center
University of Michigan Health
System
Department of Anesthesiology
PO Box 385
Ann Arbor, MI 48106
(734) 998-6939
Fax: (734) 998-6900
www.med.umich.edu

City of Hope Pain Resource
Center
1500 East Duarte Road
Duarte, CA 91010
(626) 256-4673
www.prc.coh.org

Clinical and Translational Science
Institute
PO Box 100219
Gainesville, FL 32610
(352) 273-8700
Fax: (352) 273-8703
www.ctsi.ufl.edu

Danish Pain Research Center
Aarhus University Hospital
Norrebrogade 44, Building 1A
DK-8000 Aarhus C, Denmark
+45 7846 3380
Fax: +45 7846 3269
www.dprc.dk

Department of Anesthesiology
Northwestern University
Feinberg School of Medicine
251 E. Huron Street, F5-704
Chicago, IL 60611
(312) 926-8105
Fax: (312) 926-9206
www.feinberg.northwestern.edu

Department of Pain Medicine &
Palliative Care
Beth Israel Medical Center
First Avenue at 16th Street
New York, NY 10003
(877) 620-9999
Fax: (212) 844-1503
www.stoppain.org

Faculty of Pain Medicine
The Royal College of Anesthetists

Churchill House
35 Red Lion Square
London WC1R 4SG
+44 (0) 20 7092 1500
Fax: +44 (0) 20 7092 1730
info@rcoa.ac.uk
www.rcoa.ac.uk

George Washington Pain Center
2131 K Street, NW
Washington, DC 20037
(202) 715-4599
Fax: (202) 715-4598
www.gwhospital.com

H. Lee Moffitt Cancer Center &
Research Institute
12902 Magnolia Drive
Tampa, FL 33612
(888) 663-3488
www.moffittcancercenter.com

HMC Pain Relief Service
325 9th Avenue S, Box 359724
Seattle, WA 98104
(206) 744-7065
Fax: (206) 744-7085
www.depts.washington.edu

The Hospital for Sick Children
555 University Avenue
Toronto, ON M5G 1X8
www.sickkids.ca

Institute for Hypnosis & Pain
Research
1328 River Road
Teaneck, NJ 07666
(201) 836-0033

JFK Johnson Rehabilitation Institute
65 James Street

Edison, NJ 08820
(732) 321-7000
www.njrehab.org

The Johns Hopkins Blaustein Pain
Treatment Center
The Johns Hopkins Hospital
1800 Orleans Street
Baltimore, MA 21287
(410) 955-5000
www.hopkinsmedicine.org

Krembil Neuroscience Centre
(KNC)
399 Bathurst Street
Toronto, ON M5T 2S8
(416) 603-5800
www.uhn.ca

Leeds Metropolitan University
Woodhouse Ln.
Leeds, United Kingdom, LS1
3HE
+44 113 81 21111
www.leedsmet.ac.uk

Michael G. DeGroote Institute
for Pain Research and Care
McMaster University
MDCL 2101
1280 Main Street West
Hamilton, ON L8S 4K1
(905) 525-9140, ext. 26538
www.fhs.mcmaster.ca/
paininstitute/

Murdoch Children's Research
Institute Royal Children's
Hospital
Flemington Road,
Parkville Victoria, 3052
Australia
(613) 8341-6200

Fax: (613) 9348-1391
www.mcri.edu.au

Napa Pain Institute
3434 Villa Lane, Suite 150
Napa, CA 94558
(707) 252-9660
www.napapaininstitute.com

National Pain Research Institute,
LLC
1201 S. Orlando Avenue
Winter Park, FL 32789
(407) 622-5766
Fax: (561) 372-0219
www.natpain.com

NHMRC Centre for Clinical
Research Excellence in Spinal
Pain, Injury and Health
Room 505, Level 5
SHRS, Therapies Building 84a
The University of Queensland
Brisbane, Street Lucia QLD 4072,
(617) 3365-4567
Fax: (617) 3365-1284

NHS Foundation Trust
Lower Lane, Fazakerley
Liverpool, L9 7LJ
0151 525 3611
Fax: 0151 529 5500
www.thewaltoncentre.nhs.ukf

North West Mersey Deanery
Regatta Place,
Brunswick Business Park
Summers Road
Liverpool L3 4BL
0151 285 4734
www.merseydeanery.nhs.uk

Northwestern University

Woodruff Lab
303 E Superior Street,
Suite 10-121,
Chicago, IL 60611
(312) 503-1385
www.womenshealth.
northwestern.edu/

Orthopedic Research Society
6300 N River Road, Suite 602
Rosemont, IL 60018
(847) 823-5770
ors@ors.org

Oxford Pain Relief Unit
Churchill Hospital
The Churchill
Oxford, OX3 7LJ, UK
+44 (0) 1865 225404
Fax: +44 (0) 1865 226078
maureen.woodford@pru.ox.ac.uk
www.medicine.ox.ac.uk

Pain and Anesthesia Research
Clinic
University of Adelaide
Adelaide, South Australia 5000
+61 8 8222 2712
Fax: +61 8 8222 2713
melanie.gentgall@health.sa.gov.au
www.adelaide.edu.au

Pain and Associated Symptoms
Research Fellowships
University of Iowa
College of Nursing Building
50 Newton Road
Iowa City, IA 52242
(319) 335-7018
Fax: (319) 335-9990
collegeofnursing@uiowa.edu
www.nursing.uiowa.edu

Pain Management Center
Department of Anesthesia
Stanford School of Medicine
450 Broadway Street
Pavilion A, 1st Floor, MC 5340
Redwood City, CA 94063
(650) 723-6238
Fax: (650) 320-9443
www.paincenter.stanfoRoad.edu

Pain Management Research
Institute
The University of Sydney
Royal North Shore Hospital
Street Leonardis, NSW 2065
+61(0) 2 9926-8423
Fax: +61 (0) 2 9906-4079
hmjohnst@nsccahs.health.nsw.gov
.au
www.sydney.edu.au

The Pain Relief Foundation
Clinical Sciences Centre,
University Hospital Aintree,
Lower Lane, Liverpool, L9 7AL
0151 529 5820
Fax: 0151 529 5821
www.painrelieffoundation.org.uk

Pain Research Center
Department of Anesthesiology
University of Utah
615 Arapeen Drive Suite 200
Salt Lake City, UT 84108
(801) 585-7690
www.painresearch.utah.edu

Pain Research Unit
Level 1 Campus Center
Sydney Children's Hospital
High Street
Randwick NSW 2031
Australia

+61 2 9382 1585
Fax: +61 2 9382 1008
Da-
vid.champion@sesiahs.health.nsw.
gov.au
www.sch.edu.au

The Penn Medicine Neuroscience
Center
Pain Medicine
Philadelphia, PA 19104
(800) 789-7366
www.pennmedicine.org

Pittsburgh Center for Pain
Research
200 Lothrop Street
Pittsburgh, PA 15213
(412) 383-5911
Fax: (412) 383-5466
www.paincenter.pitt.edu

The Resource Center of the
Alliance of State Pain Initiatives
(608) 262-0978
trc@mailplus.wisc.edu

The Royal College of
Anaesthetists
Faculty of Pain Medicine
35 Red Lion Square
London WC1R 4SG
020 7092 1500
Fax: 020 7092 1730
www.rcoa.ac.uk

Santa Monica Pain Management
Center
1245 16th Street, Suite 225
Santa Monica, CA 90404
(310) 794-1841
Fax: (310) 319-2263
www.anes.ucla.edu

The Scripps Research Institute
Dorris Neuroscience Center
10550 North Torrey Pines Road
La Jolla, CA 92037
(858) 784-1000
www.scripps.edu

Street John Medical Center
29000 Center Ridge Road
Westlake, OH 44145
(440) 835-8000
Fax: (440) 827-5015
www.sjws.net

Stanford Patient Education
Research Center
1000 Welch Road, Suite 204
Palo Alto, CA 94304
(650) 723-7935
Fax: (650) 725-9422
www.patienteducation.
stanfoRoadedu

Stanford University
Pain Management Center
450 Broadway Street
Pavilion A, 1st Floor, MC 5340
Redwood City, CA 94063
(650) 723-6238
Fax: (650) 320-9443
www.paincenter.stanfoRoadedu

Swedish Pain and Headache
Center
Swedish Medical Center
1101 Madison Street, Suite 200
Seattle, WA 98104
(206) 386-3806
www.swedish.org

Sydney Children's Hospital:
The Pain Research Unit

Level 1 Campus Centre
High Street
Randwick, NSW 2031
Australia
www.sch.edu.au

Translational Research Institute
on Pain in Later Life
Weill Medical College
525 East 68th Street
New York, NY 10065
(212) 746-1677
Fax: (212) 746-4888
maw2054@med.cornell.edu
www.tripll.org

UC Davis Health System
UC Davis Department of
Anesthesiology and Pain
Medicine
4150 V Street, Suite 1200
Sacramento, CA 95817
(916) 734-5028
Fax: (916) 734-7980
www.ucdmc.ucdavis.edu

UCLA Center for the
Interdisciplinary Study and
Treatment of Pain
0940 Wilshire Boulevard,
Suite 810
Los Angeles, CA 90024
(310) 794-6290
www.pain.ucla.edu

UMDNJ-Robert Wood Johnson
Medical School
Department of Anesthesia
125 Paterson Street, CAB 3100
New Brunswick, NJ 08901
(732) 235-6153
Fax: (732) 235-5100
www.rwjms.umdnj.edu

University of Aberdeen
King's College,
Aberdeen AB24 3FX
+44 (0)1224-272000
www.abdn.ac.uk

University of Alberta
Department of Anesthesiology &
Pain Medicine
8-120 Clinical Sciences Building
(CSB)
8440 112 Street NW
Edmonton, AB T6G 2G3
(780) 407-8861
Fax: (780) 407-3200
www.anesthesiology.med.
ualberta.ca

University of Liverpool
Clinical Sciences Centre,
University Hospital Aintree
Liverpool, L97AL, UK
0151 529 5820
Fax: 0151 529 5821
www.liv.ac.uk

The University of Toronto Center
for the Study of Pain
155 College Street, Suite 300,
Room 302

Toronto, ON M5T 1P8
(416) 946-8270
Fax: (416) 978-0817
www.utoronto.ca

University of Virginia
Pain Management Center
Fontaine Research Park
545 Ray C. Hunt Drive, 3rd Floor
Charlottesville, VA 22908
(434) 243-5676
Fax: (434) 243-5689
www.uvahealth.com

Washington University Pain
Management Center
10th floor, Suite A
4921 Parkview Pl
Street Louis, MO 63110
(314) 362-8820
www.pain.wustl.edu

Wasser Pain Management Centre
Mount Sinai Hospital
Joseph and Wolf Lebovic Health
Complex
600 University Avenue, 11th Floor
Toronto, ON M5G 1X5
(416) 596-4200
www.mountsinai.on.ca

Appendix C

PAIN ORGANIZATIONS

American Academy of
Family Physicians
11400 Tomahawk Creek Parkway
Leawood, KS 66211
(800) 274-2237
contactcenter@aafp.org

American Academy of
Hospice and Palliative Medicine
4700 W. Lake Avenue
Glenview, IL 60025
(847) 375-4712
info@aahpm.org

American Academy of Nurse
Practitioners
Capital Station, LBJ Building
P.O. Box 12926
Austin, TX 78711

American Academy of Pain
Management
975 Morning Star Drive, Suite A
Sonora, CA 95370
(209) 533-9744
info@aapainmanage.org

American Academy of Pain
Medicine
4700 W. Lake Avenue
Glenview, IL 60025
(847) 375-4731
info@painmed.org

American Academy of Physical
Medicine and Rehabilitation
9700 W. Bryn Mawr Avenue,
Suite 200
Rosemont, IL 60018
(847) 737-6000

American Association of
Orthopedic Medicine
555 Waterview Lane
Ridgeway, CO 81432
(888) 687-1920
aaom@aaomed.org

American Board of Pain Medicine
4700 W. Lake Avenue
Glenview, IL 60025
(847) 375-4726

American Chronic Pain
Association
PO Box 850
Rocklin, CA 95677
(800) 533-3231
ACPA@theacpa.org

American College of
Rheumatology/ARHP
2200 Lake Boulevard NE
Atlanta, GA 30319
(404) 633-3777
acr@rheumatology.org

American College of Sports
Medicine
401 West Michigan Street
Indianapolis, IN 46202
(317) 637-9200

American Council on Fitness
4851 Paramount Drive
San Diego, CA 92123
(888) 825-3636

American Headache Society
19 Mantua Road
Mount Royal, NJ 08061
(856) 423-0043
ahshq@talley.com

American Medical Association
515 N. State Street
Chicago, IL 60654
(800) 621-8335

American Migraine Foundation
19 Mantua Road
Mount Royal, NJ 08061
(856) 423-0043
amf@talley.com

American Pain Society
4700 W. Lake Avenue
Glenview, IL 60025
(847) 375-4715
info@americanpainsociety.org

American Physical Therapy
Association
1111 North Fairfax Street
Alexandria, VA 22314
(703) 683-6748

American Society of
Anesthesiologists
520 N, Northwest Highway
Park Ridge, IL 60068
(847) 825-5586
communications@asahq.org

American Society of Consultant
Pharmacists
1321 Duke Street
Alexandria, VA 22314
(703) 739-1300
info@ascp.com

American Society for Pain
Management Nursing
18000 W 105th Street
Olathe, KS 66061
aspmn@goamp.com

American Society of Regional
Anesthesia and Pain Medicine
239 Fourth Avenue, Suite 1714
Pittsburgh, PA 15222
(855) 795-ASRA

Asia-Oceanian Society of Physical
and Rehabilitation Medicine
Unit A, 2/F, Ming Tak Centre
135–137 Tung Chau Street
Kowloon, Hong Kong

852 2396 6261

Association of Professional Team
Physicians
333 City Boulevard West
Orange, CA 92668
(714) 938-3818

Arthroscopy Association of
North America
6300 North River Road, Suite 600
Rosemont, IL 60018
(847) 292-2262
susan@aana.org

Atlantic Neuroscience Institute's
Pain Management Center
99 Beauvoir Avenue
Summit, NJ 07901
(908) 522-2000

Canadian Association of Physical
Medicine & Rehabilitation
1937 Portobello Road
PO Box 17059
Ottawa, ON K4A 4W0
(613) 707-0483
info@capmr.ca

The Center to Advance
Palliative Care
1255 Fifth Avenue, Suite C-2
New York, NY 10029
(212) 201-2670
capc@mssm.edu

Centers for Disease Control and
Prevention
1600 Clifton Road
Atlanta, GA 30333
(800) 232-4636

Endo Health Solutions
1400 Atwater Drive
Malvern, PA 19355
(484) 216-0000

Hospice and Palliative Nurses
Association
One Penn Center West, Suite 229
Pittsburgh, PA 15276
(412) 787-9301

Indian Association of Physical
Medicine and Rehabilitation
J 103, Kaveri Apartments, Plot 4
Sector 6 Dwarka
New Delhi, India 110075

Institute for Healthcare
Improvement
20 University Road, 7th Floor
Cambridge, MA 02138
(617)- 301-4800
info@ihi.org

Institute for Safe Medication
Practices
200 Lakeside Drive; Suite 200
Horsham, PA 19044
(215) 947-7797

International Association for
Hospice & Palliative Care
5535 Memorial Drive Suite F,
PMB 509
Houston, TX 77007
(936) 321-9846

International Association for the
Study of Pain
1510 H Street NW, Suite 600
Washington, DC 20005
(202) 524-5300

International Federation of
Sports Medicine
Av. de Rhodanie 54
CH-1007 Lausanne, Switzerland
headquarters-ch@fims.org

International Society of Physical
and Rehabilitation Medicine
1-3 Rue de Chantepoulet
Geneva, Switzerland
(22) 908-04-83

The Japanese Association of
Rehabilitation Medicine
6-32-3 Kagurazaka
Shinjuku, Tokyo 162-0825
(813) 5206-6011

National Association for
Healthcare Quality
4700 West Lake Avenue
Glenview, IL 60025
(800) 966-9392
ssochacki@nahq.org

National Association of State
Controlled Substance Authorities
72 Brook Street
Quincy, MA 02170
(617) 471-0520
kathykeough@nascsa.org

National Center for Medical
Rehabilitation Research
31 Center Drive, Bldg. 31,
Rm. 2A32
Bethesda, MD 20892

National Headache Foundation
820 N. Orleans, Suite 411
Chicago, IL 60610
(888) 643-5552
info@headaches.org

National Hospice and Palliative
Care Organization
1731 King Street
Alexandria, VA 22314
(703) 837-1500

National Institute of Neurological
Disorders and Stroke
P.O. Box 5801
Bethesda, MD 20824
(800) 352-9424

National Pain Foundation
201 North Charles Street,
Suite 710
Baltimore, MD 21201

New York State Society of
Anesthesiologists
110 E. 40th Street, Suite 300
New York, NY 10016
(212) 867-7140
hq@nyssa-pga.org

The NIH Pain Consortium
Bethesda, MA 20892
nihpaininfo@mail.nih.gov

The North American Spine
Society
7075 Veterans Boulevard
Burr Ridge, IL 60527
(630) 230-3600

Pain and Palliative Care Resource
Center/City of Hope
1500 East Duarte Road
Duarte, CA 91010
(626) 256-HOPE
prc@coh.org

Pain and Policy Studies Group
Wisconsin University
6152 Medical Sciences Center
1300 University Avenue
Madison, WI 53706
(608) 263-7662

Pain.com/Dannemiller   Memorial
Educational Foundation
5711 Northwest Parkway
San Antonio, TX 78246
(210) 572-2512

Society for Pain Practice
Management
PO Box 7228
Overland Park, KS 66211
(913) 327-5999

Substance Abuse and Mental
Health Services Administration
P.O. Box 2345
Rockville, MD 20847
(800) 487-4889
SAMHSAInfo@samhsa.hhs.gov

Weill Cornell Physicians
1300 York Avenue
New York, NY 10065
(212) 746-5454

Appendix D

NATIONALLY RECOGNIZED PAIN CLINICS

Bay Area Orthopedic Surgery and Sports Medicine
100 Hospital Drive, Suite 303
Vallejo, CA 94589
(707) 645-7210

Brigham and Women's Hospital
850 Boylston Street
Chestnut Hill, MA 02467
(617) 732-9060
pain@zeus.bwh.harvaRoadedu

Center for Pain Management
Rehabilitation Institute of Chicago
345 E. Superior Street
Chicago, IL 60611
(312) 238-7800
www.ric.org

Center for Pain Management
The University of Toledo Medical Center
3000 Arlington Avenue
Toledo, OH 43614
(419) 383-3761
utmc.webmaster@utoledo.edu
www.utmc.utoledo.edu

Children's Hospital & Regional Medical Center
Clinical and Diagnostic Services
4800 Sand Point Way NE
Seattle, WA 98105
(206) 987-2704

Chronic Pain Management Clinic
Boston Children's Hospital
300 Longwood Avenue
Boston, MA 02115
(617) 355-7040
Fax: (617) 730-0152
www.childrenshospital.org

Chronic Pain Rehabilitation
Program
Neurological Center for Pain
9500 Euclid Avenue
Cleveland, OH 44195
(800) 223-2273

Chronic Pain Rehabilitation
Program
Courage Center
3915 Golden Valley Road
Minneapolis, MN 55422
(763) 588-0811
www.couragecenter.org

Cleveland Clinic
2049 East 100th Street
Cleveland, OH 44195
(216) 445-8904

Comprehensive Pain Center
13000 Bruce B. Downs Boulevard
Tampa, FL 33612
(813) 972-2000

Comprehensive Pain
Management
92 Nordson Overlook, Suite 205
Dawsonville, GA 30534
(678) 256-2667
www.
atlantapainmanagementcenters.
com

Comprehensive Pain Center of
Sarasota
1921 Waldermere Street
Suite 607
Sarasota, FL 34239
(941) 363-9400

Department of Pain Management
Cleveland Clinic
9500 Euclid Avenue / C25
Cleveland, OH 44195
(216) 444-7246
(800) 392-3353
www.my.clevelandclinic.org

Department of Pain Medicine and
Palliative Care
Beth Israel Medical Center
First Avenue at 16th Street
New York, NY 10003
(877) 620-9999
stoppain@chpnet.org

Doctors Pain Clinic
1011 Boardman-Canfield Road
Youngstown, OH 44512
(330) 629-2888
Fax: (330) 629-8940
www.doctorspainclinic.com

Fairview Pain Management
Center, University of Minnesota
Medical Center
606 24th Avenue S, Suite 600
Minneapolis, MN 55454
(612) 273-5400

Fraser Health
Suite 400, Central City Tower
13450 – 102nd Avenue
Surrey, BC V3T 0H1
(604) 587-4600
Fax: (604) 587-4666
www.fraserhealth.ca

Holistic Resource Center
29020 Agoura Road A-8
Agoura, CA 91301
(818) 597-0966

Jane B. Pettit Pain and Palliative Care Center
9000 West Wisconsin Avenue
Wauwatosa, WI 53226
(414) 266-2000

Kure Pain Management
The Spine Specialists
120 Sallitt Drive, Suite D
Stevensville, MD 21666
(877) 621-1269

La Jolla Whole Health Medical Clinic
8950 Villa La Jolla Drive
La Jolla, CA 92037
(858) 450-5053

Las Vegas Pain Institute and Medical Center
Centennial Medical Center
7175 N. Durango Drive, Suite 170
Las Vegas, NV 89149
(702) 880-4193
www.lasvegaspaininstitutes.com

Lawrence J. Ellison Ambulatory Care Clinic
Department of Anesthesiology and Pain Medicine
4860 Y Street, Suite 2600
Sacramento, CA 95817
(916) 734-7246

Multidisciplinary Pain Center
University of Alberta
Surgery A
Reception Area #2A1-01
Edmonic Clinic
11400 University Avenue
Edmonton, AB T6G 1Z1
(780) 407-8638
Fax: (780) 407-2736

apmcomm@ualberta.ca
www.uofpain.med.ualberta.ca

National Osteoporosis Foundation
1150 17th Street, NW Suite 850
Washington, DC 20036
(800) 231-4222

National Pain Centers
1585 Barrington Road, Doctors Office Bldg. 2, Suite 103
Hoffman Estates, IL 60169
(847) 701-3250

Natural Healing Institute
515 Encinitas Boulevard Suites 201 & 203
Encinitas, CA 92024
(760) 943.8485
enroll@naturalhealinginStreetcom

Pain Clinic
University of Colorado Hospital
1635 Aurora Court, Suite 1101
Aurora, CO 80010
(720) 848-1970
www.uch.edu

Pain Management & Rehabilitation Center
4793 Manhattan Drive
Rockford, IL 61107
(815) 398-7246
Fax: (815) 398-7276
kunli4@comcaStreetnet
www.painrehabcenter.com

Pain Management Center
University of Minnesota Medical Center, Fairview
606 24th Avenue
Minneapolis, MN 55454
(612) 273-5400

www.uofmmedicalcenter.org

Pain Management and
Rehabilitation
801 Brewster Avenue, Suite 240
Redwood City, CA 94063
(650) 366-4542

Pain Management and Rehabilitation Center
223 Stoneridge Drive
Columbia, SC 29210
(803) 296-7246
paininfo@palmettohealth.org
www.palmettohealth.org

Pain Management Center
Columbia University
622 West 168th Street
New York, NY 10032
(212) 305-7114
Fax: (212) 305-8883
www.cumc.columbia,edu

Pain Management Centers
North Shore University Health
System
Evanston Hospital
2650 Ridge Avenue
Evanston, IL 60201
(847) 570-2000
www.northshore.org

The Pain Management Center at
Stanford University Medical Center
450 Broadway Street
Pavilion A 1st Floor MC 5340
Redwood City, CA 94063
(650) 723-6238
medicalgiving@stanfoRoadedu

Pain Management Center
University of California
2255 Post Street
San Francisco, CA 94143-1654
(415) 885-7246
Fax: (415) 885-3883
www.ucsfhealth.org

Pain Management Center
University of Maryland Medical
System
Kernan Hospital
2200 Kernan Drive
Baltimore, MD 12107
(888) 453-7626
paininfo@anes.umm.edu
www.kernan.org

Pain Management Center
University of Miami Health System
Northwest 14th Street
Miami, FL 33136
(305) 243-4000
www.uhealthsystem.com

Pain Management Clinic
Lawrence J. Ellison Ambulatory
Care Clinic
Department of Anesthesiology
and Pain Medicine
4860 Y Street – Suite 2600
Sacramento, CA 95817
(916) 734-7246
www.ucdmc.ucdavis.edu

Pain Rehab Clinic
Arc Motion
55 E. Huntington Drive
Suite 219
Arcadia, CA 91006
www.arcmotionrehab.com

Pain Rehabilitation Clinic
6D-1550 South Gateway Road
Mississauga, ON L4W5G6
(905) 238-0739
Fax: (905) 602-6852
www.painrehabclinic.com

Pediatric Pain Rehabilitation
Clinic
Kennedy Krieger Institute
707 North Broadway
Baltimore, MD 21205
(443) 923-9200
Fax: (443) 923-2645
www.kennedykrieger.org

Preventive Medical Center of
Marin (PMCM)
25 Mitchell Boulevard, Suite 8
San Rafael, CA 94903
(415) 472-2343

Rehabilitation Institute of
Washington
415 1st Ave N #200
Seattle, WA 98109
(206) 859-5030

Seattle Cancer Care Alliance
825 Eastlake Avenue E
Seattle, WA 98109
(206) 288-1024

Swedish Medical Center
Pain Center
747 Broadway
Seattle, WA 98122
(206) 386-2013

United Back Care Redmond
2515 140th Avenue NE
STE E110

Bellevue, WA 98005
(425) 644-4100
info@lifeworkwellness.com

University of Rochester Pain
Treatment Center
180 Sawgrass Drive, Suite 210
Rochester, NY 14620
(585) 242-1300
www.rochesterpaincenter.com

University of Washington Medical
Center Multidisciplinary
Pain Center
1959 NE Pacific Street
Seattle, WA 98195
(206) 598-3300

University Pain Center
Rush Oak Park Hospital
610 South Maple Avenue
Suite 1500
Oak Park, IL 60304
(312) 923-9771
www.universitypaincenters.com

University Pain Consultants
6900 Brockton Avenue
Riverside, CA 92506
(951) 784-7111
Fax: (951) 823-0378
www.healthgrades.com

University Pain Medicine Center
Towne Professional Park at
Somerset
33 Clyde Road, Suites 105, 106
Somerset, NJ 08873
(732) 873-6868
Fax: (732) 873-6869
www.upmcpainmedicine.com

Virginia Mason Medical Center
Physical Medicine and
Rehabilitation
1100 9th Avenue
Seattle, WA 98101
(206) 625-7249

Washington University Pain
Management Center
4921 Parkview Place
Street Louis, MO 63110
(314) 362-8820
Fax: (314) 362-9471
paincenter@wustl.edu
www.paincenter.wustl.edu

Appendix E

FOR FURTHER READING

Andrews, James R. *Any Given Monday: Sports Injuries and How to Prevent Them for Athletes, Parents, and Coaches—Based on My Life in Sports Medicine.* New York: Scribner, 2013.
Barnard, Neal D. *Foods That Fight Pain: Proven Dietary Solutions for Maximum Pain Relief without Drugs.* Emmaus, PA: Rodale Press, 2008.
———. *Foods That Fight Pain: Revolutionary New Strategies for Maximum Pain Relief.* New York: Harmony Books, 1998.
Barsky, Arthur J., and Emily C. Deans. *Stop Being Your Symptoms and Start Being Yourself: The 6-Week Mind-Body Program to Ease Your Chronic Symptoms.* New York: William Morrow, 2006.
Bernstein, Carolyn. *The Migraine Brain: Your Breakthrough Guide to Fewer Headaches, Better Health.* New York: Free Press, 2008.
Block, Keith. *Life Over Cancer: The Block Center Program for Integrative Cancer Treatment.* New York: Bantam, 2009.
Boswell, Mark V., and B. Eliot Cole. *Weiner's Pain Management: A Practical Guide for Clinicians.* Boca Raton, FL: CRC Press, 2005.
Brady, Scott, and William Proctor. *Pain Free for Life: The 6-Week Cure for Chronic Pain—without Surgery or Drugs.* New York: Center Street, 2011.
Brownstein, Art. *Healing Back Pain Naturally: The Mind-Body Program Proven to Work.* New York: Pocket, 2001.
Bruera, Eduardo, Irene Higginson, and Charles von Gunten. *Textbook of Palliative Medicine.* Boca Raton, FL: CRC Press, 2009.
Buchholz, David. *Heal Your Headache: The 1-2-3 Program for Taking Charge of Your Pain.* New York Workman Publishing Company, 2002.
Catalano, Ellen Mohr, and Kimeron N. Hardin. *Chronic Pain Control Workbook.* Oakland, CA: New Harbinger, 1996.
Chew, Ming, and Stephanie Golden. *The Permanent Pain Cure.* New York: McGraw-Hill, 2008.
Cochran, Robert T. Jr. *Understanding Chronic Pain: A Doctor Talks to His Patients.* Franklin, TN: Hillsboro Press, 2004.
Davies, Clair, Amber Davies, and David G. Simons. *The Trigger Point Therapy Workbook.* Oakland, CA: New Harbinger Publications, 2004.
Egoscue, Pete, and Roger Gittines. *A Revolutionary Method for Stopping Chronic Pain.* New York: Bantam, 1998.
Egoscue, Pete. *Pain Free for Women: The Revolutionary Program for Ending Chronic Pain.* New York: Bantam, 2002.
Fishman, Loren M., and Carol Ardman. *Relief Is in the Stretch: End Back Pain through Yoga.* New York: W. W. Norton & Company, 2005.
Gokhale, Esther, and Adams Susan. *8 Steps to a Pain-Free Back: Natural Posture Solutions for Pain in the Back, Neck, Shoulder, Hip, Knee, and Foot.* Stanford, CA: Pendo Press, 2008.
Goodman, Eric, Peter Park, and Lance Armstrong. *Foundation: Redefine Your Core, Conquer Back Pain, and Move with Confidence.* Emmaus, PA: Rodale Books, 2011.

Hassett Dahm, Nancy. *Mind, Body, and Soul: A Guide to Living with Cancer*. Garden City, NY: Taylor Hill, 2001.

Heller, Sharon. *Too Loud, Too Bright, Too Fast, Too Tight: What to Do If You Are Sensory Defensive in an Overstimulating World*. New York: HarperCollins, 2002.

Hitzmann, Sue. *The MELT Method: A Breakthrough Self-Treatment System to Eliminate Chronic Pain, Erase the Signs of Aging, and Feel Fantastic in Just 10 Minutes a Day!* New York: HarperOne, 2013.

Hong Wang, Linda, Anne Marie McKenzie-Brown, and Allen Hord. *The Handbook of C-Arm Fluoroscopy-Guided Spinal Injections*. Boca Raton, FL: CRC Press, 2006.

Hurley, Daniel. *Facing Pain, Finding Hope: A Physician Examines Pain, Faith, and the Healing Stories of Jesus*. Chicago: Loyola Press, 2005.

Jay, Gary W. *Chronic Pain*. Boca Raton, FL: CRC Press, 2007.

Kaye, Alan D. *Understanding Pain: What You Need to Know to Take Control* (The Praeger Series on Contemporary Health and Living). Santa Barbara, CA: Praeger, 2011.

Khalsa, Dharma Singh, and Cameron Stauth. *The Pain Cure: The Proven Medical Program That Helps End Your Chronic Pain*. New York: Warner, 1999.

Klapper, Robert, and Lynda Huey. *Heal Your Knees: How to Prevent Knee Surgery and What to Do If You Need It*. New York: M. Evans & Company, 2004.

Kolster, Bernard C., and Astrid Waskowiak. *The Reflexology Atlas*. Rochester, VT: Healing Arts Press, 2005.

Jacob, Stanley W. *The Miracle of MSM : The Natural Solution for Pain*. New York: Putnam Adult, 1999.

Laliberte, Richard. *Doctors' Guide to Chronic Pain*. New York: Readers Digest, 2004.

Lehman, Thomas J. A. *It's Not Just Growing Pains: A Guide to Childhood Muscle, Bone and Joint Pain, Rheumatic Diseases, and the Latest Treatments*. New York: Oxford University Press, 2004.

McKenzie, Robin. *Treat Your Own Neck 5th ed*. Valley Stream, NY: Orthopedic Physical Therapy Products, 2011.

Melzack, Ronald, and Patrick D. Wall. *Handbook of Pain Management: A Clinical Companion to Textbook of Pain*. 1st ed. London: Churchill Livingstone, 2003.

Natelson, Benjamin H. *Your Symptoms Are Real: What to Do When Your Doctor Says Nothing Is Wrong*. Hoboken, NJ: Wiley, 2007.

Patterson, David R. *Clinical Hypnosis for Pain Control*. Washington, DC: American Psychological Association, 2010.

Petrone, Elaine. *The Miracle Ball Method: Relieve Your Pain, Reshape Your Body, Reduce Your Stress*. New York: Workman, 2003.

Sarno, John E. *Healing Back Pain: The Mind-Body Connection*. New York: Grand Central Life & Style, 2010.

Sarno, John E. *The Mindbody Prescription: Healing the Body, Healing the Pain*. New York: Warner Books, Inc., 1999.

Sarno, John E. *The Divided Mind: The Epidemic of Mindbody Disorders*. New York: Harper, 2006.

Schatman, Michael E., Alexandra Campbell, and American Academy of Pain Management. *Chronic Pain Management: Guidelines for Multidisciplinary Program Development*. Boca Raton, FL: CRC Press, 2007.

Schuler, Lou, Alwyn Cosgrove. *The New Rules of Lifting for Life: An All-New Muscle-Building, Fat-Blasting Plan for Men and Women Who Want to Ace Their Midlife Exams*. New York: Avery, 2102.

Sun Peilin. *The Treatment of Pain with Chinese Herbs and Acupuncture*. Churchill Livingstone, 2010.

Thernstrom, Melanie. *The Pain Chronicles: Cures, Myths, Mysteries, Prayers, Diaries, Brain Scans, Healing, and the Science of Suffering*. New York: Farrar, Straus and Giroux, 2010.

Vad, Vijay. *Arthritis Rx: A Cutting-Edge Program for a Pain-Free Life*. New York: Gotham, 2006.

Warson, James, and Ami Hendrickson. *The Rider's Pain-Free Back: Overcome Chronic Soreness, Injury and Aging, and Stay in the Saddle for Years to Come*. North Pomfret, VT: Trafalgar Square Books, 2007.

GLOSSARY

A

abdominal aortic aneurysm (AAA). A painful occurrence whereby the abdominal aorta has more than doubled its size and spreads severe pain from the abdomen down to the limbs.

abducens nerve. The sixth cranial nerve; it is directly responsible for the movement of the lateral rectus muscle of the eye.

accessory nerve. The eleventh cranial nerve that regulates movement on the shoulder and neck muscles.

acetylcholine. A neurotransmitter used in the motor functioning of the brain and the rest of the body.

acetylsalicylic acid. Better known as aspirin, a drug used for reduction of pain, fever and swelling.

acquired immunodeficiency syndrome (AIDS). A disorder that makes a person more susceptible to infection due to the weakening of the body's natural defense or immune system. It is caused by a virus called human immunodeficiency virus (HIV).

acupuncture. Method used in traditional Chinese medicine whereby needles are inserted into the skin to stimulate certain points in the body to promote healing. One of the most recognized forms of alternative medicine.

acute pain. A kind of pain that does not last longer than three to six months but can be more painful than chronic pain.

adjuvant pain medications. A group of drugs used to minimize pain indirectly. Examples are muscle relaxants, antidepressants, and anxiolytics.

alternative medicine. A separate body of medical practice not taught rigorously in medical school; includes acupuncture, chiropractic, and homeopathy, among others.

Alzheimer's disease. A disease that usually affects people age sixty-five and above. The memory functioning slowly degenerates, leading up to the person's death.

amenorrhea. The non-occurrence of a woman's monthly menstrual cycle.

amygdalae. A part of the brain that is significantly involved in emotional responses as well as memory processes.

analgesic. A kind of drug or medication used to relieve pain.

anaphylactic reaction. Pertaining to anaphylaxis; a dangerous and rapid allergic reaction.

anesthesiology. A branch of medical study that specializes in anesthesia and its administration.

anterior cingulate cortex. A part of the brain that is believed to be involved with decision-making tasks, problem solving, and motivation.

anterograde amnesia. The inability to form and retain a new set of memories.

anxiolytic. A kind of drug that can help prevent anxiety.

arthroplasty. A surgical procedure involving the replacement of the articular exterior of a musculoskeletal joint in order to alleviate pain.

Asperger's syndrome. A behavioral disorder consisting of social, emotional and verbal difficulties. It is within the umbrella of autism, but the person having Asperger's exhibits repetitive actions and limited interests.

astrocytes. A glial cell with a shape similar to a star whose immediate function is to repair the damage within the brain and spinal cord areas.

Attention Deficit Hyperactivity Disorder (ADHD). A behavioral disorder mostly diagnosed in children attending school who are having difficulty focusing on a single task, sitting and listening during class, and regulating their reactions to their environment.

autonomic nervous system. A part of the nervous system directly responsible for involuntary or automatic reactions of the body to both internal and external stimuli such as breathing, heartbeats, sexual arousal, and sweating, among others.

axon. The long branch of a neuron that sends out signals to nearby neurons.

B

benzodiazepine (BZD). A drug class that produces a calming effect on the body, thereby reducing anxiety. At times it can also relieve pain.

biofeedback. A process of self-awareness that is enhanced through proper control and continuous observation of the patient's bodily reaction to stress, pain, and emotions.

bone metastasis. A disease concerning the bone that develops a tumor and has cancer-like progression.

bradycardia. The slowing of the heart rate causing dizziness and fatigue.

brain stem. The lower portion of the brain that includes the medulla oblongata, pons, and midbrain.

Broca's area. An important part of the brain that has a direct function in the production of speech.

Brodmann areas. A region in the brain cortex that contains areas responsible for hearing process and understanding language.

brucellosis. The other term for rock fever or Bang's disease. Caused by drinking contaminated milk or meat portions of an animal infected with the bacteria.

bupivacaine. Pain reliever that is used during long surgical operations.

buprenorphine. Drug that is indicated for treatment on patients having opioid addiction.

C

carbuncle. Skin disease that is worse than a boil, it has two or more holes, which helps to drain the discharge.

carpal tunnel syndrome. A compression around the wrist area causing pain and numbness ranging from the wrist to the arm.

celiac disease. A dysfunction of the small intestine resulting in reduced absorbing capacity to take vital nutrients from ingested food.

central nervous system (CNS). Main part of the nervous system that specializes in receiving and processing information. The group includes the brain, spinal cord, retina, and cranial nerves.

cerebellum. A part of the brain that specializes in motor-coordination, posture, fine motor skills, and physical accuracy.

cerebrum. The uppermost region of the brain divided into two hemispheres, which are further categorized into four lobes, namely: frontal, occipital, parietal, and temporal.

chronic fatigue syndrome. A condition usually affecting women who feel severely tired, sometimes due to muscle pain on joints, arms, and legs.

chronic pain. Type of pain felt for longer than three to six months but generally less severe than acute pain.

complex regional pain syndrome (CRPS). Formerly known as causalgia, it is a disease that spreads and worsens over time. The patient experiences severe pain as well as inflammation of affected areas.

computed tomography (CT) scan. An advanced method of viewing internal parts of the body by using X-rays, computers, and film.

congenital insensitivity to pain (CIP). A rare occurrence where people are born with the inability to feel pain, thereby making them susceptible to infection due to neglected wounds or prolonged illnesses.

cordotomy. Medical procedure done by surgically severing the tracts that connect the spinal cord to the receptor that triggers pain. This method is used when the patient is in extreme pain or if no other treatment can be successfully done.

COX-2 inhibitor. A family of NSAIDs specifically used to minimize swelling and provide pain relief.

cranial nerves. The twelve pairs of nerves that branch out from the brain.

Crohn's disease. A disorder that targets the mouth all the way to the anus; it causes the gastrointestinal tract to swell and produce a variety of illnesses such as diarrhea, skin rashes, and abdominal pain among others.

D

deep brain stimulation (DBS). A medical procedure that allows a brain pacemaker to be surgically inserted into a specific area of the brain.

dementia. A mental disorder characterized by the gradual loss of mental functioning, generally caused by aging but sometimes a result of an accident.

dendrites. Short branches of a neuron that receives signals from nearby neurons.

dopamine. Natural hormone that allows for positive feelings and reward-driven learning.

drug metabolism. A process wherein the body actively uses and breaks down a drug substance.

dyslexia. A learning disorder usually observed in school children having difficulty reading. A person with dyslexia can be visually confused regarding the positioning of some alphabets with their mirror images.

E

electronic medical record (EMR). A computerized report of the patient's medical history that is easily accessible but quite costly.

endogenous opiates. Also known as endorphin, a natural hormone released by the body that can help reduce or even eliminate pain over time.

erythemalgia. A kind of disorder affecting the hands and feet that becomes painful and then changes to a purplish color.

F

facial nerve. Cranial nerve seven. Its function is to control facial muscles and the part of the tongue responsible for the sense of taste.

fibromyalgia. A disorder characterized by fluctuating reception of widespread pain.

G

gamma-aminobutyric acid. Commonly referred to as GABA; these are involuntary neurotransmitters.

H

herpes zoster. Also called shingles, this viral disorder produces blisters and painful rashes that linger on for weeks at a time.
hippocampus. Part of the brain that plays a vital role in storing memory.
hyperkinesia. An excessive use of muscles that can cause tissue damage.
hypnotherapy. Combination of hypnosis and psychotherapy that is used to help patients overcome a difficulty or a personal crisis by tapping into the unconscious mind.
hypothalamus. Emotional center of the brain.

L

laudanum. Medicine used for pain in the previous century and earlier; it can be created by adding opium and alcohol.
lysergic acid diethylamide (LSD). In short form called LSD-25; it is a drug that can change thinking states, and even perception of time and space.

M

medulla oblongata. Part of the brain responsible for basic body functions needed for survival, such as respiratory and cardiovascular activities. Called the "bulb" in older medical terminology.
metabolic rate. Sum of energy used in a specified time.
myelin sheath. Material covering an axon. It allows a stimulus to slide fast from one neuron to the next.

N

neuron. A term used for brain cells. A major part of the central nervous system.
nociceptor. A type of neuron that gives off warning signals to the brain when the body receives stimuli that can possibly harm the body.
nonsteroidal inflammatory drugs (NSAIDs). A type of drug with pain relieving effects as well as anti-inflammatory and antipyretic (anti-fever) properties.

O

occipital nerve stimulation (ONS). Can be referred to as peripheral nerve stimulation (PNS). It is a procedure that can help alleviate pain caused by chronic migraine.
oculomotor nerve. The third cranial nerve responsible for the functioning of the eye muscles and their movement.
olfactory nerve. First cranial nerve. It is directly responsible for the functioning of the nose and its sense of smell.
optic nerve. The second cranial nerve, which is responsible for the relaying of stimulus from the eyes (through the retina) to the brain.

P

palliative care. An arm of medical care that aims to lessen the pain and distress of patients in every stage of their disease.
Parkinson's disease. The easily identified symptom of this brain disorder are shaking and awkward movements due to degeneration of cells responsible for motor functioning.
peripheral nervous system (PNS). A part of the nervous system that includes the nerves and ganglia connected to the arms and legs. These nerves bring the stimulus from the extremities to the central nervous system.
physiatry. Also termed physical medicine and rehabilitation, an arm of medical study focusing on treatment for patients with physical disabilities and pain.

R

radicular pain. A kind of pain felt from the nerve root, moving along the spinal cord.
radiographic. Pertaining to radiography; a method where rays are absorbed in different levels depending on the heterogeneous substance used.
retina. A part of the eye that creates images for the brain.

S

serotonin. A naturally produced neurotransmitter that has a positive effect on the body's sense of importance and happiness.
somatic pain. Pain felt coming from within the body ("soma" = body).

T

temporomandibular joint (TMJ) disorder. Disorder characterized by reduced ability to move the jaw due to problems with the muscles of the jaw and the connecting joints.
thalamus. A part of the diencephalon that has a shape similar to a walnut, its main function is to transmit and process stimuli coming from the sensory and motor receptors up to the cerebral cortex.
tramadol. A drug indicated for moderate to slightly severe forms of pain.
transcutaneous electrical nerve stimulation (TENS). A method that uses mild electrical pulses placed on the skin to stimulate nerves, thereby adding to the relief of pain.
trigeminal nerve. The fifth cranial nerve, whose function includes facial and mandibular motor activities such as biting and chewing.
trochlear nerve. The fourth cranial nerve; the smallest among the twelve with respect to the number of axons it carries.

V

visceral pain. Kind of pain that is difficult to locate because it is spread out and within organs, possibly around pelvic areas and the abdomen.

W

Wernicke's area. Area of the brain that processes speech.

NOTES

PREFACE

1. American Pain Society (APS), *Principles of Analgesic Use in the Treatment of Acute Pain and Cancer Pain* (Glenview, IL: American Pain Society, 2003).

2. M. McCaffery and C. Pasero, *Pain: Clinical Manual* (St. Louis, MO: Mosby, 1999), 17.

3. W. Winlow and A. V. Holden, *The Neurobiology of Pain: Symposium of the Northern Neurobiology Group* (Manchester, UK: Manchester University Press, 1984), 106.

4. C. I. Ripamonti, D. A. Sichetti, C. Fanizza, and M. Romero, "Is Pain Reporting to Health Care Professionals Age-Related? A Cross Sectional Multicenter Study in a Hospital Setting," *Expert Opinions on Pharmacotherapy* 14, no. 15 (2013): 2011–17.

5. McCaffery and Pasero, *Pain: Clinical Manual*, 33.

6. American Geriatrics Society (AGS), "Clinical Practice Guidelines: The Management of Chronic Pain in Older Persons," *Journal of the American Geriatrics Society* 53, Suppl. 3 (1998): 635–51.

7. M. Stanley, K. A. Blair, and P. G. Beare, *Gerontological Nursing: Promoting Successful Aging with Older Adults* (Philadelphia: F. A. Davis, 2005), 25.

1. INTRODUCTION TO PAIN

1. "Pain Terms," International Association for the Study of Pain, accessed September 7, 2012, www.iasp-pain.org.

2. The Free Dictionary, "Definition of Pain," accessed September 7, 2012, http://medical-dictionary.thefreedictionary.com/pain.

3. The Free Dictionary, "Definition of Pain."

4. The Free Dictionary, "Definition of Pain."

5. MondoFacto, "Dolorology," accessed September 8, 2012, www.mondofacto.com/facts/dictionary?dolorology.

6. A. Honeycutt and M. E. Milliken, *Understanding Human Behavior: A Guide for Health Care Providers*, 8th ed. (New York: Delmar Cengage Learning, 2012), 373.

7. Honeycutt and Milliken, *Understanding Human Behavior*.

8. Merriam-Webster Online, "Dolorology," accessed September 8, 2012, www.merriam-webster.com/medical/dolorology.

9. M. Osterweis and A. Kleinman, *Pain and Disability: Clinical, Behavioral, and Public Policy Perspectives* (Atlanta, GA: National Academies Press, 1987).

10. J. H. Blass, *The Family Counselor* (Bloomington, IN: iUniverse, 2012).

11. MedicineNet Inc., "Pain Management," accessed September 12, 2012, www.medicinenet.com/pain_management/article.htm.

12. A. Morrow, "What Is Pain ?" About.com, accessed September 20, 2012, www.dying.about.com.

13. A. Schmeling, A. Correns, and G. Geserick, "An Unusual Autoerotic Accident: Sexual Pleasure from Peritoneal Pain" [German], *Archiv für Kriminologie* 207, nos. 5–6 (2001): 148–53; W. Sohn, "Pleasure and Pain in Sexual Relations. The Basis and Reasons for Sex Counseling by the General Practitioner" [German], *MMW Fortschritte der Medizin* 145, no. 46 (2003): 37–40.

14. Morrow, "What Is Pain."

15. P. A. McGrath, "Psychological Aspects of Pain Perception," *Archives of Oral Biology* 39, Suppl. (1994): 55S–62S.

16. R. G. Large, "Psychological Aspects of Pain," *Annals of the Rheumatic Diseases* 55, no. 6 (1996): 340–45.

17. C. J. Main and P. J. Watson, "Psychological Aspects of Pain," *Manual Therapy* 4, no. 4 (1999): 203–15.

18. Main and Watson, "Psychological Aspects of Pain."

19. M. S. Hirsch and R. M. Liebert, "The Physical And Psychological Experience of Pain: The Effects of Labeling and Cold Pressor Temperature on Three Pain Measures in College Women," *Pain* 77, no. 1 (1998): 41–48; R. Leaton "Is Emotional Pain or Physical Pain More Painful?" accessed September 9, 2012, http://goarticles.com.

20. "Pain," National Library of Medicine, accessed September 7, 2012, www.nlm.nih.gov/medlineplus/pain.html.

21. J. L. Hallenbeck, "Pain Management: Evaluation of Pain," in *Palliative Care Perspectives* (New York: Oxford University Press, 2003).

2. INTRODUCTION TO THE
NERVOUS SYSTEM

1. E. R. Kandel, J. H. Schwartz, and T. M. Jessel, eds., "Nerve Cells and Behavior," in *Principles of Neural Science* (New York: McGraw-Hill Professional, 2000).

2. "Nervous system," in *Columbia Encyclopedia* (New York: Gale Group, 2000).

3. A. Maton, J. Hopkins, C. McLaughlin, S. Johnson, M. Warner, D. La-Hart, and J. D. Wright, *Human Biology and Health* (Englewood Cliffs, NJ: Prentice Hall, 1993), 132–144.

4. S. Jacobson and E. Marcus, *Neuroanatomy for the Neuroscientist* (New York: Springer, 2008), 147.

5. M. Steriade and R. Llinás, "The Functional States of the Thalamus and the Associated Neuronal Interplay," *Physiological Reviews* 68, no. 3 (1988): 649–742.

6. M. Frank, J. Samanta, A. Moustafa, and S. Sherman, "Hold Your Horses: Impulsivity, Deep Brain Stimulation, and Medication in Parkinsonism," *Science* 318, no. 5854 (2007): 1309–12.

7. J. Godine, W. Chin, and J. Habener, "Alpha Subunit of Rat Pituitary Glycoprotein Hormones: Primary Structure of the Precursor Determined from the Nucleotide Sequence of Cloned cDNAs," *Journal of Biological Chemistry* 257, no. 14 (1982): 8368–71.

8. R. Treister, D. Pud, R. P. Ebstein, E. Laiba, Y. Raz, E. Gershon, M. Haddad, and E. Eisenberg, "Association between Polymorphisms in Serotonin and Dopamine-Related Genes and Endogenous Pain Modulation," *The Journal of Pain* 12, no. 8 (2011): 875–83.

9. U. Wolf, M. J. Rapoport, and T. A. Schweizer, "Evaluating the Affective Component of the Cerebellar Cognitive Affective Syndrome," *Journal of Neuropsychiatry and Clinical Neurosciences* 21, no. 3 (2009): 245–53.

10. E. J. Fine, C. C. Ionita, and L. Lohr, "The History of the Development of the Cerebellar Examination," *Seminars in Neurology* 22, no. 4 (2002): 375–84.

11. C. Y. Saab and W. D. Willis, "Nociceptive Visceral Stimulation Modulates the Activity of Cerebellar Purkinje Cells," *Experimental Brain Research* 140, no. 1 (2001): 122–26; Y. Q. He, Q. Chen, L. Ji, Z. G. Wang, Z. H. Bai, R. L. Stephens Jr., and M. Yang, "PKC gamma Receptor Mediates Visceral Nociception and Hyperalgesia Following Exposure to PTSD-Like Stress in the SPINAL CORD of Rats," *Molecular Pain* 9, no. 1 (2013): 35.

12. A. Siegel and H. N. Sapru, *Essential Neuroscience*, 2nd ed. (Philadelphia: Lippincott Williams & Wilkins, 2010), 190.

13. C. Habas, "Functional Imaging of the Deep Cerebellar Nuclei: A Review," *Cerebellum* 9, no. 1 (2010): 22–28.

14. D. Marr, "A Theory of Cerebellar Cortex," *Journal of Physiology* (London) 202, no. 2 (1969): 437–70.

15. W. T. Liu, Y. Han, H. C. Li, B. Adams, J. H. Zheng, Y. P. Wu, M. Henkemeyer, and X. J. Song, "An In Vivo Mouse Model of Long-Term Potentiation at Synapses between Primary Afferent C-Fibers and Spinal Dorsal Horn Neurons: Essential Role of Ephb1 Receptor," *Molecular Pain* 5 (2009): 29.

16. J. Simpson, D. Wylie, and C. De Zeeuw, "On Climbing Fiber Signals and Their Consequence(s)," *Journal of Behavioral and Brain Science* 19, no. 3 (1996): 384–98.

17. K. L. Davis, R. S. Kahn, G. Ko, and M. Davidson, "Dopamine in schizophrenia: A Review and Reconceptualization," *American Journal of Psychiatry* 148, no. 11 (1991):1474–86; R. Allen, "Dopamine and Iron in the Pathophysiology of Restless Legs Syndrome (RLS)," *Sleep Medicine* 5, no. 4 (2004): 385–91.

18. B. Ford, "Pain in Parkinson's Disease," *Movement Disorders* 25, Suppl. 1 (2010): S98–103; M. Sophie, B. Ford, "Management of Pain in Parkinson's Disease," *CNS Drugs* 26, no. 11 (2012): 937–48.

19. B. C. Jobst, P. D. Williamson, V. M. Thadani, K. L. Gilbert, G. L. Holmes, R. P. Morse, T. M. Darcey, A. C. Duhaime, K. A. Bujarski, and D. W. Roberts, "Intractable Occipital Lobe Epilepsy: Clinical Characteristics and Surgical Treatment," *Epilepsia* 51, no. 11 (2010): 2334–37; I. Taylor, C. Marini, M. R. Johnson, S. Turner, S. F. Berkovic, and I. E. Scheffer, "Juvenile Myoclonic Epilepsy and Idiopathic Photosensitive Occipital Lobe Epilepsy: Is There Overlap?" *Brain* 127, no. 8 (2004): 1878–86; G. B. Young and W. T. Blume, "Painful Epileptic Seizures," *Brain* 106, no 3 (1983): 537–54.

20. "Temporal Lobe," Rice University, accessed January 13, 2013, www.ruf. rice.edu/~lngbrain/cglidden/temporal.html.

21. K. S. Weiner and K. Grill-Spector, "Sparsely-Distributed Organization of Face and Limb Activations in Human Ventral Temporal Cortex," *Neuroimage* 52, no. 4 (2010): 1559–73.

22. J. W. Younger, Y. F. Shen, G. Goddard, and S. C. Mackey, "Chronic Myofascial Temporomandibular Pain Is Associated with Neural Abnormalities in the Trigeminal and Limbic Systems," *Pain* 149, no. 2 (2010): 222–28.

23. A. Maton, J. Hopkins, C. W. McLaughlin, S. Johnson, M. Q. Warner, D. LaHart, and J. D. Wright, *Human Biology and Health* (Englewood Cliffs, NJ: Prentice Hall, 1993), 132–44.

24. J. Krantz, "What Is Sensation and Perception?" in *Experiencing Sensation and Perception* (New York: Pearson Education, 2012).

25. "Cardiovascular system," Dorland's Medical Dictionary, accessed February 12, 2013, www.dorlands.com.

26. J. S. Dasen and M. G. Rosenfeld, "Signaling Mechanisms in Pituitary Morphogenesis and Cell Fate Determination," *Current Opinion in Cell Biology* 11, no. 6 (1999): 669–77.

27. Dasen and Rosenfeld, "Signaling Mechanisms in Pituitary Morphogenesis."

28. "Sensory Reception; Human Vision; Structure and Function of the Human Eye," in *The New Encyclopedia Britannica*, vol. 27 (Chicago: Encyclopedia Britannica Inc., 1987).

3. PHYSIOLOGY OF THE NERVOUS SYSTEM

1. D. Purves, G. J. Augustine, and D. Fitzpatrick, *Neuroscience*, 3rd ed. (Sunderland, MA: Sinauer Associates, Inc., 2004), 241.

2. E. Kandel, J. Schwartz, and T. Jessell, *Principles of the Neural Science* (New York: McGraw-Hill Companies, Inc., 2000), 52.

3. D. Longo, A. Fauci, D. Kasper, S. Hauser, J. Jameson, and J. Loscalzo, *Harrison's Principles of Internal Medicine* (New York: McGraw-Hill Professional, 2008), 111.

4. I. Majkutewicz, D. Myślińska, G. Jerzemowska, K. Plucińska, M. Listowska, B. Grembecka, M. Podlacha, and D. Wrona, "Stress-Induced Differences in the Limbic System Fos Expression Are More Pronounced in Rats Differing in Responsiveness to Novelty Than Social Position," *Brain Research Bulletin* 89, nos. 1–2 (2012): 31–40.

5. P. Rakic, "Specification of the Cerebral Cortical Areas," *Science* 248, no. 4862 (2011):170–76.

6. E. Goldberg, *The Executive Brain: Frontal Lobes and the Civilized Mind* (New York: Oxford University Press, 2001), 86.

7. M. S. Gazzaniga, *The Cognitive Neurosciences* (Cambridge, MA: MIT Press, 2004), 58.

8. L. Sherwood, *Human Physiology: From Cells to Systems* (Belmont, CA: Brooks/Cole, Cengage Learning, 2008), 41.

9. L. J. Elias and D. M. Saucier, *Neuropsychology: Clinical and Experimental Foundations* (Boston: Pearson, 2005), 95.

10. A. Peters, S. L. Palay, and H. deF. Webster, *The Fine Structure of the Nervous System* (New York: Oxford University Press, 1991), 21.

11. M. Sekiguchi, Y. Sekiguchi, S. Konno, H. Kobayashi, Y. Homma, and S. Kikuchi, "Comparison of Neuropathic Pain and Neuronal Apoptosis Following Nerve Root or Spinal Nerve Compression," *European Spine Journal* 18, no. 12, (2009): 1978–85.

4. OCCURRENCE OF PAIN

1. A. V. Apkarian, Y. Sosa, S. Sonty, R. M. Levy, R. N. Harden, T. B. Parrish, and D. R. Gitelman, "Chronic Back Pain Is Associated with Decreased Prefrontal and Thalamic Gray Matter Density," *Journal of Neuroscience* 24 (2004): 10410–15; A. Kuchinad, P. Schweinhardt, D. A. Seminowicz, P. B. Wood, B. A. Chizh, and M. C. Bushnell, "Accelerated Brain Gray Matter Loss in Fibromyalgia Patients: Premature Aging of the Brain?" *Journal of Neurosci-*

ence 27, no. 15 (2007): 4004–7; P. Y. Geha, M. N. Baliki, R. N. Harden, W. R. Bauer, T. B. Parrish, and A. V. Apkarian, "The Brain in Chronic CRPS Pain: Abnormal Gray-White Matter Interactions in Emotional and Autonomic Regions," *Neuron* 60, no. 4 (2008): 570–81; K. D. Davis, G. Pope, J. Chen, C. L. Kwan, A. P. Crawley, and N. E. Diamant, "Cortical Thinning in IBS: Implications for Homeostatic, Attention, and Pain Processing," *Neurology* 70, no. 2 (2008): 153–54; W. Valfrè, I. Rainero, M. Bergui, and L. Pinessi, "Voxel-Based Morphometry Reveals Gray Matter Abnormalities in Migraine," *Headache* 48, no. 1 (2008): 109–17.

2. V. S. Ramachandran, D. Rogers-Ramachandran, and M. Stewart, "Perceptual Correlates of Massive Cortical Reorganization," *Science* 258, no. 5085 (1992): 1159–60.

3. T. Schmidt-Wilcke, E. Leinisch, S. Gänssbauer, B. Draganski, U. Bogdahn, J. Altmeppen, and A. May, "Affective Components and Intensity of Pain Correlate with Structural Differences in Gray Matter in Chronic Back Pain Patients," *Pain* 125, nos. 1–2 (2006): 89–97.

4. C. Freudenrich, "Introduction to How Pain Works" accessed September 21, 2012, http://science.howstuffworks.com.

5. A. V. Apkarian, M. N. Baliki, B. Petre, S. Torbey, K. M. Herrmann, L. Huang, and T. J. Schnitzer, "Corticostriatal Functional Connectivity Predicts Transition to Chronic Back Pain," *Nature Neuroscience* 15, no. 8 (2012): 1117–19.

6. Z. Wiesenfeld-Hallin, "Sex Differences in Pain Perception," *Gender Medicine* 2, no. 3 (2005): 137–45; M. Al'Absi, L. E. Wittmers, D. Ellestad, G. Nordehn, S. W. Kim, C. Kirschbaum, and J. E. Grant, "Sex Differences in Pain and Hypothalamic-Pituitary-Adrenocortical Responses to Opioid Blockade," *Psychosomatic Medicine* 66, no. 2 (2004): 198–206; M. S. Cepeda and D. B. Carr, "Women Experience More Pain and Require More Morphine Than Men to Achieve a Similar Degree of Analgesia," *Anesthesia & Analgesia* 97, no. 5 (2003): 1464–68.

7. A. M. Elliot, B. H. Smith, K. I. Penny, W. C. Smith, and W. A. Chambers, "The Epidemiology of Chronic Pain in the Community," *Lancet* 354, no. 9186 (1999): 1248–52.

8. C. Leboeuf-Yde and K. Kyvik, "At What Age Does Low Back Pain Become a Common Problem?" *Spine* 23, no. 2 (1998): 228–34.

9. K. D. Watson, A. C. Papageorgiou, G. T. Jones, S. Taylor, D. P. Symmons, and A. J. Silman, "Low Back Pain in Schoolchildren: The Role of Mechanical and Psychosocial Factors," *Archives of Disease in Childhood* 88, no. 1 (2003): 12–17.

10. M. L. Taylor, D. R. Trotter, and M. E. Csuka, "The Prevalence of Sexual Abuse in Women with Fibromyalgia," *Arthritis & Rheumatism* 38, no. 2 (1995): 229–34.

11. R. W. Alexander, L. A. Bradley, G. S. Alarcón, M. Triana-Alexander, L. A. Aaron, and K. R. Alberts, "Sexual and Physical Abuse in Women with Fibromyalgia: Association with Outpatient Healthcare Utilization and Pain Medication Usage," *Arthritis Care & Research* 11, no. 2 (1998): 110215.

5. HISTORY OF PAIN

1. "Pain: Hope through Research," National Institutes of Health, updated September 4, 2012, accessed February 12, 2013, www.ninds.nih.gov/disorders/chronic_pain/detail_chronic_pain.htm.

2. "Pain: Hope through Research."

3. "Poena," A Latin Dictionary; Perseus Digital Library, Tufts University, accessed September 7, 2012, www.perseus.tufts.edu/hopper; "Pain," Online Etymology Dictionary, accessed September 8, 2012, www.etymonline.com.

4. C. Sherrington, *The Integrative Action of the Nervous System* (Oxford: Oxford University Press, 1906).

5. Linton, "Models of Pain Perception."

6. Linton, "Models of Pain Perception."

7. M. Lallanilla, "A Brief History of Pain," ABC News, accessed September 15, 2012, http://abcnews.go.com/Health/PainManagement/story?id=731553.

8. M. Booth, *Opium: A History* (London: Simon & Schuster, 1996).

9. S. J. Linton, "Models of Pain Perception," in *Understanding Pain for Better Clinical Practice: A Psychological Perspective* (Philadelphia: Elsevier Health, 2005).

10. F. Salmón, "Pain and Medieval Medicine," The Wellcome Trust, accessed September 19, 2012, www.wellcome.ac.uk/en/pain/microsite/history2.html.

11. Seeger-Weiss, L. L. P., "A Brief History of Pain Relief: From Coal Tar to Tylenol," accessed September 19,2012, http://www.tylenolliverdamages.com/timeline.html.

12. J. J. Bonica, ed., "History of Pain Concepts and Therapies," in *The Management of Pain*, 2nd ed., vol.1 (Philadelphia: Lea & Febiger, 1990).

13. C. Bell, "Idea of a New Anatomy of the Brain; Submitted for the Observation of His Friends," in *The Way In and The Way Out: François Magendie, Charles Bell and the Roots of the Spinal Nerves*, ed. P. F. Cranefield (New York: Futura, 1974).

14. R. Melzack, *The Puzzle of Pain* (New York: Basic Books; 1973), 128.

15. K. M. Dallenbach, "Pain: History and Present Status," *American Journal of Psychology* 52, no. 3 (1939): 331–47.

16. E. M. Todd and A. Kucharski, *"Pain: Historical Perspectives,"* in Z. H. Bajwa and C. A. Warfield, *Principles and Practice of Pain Medicine*, 2nd ed. (New York: McGraw-Hill, 2004).

17. R. Melzack and P. D. Wall, "Pain Mechanisms: A New Theory," *Science* 150, no. 3699 (1965): 971–79.

18. H. Merskey and N. Bogduk, eds., "Pain Terms: A Current List with Definitions and Notes on Usage," in *Classification of Chronic Pain*, 2nd ed. (Seattle, WA: International Association for the Study of Pain [IASP] Press, 1994), 209–14.

19. W. James, *Principles of Psychology* (London: Macmillan, 1892).

20. H. Martineau, *Life in the Sick-Room* (London: Edward Moxon, 1844).

21. L. Bending, "Pain in Victorian England," The Wellcome Trust, accessed September 19, 2012, www.wellcome.ac.uk/en/pain/microsite/history1.html.

22. F. Mancini, M. R. Longo, M. P. Kammers, and P. Haggard, "Visual Distortion of Body Size Modulates Pain Perception," *Psychological Science* 22, no. 3 (2011): 325–30.

23. I. Sample, "Religious Belief Can Help Relieve Pain, Say Researchers," *Guardian Online*, September 30, 2008, accessed December 5, 2013, www.theguardian.com/science/2008/oct/01/medicalresearch.humanbehaviour.

6. DIFFERENT INTERPRETATIONS OF PAIN

1. K. M. Woodrow, G. D. Friedman, A. B. Siegelaub, and M. F. Collen, "Pain Tolerance: Differences According to Age, Sex, and Race," *Psychosomatic Medicine* 34, no. 6 (1972): 548–56.

2. S. Lautenbacher, M. Kunz, P. Strate, J. Nielsen, and L. Arendt-Nielsen, "Age Effects on Pain Thresholds, Temporal Summation and Spatial Summation of Heat and Pressure Pain," *Pain* 115, no. 3 (2005): 410–18.

3. A. B. Krueger and A. A. Stone, "Assessment of Pain: A Community-Based Diary Survey in the USA," *The Lancet* 371, no. 9623 (2008): 1519–525.

4. K. Kingsbury, "Millions of Americans in Chronic Pain," *Time* online, May 2, 2008, accessed March 12, 2013, http://content.time.com/time/health/article/0,8599,1737255,00.html.

5. T. E. Dorner, J. Muckenhuber, W. J. Stronegger, E. Rasky, B. Gustorff, and W. Freidl, "The Impact of Socio-Economic Status on Pain and the Perception of Disability Due to Pain," *European Journal of Pain* 15, no. 1 (2011): 103–9.

6. M. Osterweis, A. Kleinman and D. Mechanic, eds., *Pain and Disability: Clinical, Behavioral, and Public Policy Perspectives* (Washington, DC: National Academy Press, 1987), 146–64.

7. S. Nayak, S. C. Shiflett, S. Eshun, and F. M. Levine, "Culture and Gender Effects in Pain Beliefs and the Prediction of Pain Tolerance," *Cross-Cultural Research* 34, no. 2 (2000): 135–51.

8. G-A. Galanti, *Caring for Patients from Different Cultures* (Philadelphia: University of Pennsylvania Press, 2004), 41–42.

9. Galanti, *Caring for Patients from Different Cultures*, 44–45.

10. S. Nayak, et al., "Culture and Gender Effects."

11. P. McGrath, "Children's Pain Perception: Impact of Gender and Age" (paper presented at the National Institute of Health's conference on Gender and Pain, Bethesda, Maryland, April 7–8 1998).

12. McGrath, "Children's Pain Perception."

13. J. L. Riley III, M. E. Robinson, E. A. Wise, and D. Price, "A Meta-Analytic Review of Pain Perception across the Menstrual Cycle," *Pain* 81, no. 3 (1999): 225–35.

14. T. W. Victor, X. Hu, J. C. Campbell, D. C. Buse, and R. B. Lipton, "Migraine Prevalence by Age and Sex in the United States," *Cephalalgia* 30, no. 9 (2010): 1065–72.

15. L. J. Staton, M. Panda, I. Chen, I. Genao, J. Kurz, M. Pasanen, A. J. Mechaber, M. Menon, J. O'Rorke, J. Wood, E. Rosenberg, C. Faeslis, T. Carey, D. Calleson, and S. Cykert, "When Race Matters: Disagreement in Pain Perception between Patients and Their Physicians in Primary Care," *Journal of The National Medical Association* 99, no. 5 (2007): 532–38.

7. THE CHANGING CULTURE OF PAIN

1. H. J. Gould III, *Understanding Pain: What It Is, Why It Happens, and How It's Managed* (New York: Demos Medical Publishing, 2007), 1–24.

2. Gallup Organization, *Pain in America: A Research Report* (Washington, DC: Ogilvy Public Relations, 2000).

3. K. Weiner, *Pain Issues: Pain Is an Epidemic* (Sonora, CA: American Academy of Pain Management, 2001).

4. C. P. Kottak, "What Is Culture?" in *Anthropology: The Exploration of Human Diversity* (New York: McGraw Hill, 2000), 61.

5. Kottak, "What Is Culture?," 61.

6. Kottak, "What Is Culture?," 62; E. A. Hoebel, *The Law of Primitive Man: A Study in Comparative Legal Dynamics* (Cambridge, MA: Harvard University Press, 1954).

7. L. A. White, *The Evolution of Culture: The Development of Civilization to the Fall of Rome* (New York: McGraw Hill, 1959), 3.

8. Kottak, "What Is Culture?," 67–68.

9. D. O'Neil, "Processes of Change," March 13, 2013, http://anthro.palomar.edu/change/change_2.htm.

10. Kottak, "What Is Culture?," 61.

11. D. L. Sam and J. W. Berry, "Acculturation: When Individuals and Groups of Different Cultural Backgrounds Meet," *Sage Journals* 5, no. 4 (2010): 472.

12. S. Silver, "Book review: *The Culture of Pain* by David B. Morris," *American Journal of Hospice and Palliative Care* 9, no. 1 (1992): 2.

13. D. B. Morris, *The Culture of Pain* (Berkeley: University of California Press, 1991), 77.

14. Morris, *The Culture of Pain*, 61.

15. B. Sattler, "A Time for Learning and for Counting—Egyptians, Greeks and Empirical Processes in Plato's *Timaeus*," in *One Book, the Whole Universe: Plato's "Timaeus" Today* (Las Vegas, NV: Parmenides Press, 2010), 249–66.

16. Silver, "Book Review: *The Culture of Pain*," 2.

17. Silver, "Book Review: *The Culture of Pain*," 2.

18. Morris, *The Culture of Pain*, 61.

19. Morris, *The Culture of Pain*, 61.

20. D. B. Morris, *The Culture of Pain* (Berkeley: University of California Press, 1991), 78.

21. "Laws, Regulations, Policies and Procedures for Drug Applications," Food and Drug Administration, August 31, 2010, accessed March 2, 2013, www.fda.gov/Drugs/DevelopmentApprovalProcess/ucm090410.htm.

22. "Safe Use Initiative: Collaborating to Reduce Preventable Harm from Medications," Food and Drug Administration, accessed March 3, 2013, www.fda.gov/Drugs/DrugSafety/SafeUseInitiative/.

23. "Development and Approval Process (Drugs)," Food and Drug Administration, October 27, 2009, accessed March 3, 2013, www.fda.gov/Drugs/DevelopmentApprovalProcess/.

24. "Sales of Painkillers—Help for Retailers" (Press Release), Medicines and Healthcare Products Regulatory Agency, December 10, 2009, accessed March 5, 2013, www.mhra.gov.uk/NewsCentre/Pressreleases/CON065559.

25. "Who makes the decisions?," Medicines and Healthcare products Regulatory Agency, February 7, 2008, accessed March 5, 2013, www.mhra.gov.uk/Howweregulate/Whomakesthedecisions/index.htm.

26. M. Webster, "Millions of Americans in Pain without Meds," January 12, 2010, accessed March 6, 2013,www.livescience.com/6028-millions-americans-pain-meds.html; "Doctors Hesitate to Prescribe Painkillers for Fear of Abuse," Addiction Treatment Programs, 2012, accessed March 6, 2013, www.addiction-treatment-programs.net.

27. K. Hahn, "Chronic Pain Management," *The Rx Consultant* 18, no. 11 (2009): 1–7; K. Hahn and Y. Colon, "The Roles of Pharmacists in Pain Management," *Journal of Pain and Palliative Care Pharmacotherapy* 23, no. 4 (2009): 414–15.

28. W. J. Guglielmo, "Treating Pain: Can Doctors Put Their Fears to Rest?," *Medical Economics* 4 (2000): 46.

29. D. Garets and M. Davis, *Electronic Patient Records: EMRs and EHRs* (New York: McGraw Hill, 2005), 2–3.

30. A. Haupt, "The Era of Electronic Medical Records: EMRs May Be Finally Coming to a Hospital or Doctor Near You," *US News & World Report*, July 18, 2011, accessed March 5, 2013, www.health.usnews.com.

31. M. F. Furukawa, "Electronic Medical Records and Efficiency and Productivity during Office Visits," *American Journal of Managed Care* 17, no. 4 (2011): 296–303.

32. "Electronic Medical Records," Open Clinical, September 2, 2005, accessed March 3, 2013, www.openclinical.org/emr.html.

33. M. W. Smith, "Chronic Pain: New Research, New Treatments," WebMD, accessed March 4, 2013, www.webmd.com/pain-management/features/chronic-pain-new-research-new-treatments.

8. PATHOLOGY OF PAIN

1. M. A. Allen, *Mosby's Pocket Dictionary of Medicine, Nursing and Allied Health* 4th ed. (Singapore: Elsevier, 2002), 949.

2. C. M. Porth, *Pathophysiology: Concepts of Altered Health States* 6th ed. (Philadelphia: Lippincott Williams & Wilkins, 2002), 13.

3. S. Robbins, *Robbins and Cotran Pathologic Basis of Disease* 8th ed. (Philadelphia: Saunders/Elsevier, 2010), 3121–25.

4. Porth, *Pathophysiology*, 13.

5. Porth, *Pathophysiology*, 14.

6. E. Long, *History of Pathology* (New York: Dove, 1965).

7. "Anatomical Pathology," The Royal College of Pathologists of Australia, accessed December 23, 2012, www.rcpa.edu.au/Pathology-Careers/What-is-Pathology.

8. "Chemical Pathology," The Royal College of Pathologists of Australia, accessed December 23, 2012, www.rcpa.edu.au/Pathology-Careers/What-is-Pathology.

9. "Clinical Pathology," The Royal College of Pathologists of Australia, accessed December 23, 2012, www.rcpa.edu.au/Pathology-Careers/What-is-Pathology.

10. "Forensic Pathology," The Royal College of Pathologists of Australia, accessed December 23, 2012, www.rcpa.edu.au/Pathology-Careers/What-is-Pathology.

11. "Genetic Pathology," The Royal College of Pathologists of Australia, accessed December 23, 2012, www.rcpa.edu.au/Pathology-Careers/What-is-Pathology.

12. "Haematology," The Royal College of Pathologists of Australia, accessed December 23, 2012, www.rcpa.edu.au/Pathology-Careers/What-is-Pathology.

13. "Immunopathology," The Royal College of Pathologists of Australia, accessed December 23, 2012, www.rcpa.edu.au/Pathology-Careers/What-is-Pathology.

14. "Microbiology," The Royal College of Pathologists of Australia, accessed December 23, 2012, www.rcpa.edu.au/Pathology-Careers/What-is-Pathology.

15. D. M. Anderson, *Mosby's Medical, Nursing and Allied Health Dictionary* 6th ed. (St. Louis, MO: Mosby, 2002), 1046.

16. C. M. Porth, *Pathophysiology: Concepts of Altered Health States* 6th ed. (Philadelphia: Lippincott Williams & Wilkins, 2002), 1043-1044.

17. H. Shryock, *Modern Medical Guide* (Nampa, I.D.: Pacific Press Publishing, 1990), 546-571.

18. Porth, *Pathophysiology*, 1183–87.

19. M. E. Doenges, M. F. Moorhouse, and A. C. Geissler-Murr, *Nursing Care Plans: Guidelines for Individualizing Patient Care* 6th ed. (Philadelphia: F. A. Davis Company, 2002), 198–99.

20. Porth, *Pathophysiology*, 1138–39.

21. Porth, *Pathophysiology*, 1155.

22. Doenges, Moorhouse, and Geissler-Murr, *Nursing Care Plans*, 199–200.

23. H. Shryock, *Modern Medical Guide* (Nampa, ID: Pacific Press Publishing, 1990), 565–71.

24. Shryock, *Modern Medical Guide*, 546–71.

25. Porth, *Pathophysiology*, 1208–12.

26. R. Billington and B. H. McCarberg, "Consequences of Neuropathic Pain: Quality of Life Issues and Associated Costs," *American Journal of Managed Care* 12, Suppl. 9 (2006): 263–68.

27. "Molecule," *Encyclopedia Britannica*, online, accessed December 23, 2012, www.britannica.com/EBchecked/topic/388236/molecule.

28. C. J. Woolf and M. W. Salter, "Neuronal Plasticity: Increasing the Gain in Pain," *Science* 288, no. 5472 (2000): 1765–69.

29. M. Zhuo and P. Li, "Silent Glutamergic Synapses and Nociception in Mammalian Spinal Cord," *Nature* 393, no. 6686 (1998): 695–98.

30. P. Li, G. A. Kerchner, C. Sala, F. Wei, J. E. Huettner, M. Sheng, and M. Zhuo, "AMPA Receptor-PDZ Interactions in Facilitation of Spinal Sensory Synapses," *Nature Neuroscience* 2, no. 11 (1999): 972–77.

31. A. V. Apkarian, M. C. Bushnell, R. D. Treede, and J. K. Zubieta, "Human brain mechanisms of pain perception and regulation in health and diseases," *European Journal of Pain* 9, no. 4 (2005): 463-48.

32. K. L. Casey, "Forebrain mechanisms of nociception and pain: Analysis through imaging," *Proceedings of the National Academy of Sciences USA* 96, no. 14 (1999): 7668–74.

33. A. A. Calejesan, S. J. Kim, and M. Zhuo, "Descending Facilitatory Modulation of a Behavioral Nociceptive Response by Stimulation in the Adult Rat Anterior Cingulated Cortex," *European Journal of Pain* 4, no. 1 (2000), 83–96; F. Wei, C. S. Qiu, S. J. Kim, L. Muglia, J. W. Maas, V. V. Pineda, H. M. Xu, Z. F. Chen, D. R. Storm, and L. J. Muglia, "Genetic Elimination of Behavioral Sensitization in Mice Lacking Calmodulin-Stiumalted Adenylyl Cyclases," *Neuron* 36, no. 4 (2002): 713–26; F. Wei, G. D. Wang, G. A. Kerchner, S. J. Kim, H. M. Xu, Z. F. Chen, and M. Zhuo, "Genetic Enhancement of Inflammatory Pain by Forebrain NR2B Overexpression," *Nature Neuroscience* 4, no. 2 (2001): 164–69.

34. K. R. Gogas, "Glutamate-based therapeutic approaches: NR2B receptor antagonists," *Current Opinion in Pharmacology* 6, no. 1 (2006), 68-74.

35. D. M. Anderson, *Mosby's Medical, Nursing and Allied Health Dictionary* 6th ed. (St. Louis, MO: A Harcourt Health Sciences Company, 2002), 313.

36. R. Melzack and K. L. Casey, *Sensory, Motivational, and Central Control Determinants of Pain* (Springfield, IL: Charles C. Thomas, 1968), 423–29.

37. W. D. Willis, "The Somatosensory System, with Emphasis on Structure Important for Pain," *Brain Research Reviews* 55, no. 2 (2007): 297–313.

38. C. Stein, J. D. Clark, U. Oh, M. R. Vasko, G. L. Wilcox, A. C. Overland, T. W. Vanderah, and R. H. Spencer, "Peripheral Mechanism of Pain and Analgesia," *Brain Research Reviews* 60, no. 1 (2009): 90–113.

39. M. F. Jarvis and J. M. Boyce-Rustay, "Neuropathic Pain: Models and Mechanisms," *Current Pharmaceutical Design* 15, no. 15 (2009): 1711–16.

40. E. D. Milligan and L. R. Watkins, "Pathological and Protective Roles of Glia in Chronic Pain," *Nature Reviews Neuroscience* 10, no. 1 (2009): 23–36.

41. N. Swaminathan, "Glia—the Other Brain Cells," *Discover* (January–February 2011), 1.

42. J. Mika, M. Osikowicz, E. Rojewska, M. Korostynski, A. Wawrzczak-Bargiela, R. Przewlocki, and B. Przewlocka, "Differential Activation of Spinal Microglial and Astroglial Cells in a Mouse Model of Peripheral Neuropathic Pain," *European Journal of Pharmacology* 623, nos. 1–3 (2009): 65–72.

43. W. J. Streit, R. E. Mrak, and W. S. Grifffin, "Microglia and Neuroinflammation: A Pathological Perspective," *Journal of Neuroinflammation* 1, no. 1 (2004): 14.

44. L. J. Wu, K. I. Vadakkan, and M. Zhuo: "ATP-Induced Chemotaxis of Microglial Processes Requires P2Y Receptor-Activated Initiation of Outward Potassium Current," *Glia* 55, no. 8 (2007): 810–21.

45. F. Scarano-Gonzalez and G. Baltuch, "Microglia as Mediators of Inflammatory Degenerative Diseases," *Annual Review of Neuroscience* 22, no. 2 (1999): 219–40.

46. M. Tsuda, K. Inoue, and M. W. Salter, "Neuropathic Pain and Spinal Microglia: A Big Problem from Molecules in Small Glia," *Trends in Neurosciences* 28, no. 2 (2005): 101–7.

47. A. J. Bruce-Keller, "Microglial-Neuronal Interactions in Synaptic Damage and Recovery," *Journal of Neuroscience Research* 58, no. 1 (1999): 191–201.

48. Tsuda, Inoue, and Salter, "Neuropathic Pain and Spinal Microglia."

49. U. Bingel and I . Tracey, "Imaging CNS modulation of pain in humans," *Physiology* 23 (2008): 371–80.

9. DIAGNOSTICS OF PAIN

1. G. A. Walco and K. R. Goldschneider, *Pain in Children: A Practical Guide for Primary Care* (Chicago: Springer, 2008).

2. F. Cole, *Overcoming Chronic Pain: A Self-Help Guide Using Cognitive Behavioral Techniques* (New York: Constable & Robinson, 2005).

3. B. E. Thorn, *Cognitive Therapy for Chronic Pain: A Step-by-Step Guide* (New York: Guilford Press, 2004).

4. J. Schneider, *Living with Chronic Pain: The Complete Health Guide to the Causes and Treatment of Chronic Pain*, 2nd ed. (Chicago: Hatherleigh Press, 2009).

5. S. Kassan, C. J. Vierck, Jr., and E.Vierck, *Chronic Pain for Dummies* (New York: John Wiley & Sons, 2011).

6. Schneider, *Living with Chronic Pain.*

7. J. M. Mennell, *The Musculoskeletal System: Differential Diagnosis from Symptoms and Physical Signs* (New York: Jones & Bartlett Learning, 1992).

8. J. G. Samuels, *Management Documentation: The Effects of the Perception of the Practice Environment and Clinical Expertise* (New York: ProQuest, 2007).

9. Mennell, *The Musculoskeletal System*.

10. Thorn, *Cognitive Therapy for Chronic Pain*.

11. Cole, *Overcoming Chronic Pain*.

12. Schneider, *Living with Chronic Pain*.

13. Samuels, *Management Documentation*.

14. Mennell, *The Musculoskeletal System*.

15. Thorn, *Cognitive Therapy for Chronic Pain*.

16. "Assessing Pain—Tips on Recognizing and Assessing Pain," About.com, accessed September 12, 2012, http://dying.about.com/od/assessingpain/a/painassessment.htm.

17. M. K. Kazanowski and M. S.Laccetti, *Pain* (Thorofare NJ: Slack, Inc., 2002).

18. Cole, *Overcoming Chronic Pain*.

19. Samuels, *Management Documentation*.

20. P. D. Larsen and I. M. Lubkin, "Chronic Pain," in *Chronic Illness: Impact And Interventions* (London: Jones & Bartlett Learning, 2006), 68–100.

21. Larsen and Lubkin, "Chronic Pain."

22. Cole, *Overcoming Chronic Pain*.

23. A. Rosenfeld, *The Truth about Chronic Pain: Patients and Professionals on How to Face It, Understand It, Overcome It* (New York: Basic Books, 2004).

24. Mennell, *The Musculoskeletal System*.

25. Mennell, *The Musculoskeletal System*.

26. Larsen and Lubkin, "Chronic Pain."

27. Samuels, *Management Documentation*.

28. Mennell, *The Musculoskeletal System*.

29. Schneider, *Living with Chronic Pain*.

30. Mennell, *The Musculoskeletal System*.

31. Mennell, *The Musculoskeletal System*.

32. Mennell, *The Musculoskeletal System*.

10. CAUSES OF PAIN

1. D. Pincus, "What Causes Pain," *The Chaotic Life* (blog), *Psychology Today*, accessed December 21, 2012, www.psychologytoday.com/blog/the-chaotic-life.

2. R. Ohrbach and W. D. McCall, "The stress-hyperactivity-pain theory of myogenic pain: Proposal for a revised theory," *The Journal of Pain* 5, no. 1 (1996): 51–66.

3. R. K. Portenoy, "Overview of Pain," Merck Manuals online, updated April 2007, accessed December 22, 2012, www.merckmanuals.com/home/brain_spinal_cord_and_nerve_disorders/pain/evaluation_of_pain.html.

4. L. Herzberg, "Problems of Immobility and Pain." *British Medical Journal* 281, no. 6233 (1980): 125.

5. S. J. Shettleworth, *Cognition, Evolution and Behavior* 2nd ed. (New York: Oxford, 2010).

6. K. A. Trujillo, H. Akil, "Inhibition of Morphine Tolerance and Dependence by the NMDA Receptor Antagonist MK-801," *Science* 251 (1991): 85–87.

7. L. R. Gardell, R. Wang, S. E. Burgess, M. H. Ossipov, T. W. Vanderah, T. P. Malan Jr., J. Lai, and F. Porreca, "Sustained Morphine Exposure Induces a spinal Dynorphin-Dependent Enhancement of Excitatory Transmitter Release from Primary Afferent Fibers," *Journal of Neuroscience* 22, no. 15 (2002): 6747–55.

8. J. Mao, "Opioid-Induced Abnormal Pain Sensitivity: Implications in Clinical Opioid Therapy," *Pain* 100, no. 3 (2002): 213–17.

9. M. J. Baron and P. W. McDonald, "Significant Pain Reduction in Chronic Pain Patients after Detoxification from High Dose Opioids," *Journal of Opioid Management* 2, no. 5 (2006): 277–82.

10. P. Compton, V. C. Charuvastra, and W. Ling, "Pain Intolerance in Opioid-Maintained Former Opiate Addicts: Effect of Long-Acting Maintenance Agent," *Drug and Alcohol Dependence*, 63, no. 2 (2001): 139–46.

11. "Understanding and Dealing with Stress," Mountain State Centers for Independent Living, accessed December 31, 2012, www.mtstcil.org/skills/stress-deal.html.

12. "Natural Stress Management and Alternative Medicine Stress Relief: Pain Doctors, Healers, Treatments and Therapies," Commando Communications, accessed December 31, 2012, www.painreliefprofessionals.com/stress.htm.

13. "Understanding and Dealing with Stress."

14. L. A. Cohen, A. J. Bonito, D. R. Akin, R. J. Manski, M. D. Macek, R. R. Edwards, and L. J. Cornelius, "Toothache Pain: Behavioral Impact and Self-Care Strategies," *Special Care in Dentistry* 29, no. 2 (2009): 85–95.

15. S. Cohen, D. Janicki-Deverts, W. J. Doyle, G. E. Miller, E. Frank, B. S. Rabin, and R. B. Turner, "Chronic Stress, Glucocorticoid Receptor Resistance, Inflammation, and Disease Risk," *Proceedings of the National Academy of Science U. S. A.* 109, no. 16 (2012): 5995–99.

16. Cohen et al., "Chronic Stress, Glucocorticoid Receptor Resistance."

17. R. Fink and R. Gates, "Pain Assessment," Textbook of Palliative Nursing 2nd ed. (New York: Oxford University Press, 2006), 53–75.

18. L. Burhansstipanov and W. Hollow, "Native American Cultural Aspects of Oncology Nursing Care," Seminars in Oncology Nursing 17, no. 3 (2001): 206–19.

19. K. E. Lasch, "Culture and Pain," *Pain Clinical Updates* 10, no. 5 (2002): 1–9.

20. Lasch, "Culture and Pain."

21. Lasch, "Culture and Pain."

22. D. J. Burgess, S. S. Fu, and M. Ryn, "Why Do Providers Contribute to Disparities and What Can Be Done about It?" *Journal of General Internal Medicine* 19, no. 11 (2004) : 1154–59.

23. Burgess, Fu, and Ryn, "Why Do Providers Contribute to Disparities?"

24. "Sleep, Stress and Environmental Factors," reviewed November 2012, accessed December 18, 2012, www.healthtalkonline.org/Bones_joints/Chronic_Pain/Topic/1618.

25. "Muscle Pain Relief—Environmental Factors," accessed December 31, 2012, www.sorewinners.com/muscle-pain.html.

26. D. Pud, Y. Golan, and R. Pesta, "Hand dominancy—a Feature Affecting Sensitivity to Pain," *Neuroscience Letters* 467, no. 3 (2009): 237–40.

27. W. Knight, "Redheads Suffer More Pain," *New Scientist* online, October 15, 2002, accessed March 31, 2013, www.newscientist.com/article/dn2923-red-heads-suffer-more-pain.html#.VFd8Y_nF98E.

28. T. Foulkes and J. N. Wood, "Pain Genes," *PLOS Genetics* 4, no. 7 (2008): e1000086; American Pain Society, "Biological, Psychological and Social Factors Influence Individual Pain Differences," News Wise, accessed December 29, 2012, www.newswise.com/articles/biological-psychological-and-social-factors-influence-individual-pain-differences.

29. Z. Wiesenfeld-Hallin, "Sex Differences in Pain Perception," *Gender Medicine* 2, no. 3 (2005): 137–45; M. Al'Absi, L. E. Wittmers, D. Ellestad, G. Nordehn, S. W. Kim, C. Kirschbaum, and J. E. Grant, "Sex Differences in Pain and Hypothalamic-Pituitary-Adrenocortical Responses to Opioid Blockade," *Psychosomatic Medicine* 66, no. 2 (2004): 198–206; M. S. Cepeda and D. B. Carr, "Women Experience More Pain and Require More Morphine Than Men to Achieve a Similar Degree of Analgesia," *Anesthesia & Analgesia* 97, no. 5 (2003): 1464–68.

11. DAMAGING EFFECTS

1. Institute of Medicine, *Relieving Pain in America: A Blueprint for Transforming Prevention, Care, Education, and Research.* (Washington, DC: The National Academies Press, 2011).

2. European Federation of IASP, *The Societal Impact of Pain—a Road Map for Action* (Brussels: European Federation of the International Association for the Study of Pain Chapters [EFIC], 2011).

3. K. A. Holroyd, "Assessment and Psychological Management of Recurrent Headache Disorders," *Journal of Consulting and Clinical Psychology* 70, no. 3 (2002): 656–77; H. F. Boardman, E. Thomas, D. S. Millson, and P. R. Croft, "Psychological, Sleep, Lifestyle, and Comorbid Associations with Headache," *Headache* 45, no. 6 (2005): 657–69; J. M. Nash and R. W. Thebarge, "Understanding Psychological Stress, Its Biological Processes, and Impact on Primary Headache," *Headache* 46, no. 9 (2006): 1377–86.

4. M. Gornitsky, A. M. Velly, and P. Philippe, "Contributing Factors to Chronic Myofascial Pain: A Case-Control Study," *Pain* 104, no. 3 (2003): 491–99.

5. M. A. Dawn, *Chronic Pain: A Primary Care Guide to Practical Management* (New Jersey: Humana Press, 2005).

6. S. Freud, *Three Essays on the Theory of Sexuality* (New York: Basic Books, 2000).

7. F. Malti-Douglas, ed., *Encyclopedia of Sex and Gender*, vol. 1 (Woodbridge, CT: Macmillan Reference USA, 2007).

8. A. Comfort, *The Joy of the Sex* (New York: Pocket Books, 1972).

9. K. M. Robinson, "10 Surprising Health Benefits of Sex," accessed January 2, 2013, www.webmd.com/sex-relationships/guide/sex-and-health.

10. R. A. Posner, *Sex and Reason* (Cambridge, MA: Harvard University Press, 1998).

11. J. S. Alter, "Seminal Truth: A Modern Science of Male Celibacy in North India," *Medical Anthropology Quarterly* 11, no. 3 (1997).

12. A. Schlegel, "The Chaste Adolescent," in *Celibacy, Culture, and Society: The Anthropology of Sexual Abstinence* (Madison: University of Wisconsin Press, 2001).

13. G. E. Simon, O. Gureje, and M. Von Korff, "A Cross-National Study of the Course of Persistent Pain in Primary Care," *Pain* 92, nos. 1–2 (2001): 195–200.

14. M. A. Dawn, *Chronic Pain: A Primary Care Guide to Practical Management* (New Jersey: Humana Press, 2005).

15. Institute of Medicine, *Relieving Pain in America: A Blueprint for Transforming Prevention, Care, Education, and Research* (Washington, DC: The National Academies Press, 2011).

16. A. D. Lopez and C. J. Murray, "Alternate Projections of Mortality and Disability by Cause 1990–2020: Global Burden of Disease Study," *Lancet* 349, no. 9064 (1997): 1498–504; S. Moussavi, S. Chatterji, E. Verdes, A. Tandon, V. Patel, and B. Ustun, "Depression, Chronic Diseases, and Decrements in Health: Results from the World Health Survey," Lancet 370, no. 9590 (2007): 851–58.

17. R. O'Connor, *Undoing Depression: What Therapy Doesn't Teach You and Medication Can't Give You* (New York: Berkeley Books, 1999).

18. "Depression Is a Common Illness and People Suffering from Depression Need Support and Treatment," World Health Organization, October 9, 2012, accessed Janurary 3, 2013, www.who.int/mediacentre/news/notes/2012/mental_health_day_20121009/en/.

19. B. S. Gillum and B. L. Hudson, "Advance Report of Final Mortality Statistics, 1990," *Month Vital Statisctics Reports* 41, no. 7 (1993): 1–52.

20. L. M. Prager, "Depression and Suicide in Children and Adolescents," *Pediatrics in Review* 30, no. 6 (2009): 199–205; M. Afifi, "Depression, Aggression and Suicide Ideation among Adolescents in Alexandria," *Neurosciences* 9, no. 3 (2004): 207–13.

21. R. F. Howard, "Current Status of Pain Management in Children," *Journal of the American Medical Association* 290, no. 18 (2003).

22. J. F. Greden, ed., *Treatment of Recurrent Depression* (Washington, DC: American Psychiatric Publishing, Inc., 2001).

23. B. S. Gillum and B. L. Hudson, "Advance Report of Final Mortality Statistics, 1990," *Month Vital Statisctics Reports* 41, no. 7 (1993): 1–52.

24. Malti-Douglas, *Encyclopedia of Sex and Gender*.

25. B. Major and J. Crocker, "Social Stigma and Self-Esteem: The Self-Protective Properties of Stigma," *Psychological Review* 96, no. 4 (1989): 608–30.

26. K. Yoshimasu, T. Kondo, S. Tokunaga, Y. Kanemitsu, H. Sugahara, M. Akamine, K. Fujisawa, K. Miyashita, and C. Kubo, "Mental and Somatic Symptoms Related to Suicidal Ideation in Patients Visiting a Psychosomatic Clinic in Japan," *International Journal of General Medicine* 2 (2009): 163–70.

27. M. Fuchikami, S. Morinobu, M. Segawa, Y. Okamoto, S. Yamawaki, N. Ozaki, T. Inoue, I. Kusumi, T. Koyama, K. Tsuchiyama, and T. Terao, "DNA Methylation Profiles of the Brain-Derived Neurotrophic Factor (BDNF) Gene as a Potent Diagnostic Biomarker in Major Depression," *Public Library of Science (PLOS) One* 6, no. 8 (2011): e23881.

28. Fuchikami, et al., "DNA Methylation Profiles."

29. Institute of Medicine, *Relieving Pain in America*.

30. "Depression Is a Common Illness."

31. G. Simon, P. S. Wang, and R. C. Kessler, "The Economic Burden of Depression and the Cost-Effectiveness of Treatment," *International Journal of Methods in Psychiatric Research* 12, no. 1 (2003): 22–33.

32. Institute of Medicine, *Relieving Pain in America*.

33. P. E. Greenberg, R. C. Kessler, H. G. Birnbaum, S. A. Leong; S. W. Lowe, P. A. Berglund, and P. K. Corey-Lisle, "The Economic Burden of Depression in the United States: How Did It Change between 1990 and 2000?," *Journal of Clinical Psychiatry* 64, no. 12 (2003): 1465–75.

34. J. P. Smith and G. C. Smith, "Long-Term Economic Costs of Psychological Problems during Childhood," *Social Science & Medicine* 71, no. 1 (2010): 110–15.

35. S. Morris and C. M. Thomas, "Cost of Depression among Adults in England in 2000," *British Journal of Psychiatry* 183 (2003): 514–19.

36. R. L. Leahy, "The Cost of Depression," *Huffington Post*, October 30, 2012, accessed January 5, 2013, www.huffingtonpost.com/robert-leahy-phd/the-cost-of-depression_b_770805.html.

37. "Suicides Cost Japan Economy $32BN," *BBC News* online, September 7, 2010, accessed August 12, 2013, www.bbc.com/news/world-asia-pacific-11219492.

38. "Suicides Cost Japan Economy $32BN."

12. ROLE OF INTERNISTS AND FAMILY PRACTICE PHYSICIANS

1. D. Wujastyk, ed., *The Roots of Ayurveda* (New York: Penguin, 2003).

2. "About Internal Medicine," American College of Physicians, accessed September 15, 2012, www.acponline.org/patients_families/about_internal_medicine/.

3. American Board of Internal Medicine, "About ABIM," accessed September 14, 2012, www.abim.org/about/.

4. T. S. Huddle, R. Centor, and G. R. Heudebert, "American Internal Medicine in the 21st Century," *Journal of General Internal Medicine* 18, no. 9 (2003): 764–67.

5. L. Pinheiro, "Right-Siting of Medical Care: Role of the Internist," *Annals of the Academy of Medicine, Singapore* 38, no. 2 (2009): 163–65; J. W. Burnside, "What the General Internist Does." *Archives of Internal Medicine* 137, nos. 1286–88 (1977).

6. "Adolescent Medicine," American College of Physicians, accessed September 29, 2012,www.acponline.org/patients_families/about_internal_medicine/subspecialties/adolescent_medicine/.

7. S. Husby and A. Hoost, "Recurrent Abdominal Pain, Food Allergy and Endoscopy," *Acta Paediatrica* 90, no. 1 (2001): 3–4; B. Regland, O. Zachrisson, V. Stejskal, and C. Gerhard Gottfries, "Nickel Allergy Is Found in a Majority of Women with Chronic Fatigue Syndrome and Muscle Pain—and May Be Triggered by Cigarette Smoke and Dietary Nickel Intake," *Journal of Chronic Fatigue Syndrome* 8, no. 1 (2001): 57–65.

8. "What Is Allergy and Immunology?," E.N.T. & Allergy Health Services, accessed September 29, 2012, www.entallergyhealth.com/index.php?option=com_content&view=article&id=9&Itemid=12.

9. A. Mandal, "What Is Cardiology?," *News Medical*, accessed September 29, 2012, www.news-medical.net/health/Cardiology-What-is-Cardiology.aspx.

10. C. Nordqvist, "What Is Cardiology?" *Medical News Today*, August 13, 2012, accessed September 26, 2012, www.medicalnewstoday.com/articles/248935.php.

11. "What Is an Endocrinologist?" Hormone Health Network, accessed September 24, 2012, www.hormone.org/contact-a-health-professional/what-is-an-endocrinologist.

12. "About Gastroenterology," American Gastroenterological Association, accessed September 23, 2012, www.gastro.org/patient-center/about-gastroenterology.

13. J. P. Mathews, "What Is Geriatrics?" Summit Medical Group, November 8, 2011, accessed September 29, 2012, www.summitmedicalgroup.com/article/What-is-Geriatrics/.

14. "Hematologist," *The Free Dictionary*, accessed September 24, 2012, www.medical-dictionary.thefreedictionary.com/hematologist.

15. "Defining the American Hematologist," American Society of Hematology, accessed September 29, 2012, http://www.hematology.org.

16. "Infectious Diseases," World Health Organization, accessed September 29, 2012, www.who.int/topics/infectious_diseases/en/.

17. "Infectious Disease," American College of Physicians, accessed September 28, 2012, www.acponline.org/patients_families/about_internal_medicine/subspecialties/infectious_disease/.

18. "Types of Oncologists," American Society of Clinical Oncology (ASCO), accessed September 29, 2012, www.cancer.net/navigating-cancer-care/cancer-basics/cancer-care-team/types-oncologists.

19. "What Is a Pulmonary Specialist?" *Health Communities Online*, accessed September 26, 2012, www.healthcommunities.com/copd/what-is-pulmonary-specialist.shtml.

20. "What is a Rheumatologist?" American College of Rheumatology, accessed September 26, 2012, www.rheumatology.org/Practice/Clinical/Patients/What_is_a_Rheumatologist_/.

21. M. L. Gross, "What is Sports Medicine?" *MedHelp Online*, January 31, 2011, accessed September 26, 2012, www.medhelp.org/user_journals/show/264908/What-is-Sports-Medicine-Five-questions.

22. "Choosing a Primary Care Provider," National Library of Medicine, accessed September 26, 2012, www.nlm.nih.gov/medlineplus/ency/article/001939.htm.

13. ROLE OF PHYSICAL MEDICINE AND REHAB IN PAIN CARE

1. R. Kennedy, "Physical Medicine and Rehabilitation (PM&R) (Physiatry)," Medical-Library.net, accessed September 19, 2012, www.medical-library.net/content/view/1181/41/

2. R. A. Staehler, "Physical Medicine and Rehabilitation Approach," modified September 29, 2011, accessed October 24 2012, www.spine-health.com/treatment/spine-specialists/physical-medicine-and-rehabilitation-approach.

3. W. C. Ngeow and R. Nair, "Injection of Botulinum Toxin Type A (BOTOX) into Tigger Zone of Trigeminal Neuralgia as a Means to Control Pain," *Oral Surgery, Oral Medicine, Oral Pathology, Oral Radiology and Endodontology* 109, no. 3: (2010): e47–50.

4. "What Types of Treatments and Procedures does a Physiatrist Perform?," American Academy of Physical Medicine and Rehabilitation, accessed September 19, 2012, www.aapmr.org.

5. "What Diseases Does a Physiatrist Treat?" American Academy of Physical Medicine and Rehabilitation, accessed September 19, 2012, www.aapmr.org/career/students/PMRspecialty/Pages/medical-students-guide-to-pmr_e.aspx.

6. "How Is a Physiatrist Different from a Physical Therapist?," American Academy of Physical Medicine and Rehabilitation, accessed September 20, 2012, www.aapmr.org/career/students/PMRspecialty/Pages/medical-students-guide-to-pmr_d.aspx.

7. "How Is a Physiatrist Different from a Physical Therapist?"

8. P. Hardy, *Chronic Pain Management: The Essentials* (London: Greenwich Medical Media, 1997).

9. C. J. Main and C. C. Spanswick, *Pain Management: An Interdisciplinary Approach* (London: Churchill Livingstone, 2000).

10. M. V. Boswell and B. E. Cole, *Weiner's Pain Management: A Practical Guide for Clinicians* (London: Informa Healthcare, 2005).

11. Staehler, "Physical Medicine and Rehabilitation Approach."

12. S. Spinasanta, "Your First Appointment with a Pain Management Specialist," Spineuniverse.com, updated February 16, 2010, accessed September 23, 2012, www.spineuniverse.com.

13. S. Spinasanta, "Your First Appointment with a Pain Management Specialist," Spineuniverse.com, updated February 16, 2010, accessed September 23, 2012, www.spineuniverse.com.

14. S. Spinasanta, "Questions to Ask Your Pain Medicine Specialist," Spineuniverse.com, updated October 12, 2012, accessed December 12, 2012, www.spineuniverse.com.

14. ROLE OF THE PAIN MANAGEMENT SPECIALIST

1. P. Hardy, *Chronic Pain Management: The Essentials* (London: Greenwich Medical Media, 1997).

2. A. Asher, "What Is Pain Management?" *About.com*, accessed October 26, 2012,http://backandneck.about.com/od/chronicpainconditions/f/painmanagement.htm.

3. J. P. Revord, "Pain Management Specialists," *Spine-Health*, 2012, www.spine-health.com/treatment/spine-specialists/pain-management-specialists.

4. Revord, "Pain Management Specialists."

5. M. Harder and R. C. Holdenwang, "Coding Pain Management Services," American Health Information Management Services, accessed October 29, 2012, http://campus.ahima.org/audio/2008/RB040308.pdf.

6. "Straight Talk about Pain," *PartnersAgainstPain*, accessed October 29, 2012, www.partnersagainstpain.com/pain-management/advice.aspx.

7. R. A. Staehler, "What Is a Physiatrist?" *Spine-Health*, accessed October 24, 2012, www.spine-health.com/treatment/spine-specialists/what-a-physiatrist.

15. CONGENITAL INSENSITIVITY TO PAIN

1. R. Kennedy, "Congenital Insensitivity to Pain with Anhidrosis (CIP)," Doctor's Medical Library, accessed September 25,2012,www.medical-library.net/content/view/1691/41/.

2. J. J. Cox, F. Reimann, A. K. Nicholas, G. Thornton, E. Roberts, K. Springell, G. Karbani, H. Jafri, J. Mannan, Y. Raashid, L. Al-Gazali, H. Hama-

my, E. Valente, S. Gorman, R. Williams, D. P. McHale, J. N. Wood, F. M. Gribble, and C. G. Woods, "An SCN9A Channelopathy Causes Congenital Inability to Experience Pain," *Nature* 444, no. 7121 (2006): 894–98.

3. E. M. Nagasako, A. L. Oaklander, and R. H. Dworkin, "Congenital Insensitivity to Pain: An Update," *Pain* 101, no. 3 (2003): 213–19.

4. D. Inouye, "Congenital Insensitivity to Pain with Anhidrosis," *Hohonu: A Journal of Academic Writing* 6, no. 4 (2008): 16–17.

5. Kennedy, "Congenital Insensitivity to Pain with Anhidrosis (CIP)."

6. Cox et al., "An SCN9A Channelopathy."

7. Cox, et al., "An SCN9A Channelopathy."

8. J. L. Bonkowsky, J. Johnson, J. C. Carey, A. G. Smith, and K. J. Swoboda, "An Infant with Primary Tooth Loss and Palmar Hyperkeratosis: A Novel Mutation in the NTRK1 Gene Causing Congenital Insensitivity to Pain With Anhidrosis," *Pediatrics* 112, no. 3 (2003): e237–41.

9. S. Mardy, Y. Miura, F. Endo, I. Matsuda, L. Sztriha, P. Frossard, A. Moosa, E. A. Ismail, A. Macaya, G. Andria, E. Toscano, W. Gibson, G. E. Graham, and Y. Indo, "Congenital Insensitivity to Pain with Anhidrosis: Novel Mutations in the TRKA (NTRK1) Gene Encoding A High-Affinity Receptor for Nerve Growth Factor," *American Journal of Human Genetics* 64, no. 6 (1999): 1570–79.

10. D. E. Houser and G. W. Zamponi, "Perceiving Pain: Health, Culture and Ritual,"*Antrocom: Online Journal of Anthropology* 7, no. 2 (2011): 191–96.

11. "Congenital Insensitivity to Pain with Anhidrosis (CIPA)," accessed September 25, 2012,www.livingnaturally.com/ns/DisplayMonograph.asp? StoreID=3ED1FF6A18BD42979FFF73C8E8CD4512&DocID=condition-cipa.

12. Cox et al., "An SCN9A Channelopathy."

13. Y. P. Goldberg et al., "Loss-of-Function Mutations in the Nav1.7 Gene Underlie Congenital Indifference to Pain in Multiple Human Populations," *Clinical Genetics* 71, no. 4 (2007): 311–19.

14. D. B. Chamberlain, "Babies Don't Feel Pain: A Century of Denial in Medicine," May 2, 1991, accessed September 25, 2012,www.nocirc.org/symposia/second/chamberlain.html.

15. S. I. Merkel, T. Voepel-Lewis, J. R. Shayevitz, and S. Malviya, "The FLACC: A Behavioral Scale for Scoring Postoperative Pain in Young Children," *Pediatric Nursing* 23, no. 3 (1997): 293–97.

16. L. J. Alcock, P. McGrath, J. Kay, S. B. MacMurray, and C. J. J. Dulberg, "The Development of a Tool to Assess Neonatal Plan," *Neonatal Network* 12, no. 6, (1993): 59–66.

17. Inouye, "Congenital Insensitivity to Pain with Anhidrosis."

18. Kennedy, "Congenital Insensitivity to Pain with Anhidrosis (CIPA)."

19. "Case Studies," MacAlester College Department of Psychology, accessed September 25, 2012,www.macalester.edu/psychology/whathap/UBNRP/pain/CaseStudies.htm.

20. "Case Studies," MacAlester College Department of Psychology, accessed September 25, 2012, www.macalester.edu/psychology/whathap/UBNRP/pain/CaseStudies.htm.

21. "Case Studies," MacAlester College Department of Psychology, accessed September 25, 2012, www.macalester.edu/psychology/whathap/UBNRP/pain/CaseStudies.htm.

22. "Naloxone: How Does it Work?," Netdoctor, March 20, 2007, accessed September 25, 2012,www.netdoctor.co.uk/lung-problems/medicines/naloxone.html.

23. V. Rozentsveig, A. Katz, N. Weksler, A. Schwartz, M. Schilly, M. Klein, and G. M. Gurman," The Anaesthetic Management of Patients with Congenital Insensitivity to Pain with Anhidrosis," *Paediatric Anaesthesia* 14, no. 4 (2004): 344–48.

24. T. Tomioka, Y. Awaya, K. Nihei, H. Sekiyama, S. Sawamura, and K. Hanaoka, "Anesthesia for Patients with Congenital Insensitivity to Pain and Anhidrosis: A Questionnaire Study in Japan," *Anesthesia & Analgesia* 94, no. 2 (2002): 271–74.

16. ACUTE VS. CHRONIC PAIN

1. J. D. Loeser, S. H. Butler, and J. J. Chapman, *Bonica's Management of Pain* 3rd ed. (Lippincott Williams & Wilkins, 2000), 18–25.

2. "Global Pain Management Market to Reach US$60 Billion by 2015, According to a New Report by Global Industry Analysts, Inc.," *PRWeb*, January 10, 2011, accessed January 13, 2013, www.prweb.com/releases/2011/1/prweb8052240.htm.

3. Institute of Medicine, *Relieving Pain in America: A Blueprint for Transforming Prevention, Care, Education and Research* (Washington, DC: The National Academies Press, 2011).

4. Richard S. Weiner, *Pain Management: A Practical Guide for Clinicians* (Boca Raton: FL: CRC Press, 2002).

5. P. Saastamoinen, P. Leino-Arjas, M. Laaksonen, and E. Lahelma, "Socio-Economic Differences in the Prevalence of Acute, Chronic and Disabling Chronic Pain among Ageing Employees," *Pain* 114, no. 3 (2005): 364–71.

6. Saastamoinen et al., "Socio-Economic Differences."

7. K. Strietberger, F. Stuber, I. K. Buchli, and U. M. Stamer, "Drug Therapy of Acute and Chronic Abdominal Pain" [in German], *Therapeutische Umschau, Revue Therapeutique* 68, no. 8 (2011): 435–40.

8. C. Bonezzi, L. Demartini, and M. Buonocore, "Chronic Pain: Not Only a Matter of Time," *Minerva Anestesiologica* 78, no. 6 (2012): 704–11.

9. C. Voscopoulos and M. Lema, "When Does Acute Pain become Chronic?" *British Journal of Anaesthesia* 105, no. 1 (2010): i69–85.

10. Bonezzi et al., "Chronic Pain: Not Only a Matter of Time."

11. G. Oderda, "Challenges in the Management of Acute Postsurgical Pain," *Pharmacotherapy* 32, no. 9 (2012): 6S–11S.

12. M. Galinsk, M. Ruscev, G. Gonzalez, J. Kavas, L. Ameur, D. Biens, F. Lapostolle, and F. Adnet, "Prevalence and Management of Acute Pain in Prehospital Emergency Medicine," *Prehospital Emergency Care* 14, no. 3 (2010): 334–39.

13. Galinsk et al., "Prevalence and Management of Acute Pain in Prehospital Emergency Medicine."

14. D. Vinatier, M. Cosson and P. Dufour, "Is Endometriosis an Endometrial Disease?," *European Journal of Obstetrics and Gynecology and Reproductive Biology* 91, no. 2 (2000): 113–25.

15. E. Denny, "Women's Experience of Endometriosis," *Journal of Advanced Nursing:* 46, no. 6 (2004): 641–48.

16. M. Aminoff, R. B. Daroff, M. J. Aminoff and R. B. Daroff, *eds., Encyclopedia of the Neurological Sciences* (Waltham, MA: Academic Press, 2003), 754–56.

17. R. H. Rho, R. P. Brewer, T. J. Lamer, and P. R. Wilson, "Complex Regional Pain Syndrome," *Mayo Clinic Proceedings* 77, no. 2 (2002): 174–80.

18. J. Macintyre, C. Johnson, and E. L. Schroeder, "Groin Pain in Athletes," *Current Sports Medicine Reports* 5, no. 6 (2006): 293–99.

19. D. B. McGuire, "Occurrence of Cancer Pain," *Journal of the National Cancer Institute Monographs* 32 (2004): 51–56.

20. M. H. Levy and T. A. Samuel, "Management of Cancer Pain," *Seminars in Oncology* 32, no. 2 (2005): 179–93.

21. J. N. Ablina, D. Buskilab, B. Van Houdenhovec, P. Luyten, F. Atzenie, and P. Sarzi-Puttin, "Is Fibromyalgia a Discrete Entity?," *Autoimmunity Reviews* 11, no. 8 (2012): 585–88.

22. P. Magown, R. Garcia, and I. Beauprie, "Occipital Nerve Stimulation for Intractable Occipital Neuralgia: An Open Surgical Technique," *Clinical Neurosurgery* 56, no. (2009): 119–24.

23. Magown et al., "Occipital Nerve Stimulation."

24. P. Dreyfuss, S. J. Dreyer, A. Cole, and K. Mayo, "Sacroiliac Joint Pain," *Journal of the American Academy of the Orthopaedic Surgeons* 12, no. 4 (2004): 255–65.

25. Dreyfuss et al., "Sacroiliac Joint Pain."

26. L. Brasseur, "Review of Current Pharmacologic Treatment of Pain" [in French], *Drugs* 53, no. 2 (1997): 10–17.

17. OCCUPATIONAL PAIN

1. C. Spanswick and C. Main, *Pain Management: An Interdisciplinary Approach* (Edinburgh, UK: Churchill Livingstone, 2000), 93.

2. Spanswick and Main, *Pain Management*, 102.

3. "The Enormous Burden of Poor Working Conditions," International Labour Organization, updated June 21, 2011, accessed February 2, 2013, www.ilo.org/public/english/region/eurpro/moscow/areas/safety/statistic.htm.

4. "The Enormous Burden of Poor Working Conditions."

5. K. Tuomi, J. Ilmarinen, L. Eskelinen, E. Järvinen, J. Toikkanen, M. Klockars, "Work Load and Individual Factors Affecting Work Ability among Aging Municipal Employees," *Scandinavian Journal of Work, Environment & Health* 17, Suppl. 1 (1991): 130.

6. V. G. Artamonova, "Current Problems of Diagnosis and Prevention of Occupational Diseases" [in Russian], *Meditsina Truda I Promyshlennaia Ekologiia* 5 (1996): 4–6; A. I. Levin and V.G. Artamonova, "Treatment of Occupational Diseases" [in Russian], *Klinicheskaia Meditsina* 5 (1986): 150–51.

7. G. Z. Fainburg, A. D. Ovsiankin, and V. I. Potemkin, *Occupational Safety and Health*, (Vladivostok: FGOU VPO PIGMU, 2007), 323.

8. Fainburg et al., *Occupational Safety and Health*, 243.

9. E. Rutkowski, ed., *An Ergonomics Approach to Avoiding Workplace Injury* (Fairfax, VA: American Industrial Hygiene Association [AIHA], 2012): 1–8.

18. SPORTS-RELATED PAIN

1. S. Loland, B. Skirstad, and I. Waddington, eds., *Pain and Injury in Sport Social and Ethical Analysis* (New York: Routledge 2006).

2. J. Napallacan and C. M. Asutilla, "Brain Injury Ends Boxing Career of Mandaue Prize Fighter," *Inquirer Global Nation*, November 17, 2009, accessed February 23, 2013, http://globalnation.inquirer.net/cebudailynews/news/view/20091117-236746/Brain-injury-ends-boxing-career-of-Mandaue-prize-fighter.

3. A. Dela Cruz, "Undefeated Filipino Boxer Dies after Fight Injury," *Inquirer Sports*, February 4, 2012, accessed February 24, 2013, http://sports.inquirer.net/33535/undefeated-filipino-boxer-dies-after-fight-injury.

4. K. Baxter, "Pacquiao Protege Upgraded to Stable," *L. A. Times Sports*, November 14, 2009, accessed February 24, 2013, http://latimes-blogs.latimes.com/sports_blog/2009/11/pacquiao-protege-upgraded-to-stable.html.

5. E. Malinowski, "For Athletes' Peak Performance, Age Is Everything," *Wired*, July 12, 2011, accessed February 24, 2013, www.wired.com/2011/07/athletes-peak-age/.

6. L. Ristolainen, A. Heinonen, B. Waller, U. M. Kujala, and J. A. Kettunen, "Gender Differences in Sport Injury Risk and Types of Injuries: A Retrospective Twelve-month Study on Cross-Country Skiers, Swimmers, Long-distance Runners and Soccer Players," *Journal of Sports Science and Medicine* 8, no. 3 (2009): 443–51.

7. K. Furgang, *Frequently Asked Questions about Sports Injuries* (New York: The Rosen Publishing Group, 2008).

8. Furgang, *Frequently Asked Questions about Sports Injuries*.

9. G. Solomon, K. Johnston, and M. Lovell, *The Heads-Up on Sport Concussion* (Champaign, IL: Human Kinetics 2005).

10. W. L. Kenney, J. Wilmore, D. Costill, *Physiology of Sport and Exercise* (Champaign, IL: Human Kinetics 2011).

11. L. Vicchiet and M. A. Giamberardino, *Muscle Pain, Myofascial Pain and Fibromyalgia Recent Advances* (Philadelphia, PA: Howerth Press 1999).

12. H. W. Griffith and D. Friscia, *Complete Guide to Sports Injuries: How to Treat Fractures, Sprains, Strains, Dislocations, Head Injuries* (Westminster, UK: Perigee Books 2004).

13. J. A. Rihn, D. T. Anderson, K. Lamb, P. F. Deluca, A. Bata, P. A. Marchetto, N. Neves, and A. R. Vaccaro, "Cervical Spine Injuries in American Football," *Sports Medicine* 39, no. 9 (2009): 697–708; R. Molinari and W. J. Molinari III, "Cervical Fracture with Transient Tetraplegia in a Youth Football Player: Case Report and Review of the Literature," *Journal of Spinal Cord Medicine* 33, no. 2 (2010): 163–67.

14. L. Carthwhright and W. Pitney, *Fundamentals of Athletic Training* (Champaign, IL: Human Kinetics, 1999).

15. S. Bird, N. Black, and P. Newton, *Sports Injuries Causes, Diagnosis, Treatment and Prevention* (London: Chapman and Hall, 1997).

16. R. Gotlin, *Sports Injuries Guidebook* (Champaign, IL: Human Kinetics 2007).

17. Gotlin, *Sports Injuries Guidebook*.

18. M. Hutson and C. Speed, eds., *Sports Injuries* (New York: Oxford University Press 2011).

19. Hutson and Speed, *Sports Injuries*.

20. L. Clayton, *Everything You Need to Know about Sports Injuries* (New York: The Rosen Publishing Group 1995).

21. B. Walker, *The Anatomy of Sports Injuries* (Chichester, UK: Lotus Publishing 2007).

22. Gotlin, *Sports Injuries Guidebook*.

23. M. P. Jensen, "Psychosocial Approaches to Pain Management: An Organizational Framework," *Pain* 152, no. 4 (2011): 717–25; S. Bhatnagar, D. Banerjee, S. Joshi, and R. Gupta, "Assessing Psychosocial Distress: A Pain Audit at IRCH-AIIMS," *Annals of Palliative Medicine* 2, no. 2 (2013): 76–84.

24. T. M. Mick and R. J. Dimeff, "What Kind of Physical Examination Does a Young Athlete Need before Participating in Sports?" *Cleveland Clinic Journal of Medicine* 71, no. 7 (2004): 587–97.

25. "Handout on Health: Sports Injuries," National Institute of Arthritis and Musculoskeletal and Skin Diseases, accessed February 2, 2013, www.niams. nih.gov/Health_Info/Sports_Injuries/.

19. PAIN FROM EXCESSIVE MOVEMENT

1. W. L. Calmbach and M. Hutchens, "Evaluation of Patients Presenting with Knee Pain: Part I, History, Physical Examination, Radiographs, and Laboratory Tests," *American Academy of Family Physicians* 68, no. 5 (2003): 912.

2. I. G. Stiel, G. H. Greenberg, G. A. Wells, I. McDowell, A. A. Cwinn, N. A. Smith, T. F. Cacciotti, and M. L. Sivilotti, "Prospective Validation of a Decision Rule for the Use of Radiography in Acute Knee Injuries," *Journal of the American Medical Association* 275, no. 8 (1996): 611–15.

3. "Meniscus Tear," *WebMD*, accessed February 7, 2013, www.webmd.com/a-to-z-guides/meniscus-tear-topic-overview.

4. "Knee Problems and Injuries," *WebMD*, accessed February 7, 2013, www.webmd.com/pain-management/knee-pain/knee-problems-and-injuries-topic-overview.

5. William H. Blahd Jr. and David Messenger, Fracture or Dislocation of the Knee, *WebMD*, www.webmd.com/pain-management/knee-pain/fracture-or-dislocation-of-the-knee.

6. Blahd and Messenger, "Fracture or Dislocation of the Knee."

7. C. Tidy, "Knee Fractures and Dislocations," accessed February 8, 2013, www.patient.co.uk/doctor/knee-fractures-and-dislocations.

8. Blahd and Messenger, "Fracture or Dislocation of the Knee."

9. "Knee Fractures," BetterBraces.com, accessed February 9, 2013, www.betterbraces.com/injury-info-center/knee-injury-guide/knee-fractures.

10. K. Lau and C. J. Lavernia, eds., "Tibial Tubercle Fracture," *Medscape Reference*, accessed February 9, 2013, http://emedicine.medscape.com/article/1250197-overview.

11. H. B. Tandeta, P. Shvartzman, and M. A. Stevens, "Acute Knee Injuries: Use of Decision Rules for Selective Radiograph Ordering," *American Family Physician* 60, no. 9 (1999): 2599–608.

20. PAIN FROM SEDENTARY LIFESTYLE

1. J. C. Adsuar, N. Gusi, M. Hernandez-Mocholí, J. A. Parraca, B. del Pozo-Cruz, and J. del Pozo-Cruz, "Musculoskeletal Fitness and Health-Related Quality of Life Characteristics among Sedentary Office Workers Affected by Sub-Acute, Non-Specific Low Back Pain: A Cross-sectional Study," *Physiotherapy* 99, no. 3 (2013): 194–200.

2. R. E. Andersen, S. J. Bartlet, J. M. Bathom, C. Christmas, C. J. Crespo, S. C. Franckowick, "How Common Is Hip Pain among Older Adults? Results from the Third National Health and Nutrition Examination Survey," *Journal of Family Practice* 4, no. 4 (2002): 345–46.

3. "Arthritis: Meeting the Challenge of Living Well," Centers for Disease Control and Prevention, accessed March 25, 2013, www.cdc.gov/chronicdisease/resources/publications/aag/arthritis.htm.

4. "Understanding High Blood Pressure—Symptoms," *WebMD*, accessed June 4, 2013, www.webmd.com/hypertension-high-blood-pressure/understanding-high-blood-pressure-symptoms.

5. C. Costin, "Is There Such a Thing as Too Much Exercise?" Association for Body Image Disordered Eating; University of California, accessed April 4, 2013, http://abide.ucdavis.edu/overexercise.html.

6. E. Quinn, "Muscle Pain and Soreness after Exercise," *About.com*, Sports Medicine, 2011, accessed April 4, 2013, http://sportsmedicine.about.com/cs/injuries/a/doms.htm.

7. J. Weiss, "Free Yourself from Back Pain," *GAIAM Life*, accessed April 7, 2013, http://life.gaiam.com/article/free-yourself-back-pain.

8. "High Blood Pressure Prevention," *Web MD*, accessed April 7, 2013, www.webmd.com/hypertension-high-blood-pressure/guide/preventing-high-blood-pressure.

21. AGE-RELATED PAIN

1. N. M. Omar, A. M. Hussein, H. A. Malek, M. A. Saad, D. M. Saleh, "Influence of Age on Pain Sensitivity in Response to Paw Pressure and Formalin Injection in Rats: A Role of Nitric Oxide," *General Physiology and Biophysics* 31, no. (2012): 185–94; K. M. Darchuk, C. O. Townsend, J. D. Rome, B. K. Bruce, W. M. Hooten, "Longitudinal Treatment Outcomes for Geriatric Patients with Chronic Non-Cancer Pain at an Interdisciplinary Pain Rehabilitation Program," *Pain Medicine* 11, no. 9 (2010): 1352–64.

2. World Health Organization, *The Global Burden of Disease* (Geneva: World Health Organization, 2004), 35.

3. National Arthritis Data Workgroup, "Estimates of the Prevalence of Arthritis and Other Rheumatic Conditions in the United States," *Arthritis & Rheumatism* 58, no. 1 (2008): 26–35.

4. I. Scott and S. Steer, "The Genetics of Rheumatoid Arthritis," National Rheumatoid Arthritis Society, accessed November 8, 2012, www.nras.org.uk/the-genetics-of-rheumatoid-arthritis.

5. R. W. Johnson and J. McElhaney, "Postherpetic Neuralgia in the Elderly," *International Journal of Clinical Practice* 63, no. 9 (2009): 1386–91.

6. Johnson and McElhaney, "Postherpetic Neuralgia in the Elderly."

7. A. Jemal, F. Bray, M. M. Center, J. Ferlay, E. Ward, and D. Forman, "Global Cancer Statistics," *CA: A Cancer Journal for Clinicians* 61, no. 2 (2011): 69–90.

8. World Health Organization, *Cancer Pain Relief—with a Guide to Opioid Availability*, 2nd ed. (Geneva: World Health Organization, 1996).

9. M. H. van den Beuken-van Everdingen, J. M. de Rijke, A. G. Kessels, H. C. Schouten, M. van Kleef and J. Patijn, "High Prevalence of Pain in Patients with Cancer in a Large Population-Based Study in The Netherlands," *Pain* 132, no. 3 (2007): 12–20.

10. B. M. del Pino, "Chemotherapy-Induced Peripheral Neuropathy," *NCI Cancer Bulletin* 7, no. 4 (2010): 6.

11. S. Lautenbachera, M. Kunza, P. Strateb, P. Nielsenc and L. Arendt-Nielsenc, "Age Effects on Pain Thresholds, Temporal Summation and Spatial Summation of Heat and Pressure Pain," *Pain* 115, no. 3, (2005): 410–18.

12. S. J. Gibson and R. D. Helme, "Age-Related Differences in Pain Perception and Report," *Clinics in Geriatric Medicine* 17, no. 3 (2001): 433–56; K.

M. Woodrow, G. D. Friedman, A. B. Siegelaub, and M. F. Collen, "Pain Tolerance: Differences According to Age, Sex and Race," *Psychosomatic Medicine* 34, no. 6 (1972): 548.

13. Gibson and Helme, "Age-Related Differences in Pain Perception and Report."; Woodrow et al., "Pain Tolerance."

14. "Degenerative Spinal Disorders," New York Presbyterian Hospital, accessed November 5, 2012, http://nyp.org/health/degenerative-spinal-disorders.html.

15. R. Bernabei, G. Gambassi, K. Lapane, F. Landi, C. Gatsonis, R. Dunlop, L. Lipsitz, K. Steel, and V. Mor, "Management of Pain in Elderly Patients with Cancer," *Journal of the American Medical Association* 279, no. 23, (1998): 1877–82.

16. Bernabei et al., "Management of Pain in Elderly Patients with Cancer."

22. TROUBLESHOOTING PAIN

1. D. B. Carr, "Letter to Forum Commenting on "Iceman from the Copper Age," *National Geographic Magazine* 4 (1993): 184.

2. M. Y. Dubois, R. M. Gallagher, and P. M. Lippe, "Pain Medicine Position Paper," *Pain Medicine* 10, no. 6 (2009): 972–1000.

3. B. J. Taylor, J. M. Robbins, J. I. Gold, T. R. Logsdon, T. M. Bird, and K. J. Anand, "Assessing Postoperative Pain in Neonates: A Multicenter Observational Study," *Pediatrics* 118, no. 4 (2006): e992–e1000.

4. M. Mcaffery and A. Beebe, *Pain: Clinical Manual for Nursing Practice* (London: Mosby, 1994).

5. F. Brennan, D. B. Carr, and M. J. Cousins, "Pain Management: A Fundamental Human Right," *International Anesthesia Research Society* 105, no. 1 (2007): 205–21.

6. Brennan, Carr, and Cousins, "Pain Management: A Fundamental Human Right."

7. Brennan, Carr, and Cousins, "Pain Management: A Fundamental Human Right."

8. A. Cintron and R. S. Morrison, "Pain and Ethnicity in the United States: A Systematic Review," *Journal of Palliative Medicine* 9, no. 6 (2006): 1454–73.

9. L. J. Staton, M. Panda, I. Chen, I. Genao, J. Kurz, M. Pasanen, A. J. Mechaber, M. Menon, J. O'Rorke, J. Wood, E. Rosenberg, C. Faeslis, T. Carey, D. Calleson, and S. Cykert, "When Race Matters: Disagreement in Pain Perception between Patients and Their Physicians in Primary Care," *Journal of the National Medical Association* 99, no.5 (2007): 532–38.

10. Staton et al., "When Race Matters."

11. N. Jimenez, K. Seidel, L. D. Martin, F. P. Rivara, and A. M. Lynn, "Perioperative Analgesic Treatment in Latino and Non-Latino Pediatric Patients," *Journal of Health Care for the Poor and Underserved*, 21, no. 1 (2010): 229–36.

12. R. B. Fillingim and W. Maixner, "Gender Differences in the Response to Noxious Stimuli," Pain Forum 4 (1995): 209–21; J. L. Riley III, M. E. Robinson, E. A. Wise, C. D. Myers, and R. B. Fillingim, "Sex Differences in the Perception of Noxious Experimental Stimuli: A Meta-Analysis," *Pain* 74, nos. 2–3 (1998): 181–87.

13. D. E. Hoffmann and A. J. Tarzian, "The Girl Who Cried Pain: A Bias against Women in the Treatment of Pain," Journal of Law, Medicine, and Ethics 29, no. 1 (2001): 13–27.

14. B. S. Faherty and M. R. Grier, "Analgesic Medication for Elderly People Post-Surgery," Nursing Research 33, no. 6 (1984): 369–72.

15. Faherty and Grier, "Analgesic Medication for Elderly People Post-Surgery."

16. D. A. Fishbain, M. Goldberg, B. R. Meagher, R. Steele, and H. Rosomoff, "Male and Female Chronic Pain Patients Categorized by DSM-III Psychiatric Diagnostic Criteria," Pain 26, no. 2 (1986): 181–97.

17. M. McCaffery and B. R. Ferrell, "Does the Gender Gap Affect Your Pain-Control Decisions?" Nursing 22, no. 8 (1992): 48–51.

18. T. Hadjistavropoulos, B. McMurty, and K. D. Craig, "Beautiful Faces in Pain: Biases and Accuracy in the Perception of Pain," Psychology and Health 11 (1996): 411–20.

19. J. Quiambao-Udan, *Fundamentals of Nursing* (Singapore: Educational Publishing House, 2004), 327–28.

20. "Prescribing Analgesics to the Elderly in Long-Term Care," WHO Pain and Palliative Care Communications Program, accessed March 21, 2013, www.whocancerpain.wisc.edu/?q=node/305.

21. J. W. Nickerson and A. Attaran, "The Inadequate Treatment of Pain: Collateral Damage from the War on Drugs," *PLOS Medicine* 9, no. 1 (2012): e1001153.

22. B. A. Rich, "Physicians' Legal Duty to Relieve Suffering," *Western Journal of Medicine* 175, no. 3 (September 2001): 151–52.

23. W. M. Stein and R. P. Miech, "Cancer Pain in the Elderly Hospice Patient," *Journal of Pain and Symptom Management* 8, no. (1993): 474–82.

24. R. Bernabei, G. Gambassi, K. Lapane, F. Landi, C. Gatsonis, R. Dunlop, L. Lipsitz, K. Steel, and V. Mor, "Management of Pain in Elderly Patients with Cancer," *Journal of the American Medical Association* 279, no. 23 (1998): 1877–82.

25. Rich, "Physicians' Legal Duty to Relieve Suffering."

26. B. Smedley, A. Stith, and A. Nelson, *Unequal Treatment: Confronting Racial and Ethnic Disparities in Healthcare* (Washington, DC: National Academy Press, 2002).

23. NATURAL APPROACHES TO PAIN

1. J. Hughes, *Pain Management: From Basics to Clinical Practice* (Philadelphia: Churchill Livingstone, 2008), 4.

2. O. Thienhaus and B. E. Cole. "The Classification of Pain," in *Pain Management: A Practical Guide for Clinicians,* 6th ed. (Boca Raton, FL: CRC Press, 2002), 29.

3. S. F. Nadler, "Nonpharmacologic Management of Pain," *Journal of the American Osteopathic Association* 104, Suppl. 8 (2004):S6-12; L. A. Menefee and D. A. Monti, "Nonpharmacologic and Complementary Approaches to Cancer Pain Management," *Journal of the American Osteopathic Association* 105, Suppl 5 (2005): S15-20.

4. "5 Foods That Help Manage Chronic Pain," *FitDay.com,* accessed October 26, 2012, www.fitday.com/fitness-articles/nutrition/healthy-eating/5-foods-that-help-manage-chronic-pain.html#b.

5. T. Polkki, K. Vehvilainen-Julkunen, and A. Pietila, "Nonpharmacological Methods in Relieving Children's Postoperative Pain: A Survey on Hospital Nurses in Finland," *Journal of Advanced Nursing* 34, no. 4 (2001): 483–92.

6. M. Titler and B. Rakel, "Nonpharmacologic Treatment of Pain," *Critical Care Nursing Clinics of North America* 13, no. 2. (2001): 221–32.

7. Titler and Rakel, "Nonpharmacologic Treatment of Pain"; B. Rakel K. Herr, "Assessment and Treatment of Postoperative Pain in Older Adults," *Journal of Perianesthesia Nursing* 19, no. 3 (2004): 194–208.

8. M. McCaffery, "Nursing Approaches to Nonpharmacological Pain Control," *International Journal of Nursing Studies* 27, no. 1 (1990): 1–5.

9. M. McCaffrey and C. Pasero "Practical Nondrug Approaches to Pain," in *Pain: Clinical Manual* (St. Louis: Mosby, 1999), 28.

10. Titler and Rakel, "Nonpharmacologic Treatment of Pain."

11. B. Cole and Q. Brunk, "Holistic Interventions for Acute Pain Episodes: An Integrative Review," *Journal of Holistic Nursing* 17, no. 4 (1999): 384–96.

12. Titler and Rakel, "Nonpharmacologic Treatment of Pain."

13. M. McCaffery, "Nursing Approaches to Nonpharmacological Pain Control," *International Journal of Nursing Studies* 27, no. 1 (1990): 27; M. Titler and B. Rakel, "Nonpharmacologic Treatment of Pain," *Critical Care Nursing Clinics of North America* 13, no. 2. (2001): 222.

14. M. Titler and B. Rakel, "Nonpharmacologic Treatment of Pain," *Critical Care Nursing Clinics of North America* 13, no. 2. (2001): 225.

15. McCaffery, "Nursing Approaches to Nonpharmacological Pain Control," 29.

16. "Complementary and Alternative Medicine," NIH, accessed September 14, 2012, http://report.nih.gov/nihfactsheets/ViewFactSheet.aspx?csid=85.

17. J. Bhatia, "Therapies to Try for Natural Pain Relief," *Every Day Health,* accessed September 14, 2012, www.everydayhealth.com/pain-management/alternative-treatments.aspx.

18. "Non Pharmacological Approaches," *Caresearch,* accessed October 27, 2012, www.caresearch.com.au/caresearch/ClinicalPractice/Physical/Pain/NonPharmacologicalApproaches/tabid/751/Default.aspx.

19. C. Pederson and B. Harbaugh, "Nurses' Use of Nonpharmacologic Techniques with Hospitalized Children," *Issues in Comprehensive Pediatric Nursing* 18, no. 2 (1995): 91–103.

20. M. E. Tota-Faucette, K. M. Gil, D. A. Williams, F. J. Keefe and V. Goli, "Predictors of Response to Pain Management Treatment. The Role of Family Environment and Changes in Cognitive Processes," *The Clinical Journal of Pain* 9, no. 2 (1993): 115–23.

21. S. Malenbaum, F. J. Keefe, A. Williams, R. Ulrich, and T. J. Somers, "Pain in Its Environmental Context: Implications for Designing Environments to Enhance Pain Control," *Pain* 134, no. 3 (2008): 241–44.

22. J. M. Walch, B. S. Rabin, R. Day, J. N. Williams, K. Choi, and J. D. Kang, "The Effect of Sunlight on Postoperative Analgesic Medication Use: A Prospective Study of Patients Undergoing Spinal Surgery," *Psychosomatic Medicine: Journal of Biobehavioral Medicine* 67 no. 1 (2005): 156–63.

23. Malenbaum et al., "Pain in Its Environmental Context."

24. B. L. Fredrickson and R. W. Levenson, "Positive Emotions Speed Recovery from Cardiovascular Sequelae of Negative Emotions," *Cognition and Emotion* 12, no. 2 (1998): 191–220.

25. P. Manning, "The Effect of Airplanes on Fibromyalgia," *eHow Health*, accessed September 29, 2012, www.ehow.com/facts_5619101_effect-airplanes-fibromyalgia.html.

26. "The Effect of Airplanes on Fibromyalgia."

27. "Enzymology," *The Free Dictionary: Medical Dictionary*, accessed April 2, 2013, www.medical-dictionary.thefreedictionary.com/enzymology.

28. M. S. Cook, "Treating Pain and Inflammation with Enzymes," *Care2*, accessed March 2, 2013, www.care2.com/greenliving/treating-pain-and-inflammation-with-enzymes.html.

29. T. Marcantel, "Systemic Enzyme Therapy for Pain," accessed March 3, 2013, www.drmarcantel.com/systemic-enzyme-therapy-for-pain.

30. Cook, "Treating Pain and Inflammation with Enzymes."

31. R. M. Griffin, "Vitamins and Supplements Lifestyle Guide," *WebMD*, accessed September 29, 2012, www.webmd.com/vitamins-and-supplements/lifestyle-guide-11/.

32. J. C. Maroon and J. W. Bost, "Omega-3 Fatty Acids (Fish Oil) as an Anti-inflammatory: An Alternative to Nonsteroidal Anti-inflammatory Drugs for Discogenic Pain," *Surgical Neurology* 65, no. 4 (2005): 326–31.

33. Griffin, "Vitamins and Supplements Lifestyle Guide."

34. Griffin, "Vitamins and Supplements Lifestyle Guide."

35. S. Haig, "Can Turmeric Relieve Pain? One Doctor's Opinion," *Time*, July 13, 2009, accessed September 30, 2012, http://content.time.com/time/health/article/0,8599,1910028,00.html.

36. "13+ Foods for Fighting Pain," *Reader's Digest*, accessed September 25, 2012, www.rd.com/slideshows/anti-inflammatory-foods/.

37. K. A. Ranson, ed., *Grolier International Encyclopedia* (Danbury, CT: Grolier Incorporated, 1991).

38. A. M. Bode and Z. Dong, "The Amazing and Mighty Ginger," in *Herbal Medicine: Biomolecular and Clinical Aspect*, 2nd ed. (Boca Raton, FL: CRC Press, 2011).

39. R. D. Altman and K. C. Marcussen, "Effects of a Ginger Extract on Knee Pain in Patients with Osteoarthritis," *Arthritis & Rheumatism* 44, no. 11 (2001): 2531–38.

40. "Vitamin D: A Champion of Pain Relief," *Pain Treatment Topics*, Minnesota State Academies, accessed September 30, 2012, www.msa.state.mn.us/wellnesscommittee/vitdachampionforpainrelief.pdf.

41. Griffin, "Vitamins and Supplements Lifestyle Guide."

42. Griffin, "Vitamins and Supplements Lifestyle Guide."

43. O. Dale, K. Moksnes, and S. Kaasa, "European Palliative Care Research Collaborative Pain Guidelines: Opioid Switching to Improve Analgesia or Reduce Side Effects: A Systematic Review, *Palliative Medicine* 25, no. 5 (2011):494–503; A. D. Furlan, J. A. Sandoval, A. Mailis-Gagnon, and E. Tunks, "Opioids for Chronic Noncancer Pain: A Meta-Analysis of Effectiveness and Side Effects," *Canadian Medical Association Journal* 174, no. 11 (2006): 1589–94; S. H. Chou, J. H. Kao, P. L. Tao, P. Y. Law, and H. H. Loh, "Naloxone Can Act as an Analgesic Agent without Measurable Chronic Side Effects in Mice with a Mutant Mu-opioid Receptor Expressed in Different Sites of Pain Pathway," *Synapse* 66, no. 8 (2012): 694–704.

24. DIETS FOR PAIN RELIEF

1. "5 Foods That Help Manage Chronic Pain," FitDay.com, accessed October 26, 2012, www.fitday.com/fitness-articles/nutrition/healthy-eating/5-foods-that-help-manage-chronic-pain.html#b.

2. W. Myers, "6 Food Additives to Subtract from Your Diet," *Everyday Health*, modified September 20, 2011, accessed October 27, 2012, www.everydayhealth.com/pain-management/6-food-additives-to-subtract-from-your-diet.aspx.

3. P. Bayer, K. Fairchild, B. Feinberg, S. C. Monje, L. Stalter, V. F. Towers, and C. B. Waff, *eds.*, "Diet," in *The Encyclopedia Americana International Edition* (Danbury, CT: Grolier Incorporated, 2001).

4. B. V. McGoey, M. Deitel, R. Saplys, and M. E. Kliman, "Effect of Weight Loss on Musculoskeletal Pain in the Morbidly Obese," *Journal of Bone and Joint Surgery* 72, no. 2 (1990): 322.

5. S. P. Messier, R. F. Loeser, M. N. Mitchell, G. Valle, T. P. Morgan, W. J. Rejeski, and W. H. Ettinger, "Exercise and Weight Loss in Obese Older Adults with Knee Osteoarthritis: A Preliminary Study," *Journal of the American Geriatrics Society* 48, no. 9 (2000): 1062.

6. R. E. Andersen, C. J. Crespo, S. J. Bartlett, J. M. Bathon, and K. R. Fontaine, "Relationship between Body Weight Gain and Significant Knee, Hip, and Back Pain in Older Americans," *Obesity Research* 11, no. 10 (2003): 1159.

7. U. E. Larsson, "Influence of Weight Loss on Pain, Perceived Disability and Observed Functional Limitations in Obese Women," *International Journal of Obesity* 28, no. 2 (2004): 269.

8. I. J. Hickman, J. R. Jonsson, J. B. Prins, S. Ash, D. M. Purdie, A. D. Clouston, and E. E. Powell, "Modest Weight Loss and Physical Activity in Overweight Patients with Chronic Liver Disease Results in Sustained Improvements in Alanine Aminotransferase, Fasting Insulin, and Quality of Life," *Gut* 53, no. 3 (2004): 413.

9. P. Dessein, E. Shipton, A. Stanwix, B. Joffe, and J. Ramokgadi, "Beneficial Effects of Weight Loss Associated with Moderate Calorie/Carbohydrate Restriction, and Increased Proportional Intake of Protein and Unsaturated Fat on Serum Urate and Lipoprotein Levels in Gout: A Pilot Study," *Annals of the Rheumatic Diseases* 59, no. 7 (2000): 539–41.

10. "7 Foods for Fighting Pain," *Reader's Digest*, accessed September 25, 2012, www.readersdigest.ca/food/healthy-food/7-foods-fighting-pain/.

11. K. Wright, *Guide to Wellbeing* (New Lanark, Scotland: Geddes and Grosset, 2004), 122.

12. Wright, *Guide to Wellbeing*, 125.

13. Wright, *Guide to Wellbeing*, 127.

14. "7 Foods for Fighting Pain."

15. Wright, *Guide to Wellbeing*, 126.

16. R. J. Wagman, ed., "Heat Exhaustion," in *The New Complete Medical and Health Encyclopedia* (New York: Ferguson Publishing Company, 1994).

17. "7 Foods for Fighting Pain."

18. M. H. Zubair, M. N. Zubair, M. M. Zubair, T. Aftab, and F. Asad, "Augmentation of Anti-Platelet Effects of Aspirin by Chocolate," *Journal of the Pakistan Medical Association* 61, no. 3 (2011): 304–7.

19. Wright, *Guide to Wellbeing*, 132.

20. J. Rhode, S. Fogoros, S. Zick, H. Wahl, K. A. Griffith, J. Huang, and J. R. Liu, "Ginger Inhibits Cell Growth and Modulates Angiogenic Factors in Ovarian Cancer Cells," *BioMedCentral (BMC) Complementary and Alternative Medicine* 7 (2007): 44.

21. "7 Foods for Fighting Pain."

22. "7 Foods for Fighting Pain."

23. Wright, *Guide to Wellbeing*, 127.

24. "7 Foods for Fighting Pain."

25. K. A. Ranson, ed., "Artichoke," in *Grolier International Encyclopedia*, (Danbury, CT: Grolier Incorporated, 1991); Wright, *Guide to Wellbeing*, 124.

26. Wright, *Guide to Wellbeing*, 125.

27. Wright, *Guide to Wellbeing*, 126.

28. Wright, *Guide to Wellbeing*, 126.

29. Wright, *Guide to Wellbeing*, 126.

30. C. Dunford, R. Cooper, and P. Molan, "Using Honey as a Dressing for Infected Skin Lesions," *Nursing Times* 96, Suppl. 14 (2000): 7–9; A. K. Ahmed, M. J. Hoekstra, J. J. Hage, and R. B. Karim, "Honey-Medicated Dressing: Transformation of an Ancient Remedy into Modern Therapy," *Annals of Plastic Surgery* 50, no. 2 (2003): 143–47.

31. B. Biglari, P. H. Linden, A. Simon, S. Aytac, H. J. Gerner, and A. Moghaddam, "Use of Medihoney as a Non-surgical Therapy for Chronic Pres-

sure Ulcers in Patients with Spinal Cord Injury," *Spinal Cord* 50, no. 2 (2012): 165–69.

32. J. H. Kim, "Anti-Bacterial Action of Onion (Allium Cepa L.) Extracts against Oral Pathogenic Bacteria," *Journal of Nihon University School of Dentistry* 39, no. 3 (1997): 136–41; J. B. Lee, S. Miyake, R. Umetsu, K. Hayashi, T. Chijimatsu, and T. Hayashi, "Anti-Influenza A Virus Effects of Fructan from Welsh Onion (Allium Fistulosum L.)," *Food Chemistry* 134, no. 4 (2012): 2164–68.

33. E. Ben-Arye, E. Goldin, D. Wengrower, A. Stamper, R. Kohn, and E. Berry, "Wheat Grass Juice in the Treatment of Active Distal Ulcerative Colitis: A Randomized Double-Blind Placebo-Controlled Trial," *Scandinavian Journal of Gastroenterology*, 37, no. 4 (2002): 444–49.

34. Wright, *Guide to Wellbeing*, 123.

35. Wright, *Guide to Wellbeing*, 127.

36. Wright, *Guide to Wellbeing*, 130.

37. Wright, *Guide to Wellbeing*, 131.

38. Wright, *Guide to Wellbeing*, 132.

39. P. Bayer, K. Fairchild, B. Feinberg, S. C. Monje, L. Stalter, V. F. Towers, and C. B. Waff, eds., "Diet," in *The Encyclopedia Americana International Edition* (Danbury, C T: Grolier Incorporated, 2001).

40. D. W. Smithemail and S. L. McFall, "The Relationship of Diet and Exercise for Weight Control and the Quality of Life Gap Associated with Diabetes," *Journal of Psychosomatic Research* 59, no. 6 (2005): 385–92.

41. W. Myers, "6 Food Additives to Subtract from Your Diet," *Everyday Health*, accessed October 27, 2012, www.everydayhealth.com/pain-management/6-food-additives-to-subtract-from-your-diet.aspx.

42. R. J. Wagman, ed., "How Food Relates to Diseases," in *The New Complete Medical and Health Encyclopedia* (New York: Ferguson Publishing Company, 1994).

43. N. D. Barnard, A. R. Scialli, D. Hurlock, and P. Bertron, "Diet and Sex-Hormone Binding Globulin, Dysmenorrhea, and Premenstrual Symptoms," *Obstetrics and Genecology* 95, no. 2 (2000): 245–49.

44. J. E. Markowitz, J. M. Spergel, E. Ruchelli, and C. A. Liacouras, "Elemental Diet Is an Effective Treatment for Eosinophilic Esophagitis in Children and Adolescents," *American Journal of Gastroenterology* 98, no. 4 (2003): 777–81.

45. K. A. Ranson, "Crohn's Disease," in *"Grolier International Encyclopedia* (Danbury, CT: Grolier Incorporated, 1991).

46. C. Ó' Moráin, A. W. Segal, and A. J. Levi, "Elemental Diet as Primary Treatment of Acute Crohn's Disease: A Controlled Trial," *British Medical Journal* 288 (1984): 1859–62.

47. T. H. Wu, T. Y. Chiu, J. S. Tsai, C. Yu. Chen, L. C. Chen, and L. L. Yang, "Effectiveness of Taiwanese Traditional Herb Diet for Pain Management in Terminal Cancer Patients," *Asia Pacific Journal of Clinical Nutrition* 17, no. 1 (2008): 18–20.

48. L. Sköldstam, L. Larsson, and F. D. Lindström, "Effects of Fasting and Lactovegetarian Diet on Rheumatoid Arthritis," *Scandinavian Journal of Rheumatology* 8, no. 4 (1979): 253–54.

49. R. J. Wagman, ed., "Diet and Disease Prevention," in *The New Complete Medical and Health Encyclopedia* (New York: Ferguson Publishing Company, 1994).

50. R. J. Wagman, ed., "Other Disease Requiring Special Diets," in *The New Complete Medical and Health Encyclopedia* (New York: Ferguson Publishing Company, 1994).

51. J. A. Murray, T. Watson, B. Clearman, and F. Mitros, "Effect of a Gluten-Free Diet on Gastrointestinal Symptoms in Celiac Disease," *The American Journal of Clinical Nutrition* 79, no. 4 (2004): 670–72.

25. EXERCISES FOR PAIN RELIEF

1. World Cancer Research Fund, *Food, Nutrition, Physical Activity, and the Prevention of Cancer: A Global Perspective* (Washington, DC: American Institute for Cancer Research, 2007).

2. American Diabetes Association, "Standards of Medical Care in Diabetes—2012 (Position Statement)," *Diabetes Care* 35, Suppl. 1 (2012): S11–S63.

3. K. T. Hoiriis, B. Pfleger, F. C. McDuffie, G. Cotsonis, O. Elsangak, R. Hinson, and G. T. Verzosa, "A Randomized Clinical Trial Comparing Chiropractic Adjustments to Muscle Relaxants for Subacute Low Back Pain," *Journal of Manipulative and Physiological Therapeutics* 27, no. 6 (2004): 388–98.

4. D. Critchley and M. Hurley, "Management of Back Pain in Primary Care. Hands On Practical Advice on Management of Rheumatic Disease," *Reports on the Rheumatic Diseases* 5, no. 13 (2007): 3.

5. "Nonspecific Neck Pain" Egton Medical Information Systems Limited, accessed July 8, 2013, www.patient.co.uk/health/nonspecific-neck-pain.

6. S. Schneider, D. Randoll, and M. Buchner, "Why Do Women Have Back Pain More Than Men? A Representative Prevalence Study in the Federal Republic of Germany," *Clinical Journal of Pain* 22, no. 8 (2006): 738–47.

7. M. Battersby, "The Power of the Stretch," *The Independent UK*, August 7, 2012, accessed March 20, 2013, www.independent.co.uk/life-style/health-and-families/features/the-power-of-the-stretch-8010034.html.

8. "10 Exercises for People in Pain: Yoga," Health Media Ventures, accessed March 29, 2013, www.health.com/health/gallery/0,,20436269_4,00.html.

9. P. M. Barnes, B. Bloom, and R. L. Nahin, *Complementary and Alternative Medicine Use among Adults and Children: United States, 2007*, National Health Statistics Reports, no. 12, pp. 1–23, 2009, www.cdc.gov/nchs/nhis/nhis_nhsr.htm.

10. "10 Exercises for People in Pain: Aerobic Activity," Health Media Ventures, accessed March 29, 2013, www.health.com/health/gallery/0,,20436269_4,00.html.

26. ADDRESSING THE MENTAL ASPECTS

1. M. Thernstrom, "My Pain, My Brain," *New York Times Magazine*, May 14, 2006, accessed October 29, 2012, www.nytimes.com/2006/05/14/magazine/14pain.html?pagewanted=all.

2. K. H. Brodersen, K. Wiech, E. I. Lomakina, C. S. Lin, J. M. Buhmann, U. Bingel, M. Ploner, K. E. Stephan, and I. Tracey, "Decoding the Perception of Pain from fMRI Using Multivariate Pattern Analysis," *Neuroimage* 63, no. 3 (2012): 1162–70; K. Davis, "Neuroimaging of Pain: What Does It Tell Us?" *Current Opinion in Supportive and Palliative Care* 5, no. 2 (2011): 116–21.

3. D. E. Drum, *The Chronic Pain Management Sourcebook* (Los Angeles: Lowell House, 1999), 18–19.

4. Drum, *The Chronic Pain Management Sourcebook*, 21–22.

5. C. S. Lewis, *The Problem of Pain* (New York: HarperOne, 2001), 136–39.

6. L. Manchikanti, K. S. Damron, C. D. Beyer, and V. Pampati, "A Comparative Evaluation of Illicit Drug Use in Patients with or without Controlled Substance Abuse in Interventional Pain Management," *Pain Physician* 6, no. 3 (2003): 281–85; L. Manchikanti, K. A. Cash, K. S. Damron, R. Manchukonda, V. Pampati, and C. D. McManus, "Controlled Substance Abuse and Illicit Drug Use in Chronic Pain Patients: An Evaluation of Multiple Variables," *Pain Physician* 9, no. 3 (2006): 215–25.

7. P. J. Norton and G. J. Asmundson, "Anxiety Sensitivity, Fear, and Avoidance Behavior in Headache Pain," *Pain* 111, nos. 1–2 (2004): 218–23; Anxiety Sensitivity in the Prediction of Pain-Related Fear and Anxiety in a Heterogeneous Chronic Pain Population," *Behavior Research and Therapy* 39, no. 6 (2001): 683–96.

8. M. Birket-Smith and E. Mortensen, "Pain in Somatoform Disorders: Is Somatoform Pain Disorder a Valid Diagnosis?" *Acta Psychiatrica Scandinavica* 106, no. 2 (2002): 103–8; H. Grabe, C. Meyer, U. Hapke, H. Rumpf, H. Freyberger, H. Dilling, and U. John, "Somatoform Pain Disorder in the General Population," *Psychotherapy and Psychosomatics* 72, no. 2 (2003): 88–94.; U. Ehlert, C. Heim,and D. Hellhammer, "Chronic Pelvic Pain as a Somatoform Disorder," *Psychotherapy and Psychosomatics* 68, no. 2 (1999): 87–94.

9. S. Skevington, *Psychology of Pain* (Hoboken, NJ: Wiley, 1995), 94–101.

10. N. Meinhart and M. McCaffery, *Pain, A Nursing Approach to Assessment and Analysis* (Norwalk, CT: Appleton-Century-Crofts, 1983), 237–38.

11. B. Calandra, "Gender: Some Painstaking Differences," *MedicineNet*, April 30, 2001, accessed March 22, 2013, www.medicinenet.com/script/main/art.asp?articlekey=51160.

12. Calandra, "Gender: Some Painstaking Differences."

13. R. Roy, *Social Relations and Chronic Pain* (New York: Kluwer Academic Publishers, 2002), 248–50.

14. S. Segerstrom and G. Miller, "Psychological Stress and the Human Immune System: A Meta-analytic Study of 30 Years of Inquiry," *Psychological Bulletin* 130, no. 4 (2004): 601-30.

15. L. Teri, L. Gibbons, S. M. McCurry, R. G. Logsdon, D. M. Buchner, W. E. Barlow, W. A. Kukull, A. Z. LaCroix, W. McCormick, and E. B. Larson, "Exercise Plus Behavioral Management in Patients with Alzheimer Disease: A Randomized Controlled Trial," *Journal of the American Medical Association* 290, no. 15 (2003): 2015–22; M. Gatz, "Educating the Brain to Avoid Dementia: Can Mental Exercise Prevent Alzheimer Disease?" *Public Library of Medicine (PLOS)* 2, no. 1 (2005): e7.

16. J. A. Blumenthal, M. A. Babyak, C. O'Connor, S. Keteyian, J. Landzberg, J. Howlett, W. Kraus, S. Gottlieb, G. Blackburn, A. Swank, and D. J. Whellan, "Effects of Exercise Training on Depressive Symptoms in Patients with Chronic Heart Failure: The HF-ACTION Randomized Trial," *Journal of the American Medical Association* 308, no. 5 (2012): 465–74.

17. P. A. Hardy, *Chronic Pain Management: The Essentials* (London: Greenwich Medical Media, 1997), 74–79.

18. F. Vertosick, *Why We Hurt: The Natural History of Pain* (New York: Harcourt, 2000), 198.

19. Vertosick, *Why We Hurt*, 200.

27. SURGERY AND OTHER NONPHARMACOLOGICAL APPROACHES

1. R. Chou, J. Baisden, E. J. Carragee, D. K. Resnick, W. O. Shaffer, J. D. Loeser, "Surgery for Low Back Pain: A Review of the Evidence for an American Pain Clinical Practice Guideline." *Spine* 34, no.10 (2009):1097.

2. F. Meyer, W. Börm, and C. Thomé, "Degenerative Cervical Spinal Stenosis: Current Strategies in Diagnosis and Treatments," *Deutsches Arzteblatt International* 105, no. 20 (2008): 366.

3. M. Greenburg, *Handbook of Neurosurgery* 7th ed., (New York: Thieme Publishing, 2010), 484.

4. J. K. MacGraw, J. A. Lippert, K. D. Minkus, P. M. Rami, T. M. Davis, and R. F. Budzik, "Prospective Evaluation of Pain Relief in 100 Patients Undergoing Percutaneous Vertebroplasty: Results and Follow-up," *Journal of Vascular and Interventional Radiology* 13, no. 9 (2002): 885.

5. S. Siegel, E. Paszkiewicz, C. Kirkpatrick, B. Hinkel, and K. Oleson, "Sacral Nerve Stimulation in Patients with Chronic Intractable Pelvic Pain," *Journal of Urology* 166, no. 5 (2001): 1742.

6. M. C. Schubert, S. Sridhar, R. R. Schade, and S. D. Wexner, "What Every Gastroenterologist Needs to Know about Common Anorectal Disorders," *World Journal of Gastroenterology* 15, no. 26 (2009): 3201.

7. P. Mantyh, D. Clohisy, M. Koltzenburg, and S. Hunt, "Molecular Mechanism of Cancer Pain," *Nature Reviews: Cancer* 2, no. 3 (2002): 203.

8. G. Di Lorenzo, R. Autorino, F. Ciardello, D. Raben, C. Bianco, T. Troiani, C. Pizza and S. Di Placido, "External Beam Radiotherapy in Bone Metastatic Prostate Cancer: Impact on Patients' Pain Relief and Quality of Life," *Oncology Reports* 10, no. 2 (2003): 399–404.

9. B. B. Bruce, K. D. Foote, J. Rosenbek, C. Sapienza, J. Romrell, G. Crucian, and M. S. Okun, "Aphasia and Thalamotomy: Important Issues," *Stereotactic and Functional Neurosurgery* 82, no. 4 (2004): 187.

10. K. Kumar, R. S. Taylor, and L. Jacques, "Spinal Cord Stimulation versus Conventional Medical Management for Neuropathic Pain," *Pain* 132, nos. 1–2 (2007): 181.

11. T. Zwas, R. Elkanovitch, and F. George, "Interpretation and Classification of Bone Scintigraphic Findings in Stress Fractures," *Journal of Nuclear Medicine* 28, no. 4 (1987): 454.

12. J. N. Fields and A. I. Tröster, "Cognitive Outcomes after Deep Brain Stimulation for Parkinson's Disease: A Review of Initial Studies and Recommendations for Future Research," *Brain and Cognition* 42, no. 2 (2000): 270.

28. PHARMACOLOGICAL APPROACHES

1. "Pharmacologic Pain Management," Michigan Institute of Pain Management, accessed May 12, 2013, www.mipmpc.com/pharmacologic-pain-management/.

2. C. F. Von Gunten and F. D. Ferris, "Pharmacological Management of Pain," Northwestern University Feinberg School of Medicine, accessed October 25, 2012, www.galter.northwestern.edu; L. Leung, "From Ladder to Platform: A New Concept for Pain Management," *Journal of Primary Health Care* 4, no. 3 (2012): 254–58.

3. A. Roden and E. Sturman, "Assessment and Management of Patients with Wound-Related Pain," *Nursing Standard* 23, no. 45 (2009): 53–62; "South West Regional Wound Care Toolkit: WHO Pain Ladder with Pain Management Guidelines," accessed May 5, 2013, www.southwesthealthline.ca/healthlibrary_docs/B.5.3.WHOPainLadder.pdf.

4. "South West Regional Wound Care Toolkit."

5. H. Smith, S. Datta, and L. Manchikanti, "Evidence-Based Pharmacotherapy of Chronic Pain," in *Handbook of Pain and Palliative Care* (New York: Springer, 2012), 471.

6. J. Ellis, "Initial Management of Acute Pain," in *Decision Making In Pain Management*, 2nd ed. (Philadelphia: Mosby, 2006), 4.

7. C. Ventola, "Direct-to-Consumer Pharmaceutical Advertising: Therapeutic or Toxic?" *Pharmacy and Therapeutics* 36, no. 10 (2011): 671–73.

8. Ventola, "Direct-to-Consumer Pharmaceutical Advertising."

9. Ventola, "Direct-to-Consumer Pharmaceutical Advertising."

10. L. Milligan, "25 Shocking Facts about the Pharmaceutical Industry," *African Executive*, www.africanexecutive.com/modules/magazine/article_print.php?article=4004.

11. A. Laycock and G. Todd, "Alcohol and Other Drugs," in *The Public Health Bush Book: A Resource for Working in Community Settings in the Northern Territory* (Darwin, Australia: Territory Health Services, 1999).

12. E. L. Riddle, A. E. Fleckenstein, and G. R. Hanson, "Role of Monoamine Transporters in Mediating Psychostimulant Effects," *American Association of Pharmaceutical Scientists (AAPS) Journal* 7, no. 4 (2005): E847–51.

13. World Health Organization, *Neuroscience of Psychoactive Substance Use and Dependence* (Geneva: World Health Organization, 2004).

14. World Health Organization, *Neuroscience of Psychoactive Substance Use*.

15. R. A. Glennon, "Classical Drugs: An Introductory Overview," *Hallucinogens: An Update* (Rockville, MD: National Institute on Drug Abuse, 1994).

16. World Health Organization, *Neuroscience of Psychoactive Substance Use*; Milligan, "25 Shocking Facts."

17. G. G. Graham and K. F. Scott, "Mechanism of Action of Paracetamol," *American Journal of Therapeutics* 12, no. 1 (2005): 46–55.

18. M. Loes, "Acetaminophen and Nonsteroidal Anti-inflammatory Drugs," in *Pain Medicine and Management: Just the Facts* (New York: McGraw-Hill, 2005), 46.

19. Loes, "Acetaminophen and Nonsteroidal Anti-inflammatory Drugs," 46.

20. "Before Using Aspirin to Lower Your Risk of Heart Attack or Stroke, Here Is What You Should Know," U.S. Food and Drug Administration, accessed May 27, 2013, www.fda.gov/Drugs/ResourcesForYou/Consumers/BuyingUsingMedicineSafely/UnderstandingOver-the-CounterMedicines/SafeDailyUseofAspirin/ucm291434.htm.

21. C. Balita, *Ultimate Learning Guide to Nursing Review* (Manila: Flipside Publishing 2004), 302–3.

22. D. Anderson and J. Beyer, "Local Anesthetic Choice," in *Decision Making in Pain Management*, 2nd ed. (Philadelphia: Mosby, 2006), 238.

23. D. Marks, M. Shah, A. Patkar, P. Masand, G. Park, and C. Pae, "Serotonin-Norepinephrine Reuptake Inhibitors for Pain Control: Premise and Promise," *Current Neuropharmacology* 7, no. 4 (2009): 331–36.

24. T. Jensen, "Anticonvulsants in Neuropathic Pain: Rationale and Clinical Evidence," *European Journal of Pain* 6, Suppl. A (2002): 61–68.

25. World Health Organization, *WHO Guidelines on the Pharmacological Treatment of Persisting Pain in Children with Medical Illnesses* (France: World Health Organization, 2012).

26. Loes, "Acetaminophen and Nonsteroidal Anti-inflammatory Drugs," 46.

27. D. Chau, V. Walker, L. Pai, and L. Cho, "Opiates and Elderly: Use and Side Effects," in *Clinical Interventions in Aging* 3, no. 2 (2008): 273.

28. Ventola, "Direct-to-Consumer Pharmaceutical Advertising," 674.

29. "Don't Be Tempted to Use Expired Medicines," U.S. Food and Drug Administration, accessed March 23, 2013, www.fda.gov/Drugs/ ResourcesForYou/SpecialFeatures/ucm252375.htm.

30. "FDA Targets Drug Side Effects," U.S. Food and Drug Administration, accessed May 24, 2013, www.fda.gov/ForConsumers/ConsumerUpdates/ ucm317496.htm.

31. "FDA's Efforts to Address the Misuse and Abuse of Opioids," U.S. Food and Drug Administration, accessed May 24, 2013, www.fda.gov/Drugs/ DrugSafety/InformationbyDrugClass/ucm337852.htm.

32. "Pharmacologic Pain Management."

29. SECOND OPINIONS

1. B. E. Cole, "Prescribing Opioids Wisely," in *Opioid Agreements and Contracts* (Sonora, CA: American Academy of Pain Management, 2003), 11.

2. "Care for Illnesses," California Department of Managed Health Care, accessed June 12, 2013, www.dmhc.ca.gov/HealthCareLawsRights/ Howdoyougetthebestcare/CareofIllnesses.aspx#.VGaY7fnF98E.

3. "The Fight against Pain Counts on Doctor-Patient Communication," International Association for the Study of Pain, accessed June 23, 2013, www. healthprzone.com/company/X97319-international-association-for-the-study- of-pain-iasp/105-the-fight-against-pain-counts-on-doctorpatient- communication.

4. "How to Find a Doctor or Treatment Facility If You Have Cancer," National Cancer Institute, June 29, 2009, accessed June 12, 2013, www.cancer. gov/cancertopics/factsheet/Therapy/doctor-facility.

5. J. E. Brody, "Chronic Pain: A Burden Often Shared," *New York Times*, November 13, 2007, accessed June 14, 2013, www.nytimes.com/2007/11/13/ health/13brod.html?_r=0.

6. "Living with Chronic Pain: Impact on the Family," The Health Experi- ences Research Group and Oxford University's Department of Primary Care, reviewed November 2010, accessed June 25, 2013.

7. "Living with Chronic Pain: Impact on the Family," The Health Experi- ences Research Group and Oxford University's Department of Primary Care, accessed June 25, 2013, www.healthtalk.org/peoples-experiences/chronic- health-issues/chronic-pain/impact-family.

8. "How Do I Get a Second Opinion?," National Health Service UK, ac- cessed June 28, 2013, www.nhs.uk/chq/Pages/910.aspx?CategoryID=68.

9. "Why Get a Second Opinion?," Partners HealthCare System, Inc, ac- cessed June 29, 2013, https://econsults.partners.org.

10. "Getting a Second Opinion," accessed June 29, 2013,www.macmillan. org.uk/Cancerinformation/Cancertreatment/Gettingtreatment/ Gettingasecondopinion.aspx.

11. "Getting a Second Opinion."

12. "Getting a Second Opinion."

13. "Diseases & Conditions: Second Opinions," Cleveland Clinic, accessed June 23, 2013, https://my.clevelandclinic.org/health/diseases_conditions/hic_breast_cancer_an_overview/hic_the_diagnosis_is_breast_cancer/hic_breast_cancer_qanda_second_opinion.

30. CONCLUSION

1. "Alternative Treatments for Chronic Pain," *WebMD*, accessed March 9, 2013, www.webmd.com/pain-management/guide/different-treatments-chronic-pain.

2. K. Kam, "Is Your Pain Acute or Chronic?," *WebMD*, accessed February 18, 2013, www.webmd.com/pain-management/chronic-pain-11/types-pain.

3. J. Black and J. H. Hawks, *Medical-Surgical Nursing Clinical Management for Positive Outcomes* (New York: Elsevier), 356–84; C. Balita, *Ultimate Learning Guide to Nursing Review* (Manila: Flipside Publishing 2004), 302–3.

BIBLIOGRAPHY

PREFACE

American Geriatrics Society (AGS). "Clinical Practice Guidelines: The Management of Chronic Pain in Older Persons." *Journal of the American Geriatrics Society* 46 (1998): 635–51.

Bines, A., and Paice, J. A. "Are Your Pain Management Skills Up-to-Date?" *Nursing* 35 (1996), 36–37.

Bergh, I., and Sjostrom, B. "A Comparative Study of Nurses' and Elderly Patients' Ratings of Pain and Pain Tolerance." *Journal of Gerontological Nursing* 25 (1999), 30–36.

Jensen, M. P., Martin, S. A., and Cheung, R. "The Meaning of Pain Relief in a Clinical Trial." *Journal of Pain* 6 (2005), 400–406.

CHAPTER I

Brookoff, D. "Chronic Pain: 1. A New Disease." *Hospital Practice* 35, no. 7 (2000): 45–52, 59.

Cohen, M., Quintner, J., and Buchanan, D. "Is Chronic Pain a Disease?" *Pain Medicine* 14 no. 9 (2013): 1284–88.

Georgesen J., and Dungan, J. "Managing Spiritual Distress in Patients with Advanced Cancer Pain." *Cancer Nursing* 19, no. 5 (1996): 376–83.

Niv D., and Devor, M. "Chronic Pain as a Disease in its Own Right." *Pain Practice* 4, no. 3 (2004): 179–81.

CHAPTER 2

Fraser, E. "The Development of the Vertebrate Excretory System." *Biological Reviews of the Cambridge Philosophical Society* 25, no. 2 (1950): 159–87.

Goldstein, B. "Anatomy of the Peripheral Nervous System." *Physical Medicine and Rehabilitation Clinics of North America* 12, no. 2 (2001): 207–36.

Sakka, L., and Vitte, E. "Anatomy and Physiology of the Vestibular System: Review of the Literature" [French]. *Morphologie* 88, no. 282 (2004): 117–26.

CHAPTER 3

Bullock, T., Orkand, R., and Grinnell, A. *Introduction to Nervous Systems*. New York: W. H. Freeman, 1977.
Johnston., D., and Miao-Sin Wu, S. *Foundations of Cellular Neurophysiology*. Cambridge, MA: The MIT Press, 1995.
Krainik, A., Feydy, A., Colombani, J., Hélias, A., and Menu, Y. "Functional Anatomy of the Central Nervous System" [French]. *Journal of Radiology* 84, no. 3 (2003): 285–97.
Shields, R. Jr. "Functional Anatomy of the Autonomic Nervous System." *Journal of Clinical Neurophysiology* 10, no. 1 (1993): 2–13.
Schmidt-Nielsen, K. *Animal Physiology: Adaptation and Environment*. Cambridge: Cambridge University Press, 1997.
Silverthorn, A., Ober, W., and Garrison, C. *Human Physiology: An Integrated Approach*. San Francisco: Benjamin-Cummings, 2007.

CHAPTER 4

Croft, P., Blyth, F., and Van Der Windt, D. *Chronic Pain Epidemiology from Aetiology to Public Health*. New York: Oxford University Press, 2010.
Grichnik, K., and Ferrante, F. "The Difference between Acute and Chronic Pain." *Mount Sinai Journal of Medicine* 58, no. 3 (1991): 217–20.
Jessell, T., Kandel, E., and Schwartz, J. "*Principles of Neural Science*." Norwalk, CT: Appleton & Lange, 1991: 472–79.
Rollin, B., *The Unheeded Cry: Animal Consciousness, Animal Pain, and Science*. New York: Oxford University Press, 1989.
Voscopoulos, C., and Lema, M. "When Does Acute Pain Become Chronic?" *British Journal of Anaesthesiology* 105, no. 1 (2010): 69–85.

CHAPTER 5

Andrade, C., and Radhakrishnan, R. "Prayer and Healing: A Medical and Scientific Perspective on Randomized Controlled Trials." *Indian Journal of Psychiatry* 51, no. 4 (2009): 247–53.
H. Van Aken, and H. Buerkle. "Acute Pain Services: Transition from the Middle Ages to the 21st Century." *European Journal of Anaesthesiology* 15, no. 3 (1998): 253–54.
Whitman, S. "Pain and Suffering as Viewed by the Hindu Religion." *Journal of Pain* 8, no. 8 (2007): 607–13.

CHAPTER 6

Fillingim, R., King, C., Ribeiro-Dasilva, M., Rahim-Williams, B., and Riley III, J. "Sex, Gender, and Pain: A Review of Recent Clinical and Experimental Findings." *Journal of Pain* 10, no. 5 (2009): 447–85.
Greenspan, J., Craft, R., LeResche, L., Arendt-Neilsen, L, Berkley, K., Fillingim, R., Gold, M., Holdcroft, A., Lautenbacher, S., Mayer, E., Mogil, J., Murphy, A., and Traub, R. "Studying Sex and Gender Differences in Pain and Analgesia: A Consensus Report." *Pain* 132, no. 1 (2007): S26–S45.
Moffett, J., Underwood, M., and Gardiner, E. "Socioeconomic Status Predicts Functional Disability in Patients Participating in a Back Pain Trial" *Disability and Rehabilitation* 31, no. 10 (2009): 783–90.
Nayak, S., Shiflett, S., Eshun, S., and Levine, F. "Culture and Gender Effects in Pain Beliefs and the Prediction of Pain Tolerance." *Cross-Cultural Research* 34, no. 2 (2000): 135–51.
Narayan, M. "Culture's Effects on Pain Assessment and Management." *American Journal of Nursing* 110, no. 4 (2010): 38–47.

Swaminath, G. "Doctor-Patient Communication: Patient Perception." *Indian Journal of Psychiatry* 49, no. 3 (2007): 150–53.
Wiesenfeld-Hallin, Z. "Sex Differences in Pain Perception." *Gender Medicine* no. 3 (2005): 137–45.

CHAPTER 7

Lasch, K. "Culture, Pain, and Culturally Sensitive Pain Care." *Pain Management Nursing* 1, no. 3 (2000): 16–22.
Rich, B. "A Legacy of Silence: Bioethics and the Culture of Pain." *Journal of Medical Humanities* 18, no. 4 (1997): 233–59.
Villarruel, A., and Ortiz de Montellano, B. "Culture and Pain: A Mesoamerican Perspective." *Advances in Nursing Science* 15, no. 1 (1992): 21–32.
Walker, A., Tan, L, and George, S. "Impact of Culture on Pain Management: An Australian Nursing Perspective." *Holistic Nursing Practice* 9, no. 2 (1995): 48–57.

CHAPTER 8

Cross, S. "Pathophysiology of Pain." *Mayo Clinic Proceedings* 69, no. 4 (1994): 375–83.
Vanderah, T. "Pathophysiology of Pain." *Medical Clinics of North America* 91, no. 1 (2007): 1–12.
Wieseler-Frank, J., Maier, S., and Watkins, L. "Glial Activation and Pathological Pain." *Neurochemistry International* 45, no. 2 (2004): 389–95.

CHAPTER 9

Carragee, E., and Hannibal, M. "Diagnostic Evaluation of Low Back Pain." *Orthopedic Clinics of North America* 35, no. 1 (2004): 7–16.
Dinnes, J., Loveman, E., McIntyre, L., and Waugh, N. "The Effectiveness of Diagnostic Tests for the Assessment of Shoulder Pain Due to Soft Tissue Disorders: A Systematic Review." *Health Technology Assessment* 7, no. 29 (2003): iii, 1–166.
Forman, T., Forman, S., and Rose, N. "A Clinical Approach to Diagnosing Wrist Pain." *American Family Physician* 72, no. 9 (2005): 1753–58.

CHAPTER 10

Clark, G., Sakai, S., Merrill, R., Flack, V., and McCreary, C. "Cross-Correlation between Stress, Pain, Physical Activity, and Temporalis Muscle EMG in Tension-Type Headache." *Cephalalgia* 15, no. 6 (1995): 511–18.
Feuerstein, M., Sult, S., and Houle, M. "Environmental Stressors and Chronic Low Back Pain: Life Events, Family and Work Environment." *Pain* 22, no. 3 (1985): 295–307.
McFarlane, A. "The Long-Term Costs of Traumatic Stress: Intertwined Physical and Psychological Consequences." *World Psychiatry* 9, no. 1 (2010): 3–10.
Narayan, M., "Culture's Effects on Pain Assessment and Management." *American Journal of Nursing* 110, no. 4 (2010): 38–47.
Stahl, M., El-Metwally, A., Mikkelsson, M., Salminen, J., Pulkkinen, L., Rose, R., Kaprio, A. "Genetic and Environmental Influences on Non-specific Neck Pain in Early Adolescence: A Classical Twin Study." *European Journal of Pain* 17, no. 6 (2013): 791–98.
Vandenkerkhof, E., Macdonald, H., Jones, G., Power, C., and Macfarlane, G. "Diet, Lifestyle and Chronic Widespread Pain: Results from the 1958 British Birth Cohort Study." *Pain Research & Management* 16, no. 2 (2011): 87–92.

Williams, F., Scollen, S., Cao, D., Memari, Y., Hyde, C., Zhang, B., Sidders, B., Ziemek, D., Shi, Y., Harris, J., Harrow, I., Dougherty, B., Malarstig, A., McEwen, R., Stephens, J., Patel, K., Menni, C., Shin, S., Hodgkiss, D., Surdulescu, G., He, W., Jin, X., McMahon, S., Soranzo, N., John, S., Wang, J., and Spector, T. "Genes Contributing to Pain Sensitivity in the Normal Population: An Exome Sequencing Study." *Public Library of Science (PLOS) Genetics* 8, no. 12 (2012): e1003095.

Wilson B. "Can Patient Lifestyle Influence the Management of Pain?" *Journal of Clinical Nursing* 18, no. 3 (2009): 399–408.

Wuitchik, M., and Feehan, G. "Opioid Withdrawal versus Opioid Maintenance for Persons with Chronic Non-cancer Pain. The Experience of the Canmore Pain Clinic." *Rehab in Review* 2 (2006): 19–21.

CHAPTER 11

Ambler, N., Williams, A., Hill, P., Gunary, R., and Cratchley, G. "Sexual Difficulties of Chronic Pain Patients." *Clinical Journal of Pain* 17, no. 2 (2001): 138–45.

Boardman, L. A., and Stockdale, C. K. "Sexual Pain." *Clinical Obstetrics and Gynecology* 52, no. 4 (2009): 682–90.

Chen, Z., Williams, K., Fitness, J., and Newton, N. "When Hurt Will Not Heal: Exploring the Capacity to Relive Social and Physical Pain." *Psychological Science* 19, no. 8 (2008): 789–95.

Eisenberger, N. "The Neural Bases of Social Pain: Evidence for Shared Representations with Physical Pain." *Psychosomatic Medicine* 74, no. 2 (2012): 126–35.

CHAPTER 12

Bishop, P., and Wing, P. "Knowledge Transfer in Family Physicians Managing Patients with Acute Low Back Pain: A Prospective Randomized Control Trial." *Spine Journal* 6, no. 3 (2006): 282–88.

Bope, E., Douglass, A., Gibovsky, A., Jones, T., Nasir, L., Palmer, T., Panchal, S., Rainone, F., Rives, P., Todd, K., and Toombs, J. "Pain Management by the Family Physician: The Family Practice Pain Education Project." *Journal of the American Board of Family Medicine* 17 (2004): S1–S12.

Chen, J., Fagan, M., Diaz, J., and Reinert, S. "Is Treating Chronic Pain Torture? Internal Medicine Residents' Experience with Patients with Chronic Nonmalignant Pain." *Teaching and Learning in Medicine* 19, no. 2 (2007): 101–5.

Clark, L., and Upshur, C. "Family Medicine Physicians' Views of How to Improve Chronic Pain Management." *Journal of the American Board of Family Medicine* 20, no. 5 (2007): 479–82.

Fabbian, F., De Giorgi, A., Pala, M., Mallozzi Menegatti, A., Gallerani, M., and Manfredini, R. "Pain Prevalence and Management in an Internal Medicine Setting in Italy." *Pain Research and Treatment* 2014 (2014): 1–5.

Scott, E., Borate, U., Heitner, S., Chaitowitz, M., Tester, W., and Eiger, G. "Pain Management Practices by Internal Medicine Residents—a Comparison Before and After Educational and Institutional Interventions." *American Journal of Hospice & Palliative Care* 25, no. 6 (2008): 431–39.

Yanni, L., Weaver, M., Johnson, B., Morgan, L., Harrington, S., and Ketchum, J. "Management of Chronic Nonmalignant Pain: A Needs Assessment in an Internal Medicine Resident Continuity Clinic." *Journal of Opioid Management* 4, no. 4 (2008): 201–11.

CHAPTER 13

Greenwald, B., Narcessian, E., and Pomeranz, B. "Assessment of Physiatrists' Knowledge and Perspectives on the Use of Opioids: Review of Basic Concepts for Managing Chronic Pain." *American Journal of Physical Medicine & Rehabilitation* 78, no. 5 (1999): 408–15.

Kim, Y. "A View of Policies for Persons with Disabilities as a Physiatrist" [Korean]. *American Academy of Physical Medicine and Rehabilitation* 27, no. 2 (2003): 157–63.
Neal, L. "Complex Regional Pain Syndrome: The Role of the Psychiatrist as an Expert Witness." *Medicine, Science and the Law* 49, no. 4 (2009): 241–46.
Press, J. "Physiatrist 2007: Who Are We and Where Are We Going?" *Archives of Physical Medicine and Rehabilitation* 89, no. 1 (2008): 1–3.

CHAPTER 14

American Society of Anesthesiologists Task Force on Chronic Pain Management, American Society of Regional Anesthesia and Pain Medicine. "Practice Guidelines for Chronic Pain Management: An Updated Report by the American Society of Anesthesiologists Task Force on Chronic Pain Management and the American Society of Regional Anesthesia and Pain Medicine." *Anesthesiology* 112, no. 4 (2010): 810–33.
Brennan F., Carr D., Cousins, M. "Pain Management: A Fundamental Human Right." *Anesthesia & Analgesia* 105, no. 1 (2007): 205–21.
Brink-Huis, A., Van-Achterberg, T., Schoonhoven, L. "Pain Management: A Review of Organisation Models with Integrated Processes for the Management of Pain in Adult Cancer Patients." *Journal of Clinical Nursing* 17, no. 15 (2008): 1986–2000.
Hansen, G. "Management of Chronic Pain in the Acute Care Setting." *Emergency Medicine Clinics of North America* 23, no. 2 (2005): 307–38.
Sherlekar, S. "Pain Management Clinics." *Clinics in Podiatric Medicine and Surgery* 25, no. 3 (2008): 477–91.
Sohn, D. "Who Is Pain Management Specialist?" *Missouri Medicine Journal* 102, no. 6 (2005): 529.

CHAPTER 15

Indo Y. "Genetics of Congenital Insensitivity to Pain with Anhidrosis (CIPA) or Hereditary Sensory and Autonomic Neuropathy Type IV. Clinical, Biological and Molecular Aspects of Mutations in TRKA(NTRK1) Gene Encoding the Receptor Tyrosine Kinase for Nerve Growth Factor." *Clinical Autonomic Research* 12, no. 1 (2002): 120–32.
Mardy, S., Miura, Y., Endo, F., Matsuda, I., Sztriha, L., Frossard, P., Moosa, A., Ismail, E., Macaya, A., Andria, G., Toscano, E., Gibson, W., Graham, G., and Indo, Y. "Congenital Insensitivity to Pain with Anhidrosis: Novel Mutations in the TRKA (NTRK1) Gene Encoding a High-Affinity Receptor for Nerve Growth Factor." *American Journal of Human Genetics* 64, no. 6 (1999): 1570–79.
Protheroe, S. "Congenital Insensitivity to Pain." *Journal of the Royal Society of Medicine* 84, no. 9 (1991): 558–59.
Sasnur, A., Sasnur, P., Ghaus-Ul, R. "Congenital Insensitivity to Pain and Anhidrosis." *Indian Journal of Orthopaedics* 45, no. 3 (2011): 269–71.

CHAPTER 16

Carr, D., and Goudas, L. "Acute Pain." *Lancet* 353, no. 9169: 2051–58.
De Pinto, M., and Cahana, A. "Medical Management of Acute Pain in Patients with Chronic Pain." *Expert Review of Neurotherapeutics* 12, no. 11 (2012): 1325–38.
Sadler, A., Wilson, J., and Colvin, L. "Acute and Chronic Neuropathic Pain in the Hospital Setting: Use of Screening Tools." *Clinical Journal of Pain* 29, no. 6 (2013): 507–11.
Shipton, E., and Tait, B. "Flagging the Pain: Preventing the Burden of Chronic Pain by Identifying and Treating Risk Factors in Acute Pain." *European Journal of Anaesthesiology* 22, no. 6 (2005): 405–12.

CHAPTER 17

Cassou, B., Derriennic, F., Monfort, C., Norton, J., and Touranchet, A. "Chronic Neck and Shoulder Pain, Age, and Working Conditions: Longitudinal Results from a Large Random Sample in France." *Occupational and Environmental Medicine* 59, no. 8 (2002): 537–44.

Damkot, D., Pope, M., Lord, J., and Frymoyer, J. "The Relationship between Work History, Work Environment and Low-Back Pain in Men." *Spine* 9, no. 4 (1984): 395–99.

Johnston, J., Landsittel, D., Nelson, N., Gardner, L., and Wassell, J. "Stressful Psychosocial Work Environment Increases Risk for Back Pain among Retail Material Handlers." *American Journal of Industrial Medicine* 43, no. 2 (2003): 179–87.

Juhl, M., Andersen, P., Olsen, J., and Andersen, A. "Psychosocial and Physical Work Environment, and Risk of Pelvic Pain in Pregnancy. A Study within the Danish National Birth Cohort." *Journal of Epidemiology & Community Health* 59, no. 7 (2005): 580–85.

Xu, Y., Bach, E., and Orhede, E. "Work Environment and Low Back Pain: The Influence of Occupational Activities." *Occupational and Environmental Medicine* 54, no. 10 (1997): 741–45.

CHAPTER 18

Bahr, R. "No Injuries, But Plenty of Pain? On the Methodology for Recording Overuse Symptoms in Sports."*British Journal of Sports Medicine* 43, no. 13 (2009): 966–72.

Baums, M., Kahl, E., Schultz, W., and Klinger, H. "Clinical Outcome of the Arthroscopic Management of Sports-Related Anterior Ankle Pain: A Prospective Study." *Knee Surgery, Sports Traumatology, Arthroscopy* 14, no. 5 (2006): 482–86.

Cavalli, M., Bombini, G., and Campanelli, G. "Pubic Inguinal Pain Syndrome: The So-Called Sports Hernia." *Surgical Technology International* 24 (2014): 189–94.

Mortimer, M., Wiktorin, C., Pernol, G., Svensson, H., and Vingard, E. "Musculoskeletal Intervention Center. Sports Activities, Body Weight and Smoking in Relation to Low-Back Pain: A Population-Based Case-Referent Study." *Scandinavian Journal of Medicine & Science in Sports* 11, no. 3 (2001): 178–84.

Neumaier, J. "Sports Injuries. What You Can do for Muscle and Joint Pain" [German]. *Fortschritte der Medizin* 153, no. 19 (2011): 24–25.

CHAPTER 19

Almekinders, L., and Almekinders, S. "Outcome in the Treatment of Chronic Overuse Sports Injuries: A Retrospective Study." *Journal of Orthopaedic & Sports Physical Therapy* 19, no. 3 (1994): 157–61.

Niemuth, P., Johnson, R., Myers, M., and Thieman, T. "Hip Muscle Weakness and Overuse Injuries in Recreational Runners." *Clinical Journal of Sport Medicine* 15, no. 1 (2005): 14–21.

Ostlie, K., Franklin, R., Skjeldal, O., Skrondal, A., and Magnus, P. "Musculoskeletal Pain and Overuse Syndromes in Adult Acquired Major Upper-Limb Amputees." *Archives of Physical Medicine and Rehabilitation* 92, no. 12 (2011): 1967–1973.e1.

Tenforde, A., Sayres, L., McCurdy, M., Collado, H., Sainani, K., and Fredericson, M. "Overuse Injuries in High School Runners: Lifetime Prevalence and Prevention Strategies." *Physical Medicine and Rehabilitation (P.M.&R.)* 3, no. 2 (2011): 125–31.

Von Korff, M. "Health Care for Chronic Pain: Overuse, Underuse, and Treatment Needs: Commentary on: Chronic Pain and Health Services Utilization—Is There Overuse of Diagnostic Tests and Inequalities in Nonpharmacologic Methods Utilization?" *Medical Care* 51, no. 10 (2013): 857–58.

CHAPTER 20

Chen, S., Liu, M., Cook, J., Bass, S., and Lo, S. "Sedentary Lifestyle as a Risk Factor for Low Back Pain: A Systematic Review." *International Archives of Occupational and Environmental Health* 82, no. 7 (2009): 797–806.

Ellingson, L., Shields, M., Stegner, A., and Cook, D. "Physical Activity, Sustained Sedentary Behavior, and Pain Modulation in Women with Fibromyalgia." *Journal of Pain* 13, no. 2 (2012): 195–206.

Fukuda, T., Melo, W., Zaffalon, B., Rossetto, F., Magalhães, E., Bryk, F., and Martin, R. "Hip Posterolateral Musculature Strengthening in Sedentary Women with Patellofemoral Pain Syndrome: A Randomized Controlled Clinical Trial with 1-Year Follow-Up." *Journal of Orthopaedic & Sports Physical Therapy* 42, no. 10 (2012): 823–30.

Vitta, A., Canonici, A., Conti, M., and Simeao, S. "Prevalence and Factors Associated with Musculoskeletal Pain in Professionals of Sedentary Activities." *Fisioterapia em Movimento* 25, no. 2 (2012): 273–80.

CHAPTER 21

Araujo, L., Macintyre, C., and Vujacich, C., "Epidemiology and Burden of Herpes Zoster and Post-Herpetic Neuralgia in Australia, Asia and South America." *Herpes* 14, no. 2 (2007): 40–44.

Donahue, J. Choo, P., Manson, J., and Platt, R. "The Incidence of Herpes Zoster." *Archives of Internal Medicine* 155, no. 15 (1995): 1605–9.

Gagliese, L., Katz, L., Gibson, M., Clark, A., Lussier, D., Gordon, A., and Salter, M. "A Brief Educational Intervention about Pain and Aging for Older Members of the Community and Health Care Workers." *Journal of Pain* 13, no. 9 (2012): 849–56.

Gibson, S., and Lussier, D. "Prevalence and Relevance of Pain in Older Persons." *Pain Medicine* 13, no. 2 (2012): S23–S26.

Glare, P., Virik, K., Jones, M., Hudson, M., Eychmuller, S. Simes, J., Christakis, N. "A Systematic Review of Physicians' Survival Predictions in Terminally Ill Cancer Patients." *British Medical Journal* 327, no. 7408 (2003): 195–98.

Hayden, E. "Cutting off Cancer's Supply Lines." *Nature* 458, no. 7239 (2009): 686–87.

Molton, I., Cook, K., Smith, A., Amtmann, D., Chen, W., and Jensen, M. "Prevalence and Impact of Pain in Adults Aging with a Physical Disability: Comparison to a US General Population Sample." *Clinical Journal of Pain* 30, no. 4 (2014): 307–15.

Rustoen, T., Wahl, A., Hanestad, B., Lerdal, A., Paul, S., and Miaskowski, C. "Age and the Experience of Chronic Pain: Differences in Health and Quality of Life among Younger, Middle-Aged, and Older Adults." *Clinical Journal of Pain* 21, no. 6 (2005): 513–23.

Widerström-Noga, E., and Finlayson, M. "Aging with a Disability: Physical Impairment, Pain, and Fatigue." *Physical Medicine & Rehabilitation Clinics of North America* 21, no. 2 (2010): 321–37.

CHAPTER 22

Bates, M., Edwards, W., and Anderson, K. "Ethnocultural Influences on Variation in Chronic Pain Perception." *Pain* 52, no. 1 (1993): 101–12.

Brennan, F., Carr, D., and Cousins, M., "Pain Management: A Fundamental Human Right." *Pain Medicine* 105, no. 1 (2007): 205–21.

Cepeda, M., and Carr, D. "Overview of Pain Management." In *Approaches to Pain Management: An Essential Guide for Clinical Leaders.* Oakbrook Terrace, IL: Jount Commission Resources, 2003: 1–20.

Hyman, C. "Pain Management and Disciplinary Action: How Medical Boards Can Remove Barriers to Effective Treatment." *Journal of Law, Medicine, and Ethics* 24, no. 4 (1996): 338–43.

Rupp, T., and Delaney, K. Inadequate Analgesia in Emergency Medicine." *Annals of Emergency Medicine* 43, no. 4 (2004): 494–503.

CHAPTER 23

Hermann, C., and Blanchard, E. "Biofeedback in the Treatment of Headache and other Childhood Pain." *Applied Psychophysiology and Biofeedback* 27, no. 2 (2002): 143–62.
Latimer, E., Crabb, M., Roberts, J., Ewen, M., and Roberts, J. "The Patient Care Travelling Record in Palliative Care: Effectiveness and Efficiency." *Journal of Pain and Symptom Management* 16, no. 1 (1998): 41–51.
Norton, S., Hogan, L., Holloway, R., Temkin-Greener, H., Buckley, M., and Quill, T. "Proactive Palliative Care in the Medical Intensive Care Unit: Effects on Length of Stay for Selected High-Risk Patients." *Critical Care Medicine* 35, no. 6 (2007): 1530–35.
Tatsumi, S., Mabuchi, T., Abe, T., Xu, L., Minami, T., and Ito, S. "Analgesic Effect of Extracts of Chinese Medicinal Herbs Moutan Cortex and Coicis Semen on Neuropathic Pain in Mice." *Neuroscience Letters* 370, nos. 2–3 (2004): 130–34.

CHAPTER 24

Black, C., and O'Connor, P. "Acute Effects of Dietary Ginger on Muscle Pain Induced by Eccentric Exercise." *Phytotherapy Research* 24, no. 11 (2010): 1620–26.
Galland, L. "Diet and Inflammation." *Nutrition in Clinical Practice* 25, no. 6 (2010): 634–40.
Masino, S., and Ruskin, D. "Ketogenic Diets and Pain." *Journal of Child Neurology* 28, no. 8 (2013): 993–1001.
Nieman, D., Shanely, R., Luo, B., Dew, D., Meaney, M., Sha, W. "A Commercialized Dietary Supplement Alleviates Joint Pain in Community Adults: A Double-Blind, Placebo-Controlled Community Trial." *Nutrition Journal* 12, no. 1 (2013): 154.
Tall, J., and Raja, S. "Dietary Constituents as Novel Therapies for Pain." *Clinical Journal of Pain* 20, no. 1 (2004): 19–26.
Vandenkerkhof, E., Macdonald, H., Jones, G., Power, C., and Macfarlane, G. "Diet, Lifestyle and Chronic Widespread Pain: Results from the 1958 British Birth Cohort Study." *Pain Research & Management* 16, no. 2 (2011): 87–92.
Yehuda, S., Leprohon-Greenwood, C., Dixon, L., Coscina, D. "Effects of Dietary Fat on Pain Threshold, Thermoregulation and Motor Activity in Rats." *Pharmacology Biochemistry and Behavior* 24, no. 6 (1986): 1775–77.

CHAPTER 25

Miller, J., Gross, A., D'Sylva, J., Burnie, S., Goldsmith, C., Graham, N., Haines, T., Bronfort, G., and Hoving, J. "Manual Therapy and Exercise for Neck Pain: A Systematic Review." *Manual Therapy* 15, no. 4 (2010): 334–54.
Mior, S. "Exercise in the Treatment of Chronic Pain." *Clinical Journal of Pain* 17, no. 4 (2001): S77–S85.
O'Reilly, S., Muir, K., and Doherty, M. "Effectiveness of Home Exercise on Pain and Disability from Osteoarthritis of the Knee: A Randomised Controlled Trial." *Annals of the Rheumatic Diseases* 58, no. 1 (1999): 15–19.
Rydeard, R., Leger, A., and Smith, D. "Pilates-Based Therapeutic Exercise: Effect on Subjects with Nonspecific Chronic Low Back Pain and Functional Disability: A Randomized Controlled Trial." *Journal of Orthopaedic and Sports Physical Therapy* 36, no. 7 (2006): 472–84.
Tanaka, R., Ozawa, J., Kito, N., and Moriyama, H. "Efficacy of Strengthening or Aerobic Exercise on Pain Relief in People with Knee Osteoarthritis: A Systematic Review and Meta-Analysis of Randomized Controlled Trials." *Clinical Rehabilitation* 27, no. 12 (2013): 1059–71.
Van Middelkoop, M., Rubinstein, S., Verhagen, A., Ostelo, R., Koes, B., and van Tulder, M. "Exercise Therapy for Chronic Nonspecific Low-Back Pain." *Best Practice & Research Clinical Rheumatology* 24, no. 2 (2010): 193–204.

CHAPTER 26

Hansen, G., and Streltzer, J. "The Psychology of Pain." *Emergency Medicine Clinics of North America* 23, no. 2 (2005): 339–48.

Keefe, F., Abernethy, A., Campbell, C. "Psychological Approaches to Understanding and Treating Disease-related Pain." *Annual Review of Psychology* 56 (2005): 601–30.

Keefe, F., Rumble, M., Scipio, C., Giordano, L., and Perri, L. "Psychological Aspects of Persistent Pain: Current State of the Science." *Journal of Pain* 5, no. 4 (2004): 195–211.

Kerns, R., Sellinger, J., and Goodin, B. "Psychological Treatment of Chronic Pain." *Annual Review of Clinical Psychology* 7 (2011): 411–34.

Meerwijk, E., Ford, J., and Weiss, S. "Brain Regions Associated with Psychological Pain: Implications for a Neural Network and its Relationship to Physical Pain." *Brain Imaging and Behavior* 7, no. 1 (2013): 1–14.

Turk, D., and Okifuji, A. "Psychological Factors in Chronic Pain: Evolution and Revolution." *Journal of Consulting and Clinical Psychology* 70, no. 3 (2002): 678–90.

CHAPTER 27

Buchbinder, R., Green, S., Bell, S., Barnsley, L., Smidt, N., and Assendelft, W. "Surgery for Lateral Elbow Pain." *Cochrane Database of Systematic Reviews* 1 (2002): CD003525.

Carter, J. "Surgical Treatment for Chronic Pelvic Pain." *Journal of the Society of Laparoendoscopic Surgeons* 2, no. 2 (1998): 129–39.

Chou, R., Baisden, J., Caragee, E., Resnick, D., Shaffer, W., and Loeser, J. "Surgery for Low Back Pain: A Review of the Evidence for an American Pain Clinical Practice Guideline." *Spine* 82, no. 10 (2009): 1094–1109.

Kumar, K., Taylor, R., Jacques, L., Eldabe, S., Meglio, M., Molet, J., and Thomson, S. "Spinal Cord Stimulation versus Conventional Medical Management for Neuropathic Pain." *Pain* 132, nos. 1–2 (2007): 179–188.

MacGraw, J., Lippert, J., Minkus, K., Rami, P., Davis, T., and Budzik, R. "Prospective Evaluation of Pain Relief in 100 Patients Undergoing Percutaneous Vertebroplasty: Results and Follow-Up." *Journal of Vascular and Interventional Radiology* 13, no. 9 (2002) 883–86.

Perkins, F., and Kehlet, H. "Chronic Pain as an Outcome of Surgery. A Review of Predictive Factors." *Anesthesiology* 93, no. 4 (2000): 1123–33.

Wieser, E., and Wang, J. "Surgery for Neck Pain." *Neurosurgery* 60, no. 1 (2007): S51–S56.

CHAPTER 28

Ansari, Z. "Evidence-Based Pharmacological Management of Chronic Neuropathic Pain." *International Journal of Basic & Clinical Pharmacology* 2, no. 3 (2013): 229–36.

Dworkin, R., O'Connor, A., Audette, J., Baron, R., Gourlay, G., Haanpa, M., Kent, J., Krane, E., Lebel, A., Levy, R., Mackey, S., Mayer, J., Miaskowski, C., Raja, S., Rice, A., Schmader, K., Stacey, B., Stanos, S., Treede, R., Turk, D., Walco, G., and Wells, C. "Recommendations for the Pharmacological Management of Neuropathic Pain: An Overview and Literature Update." *Mayo Clinic Proceedings* 85, no. 3 (2010): S3–S14.

Inturrisi, C. "Clinical Pharmacology of Opioids for Pain." *Clinical Journal of Pain* 18, no. 4 (2002): S3–S13.

Park, H., and Moon, D. "Pharmacologic Management of Chronic Pain." *Korean Journal of Pain* 23, no. 2 (2010): 99–108.

Varrassi, G., Müller-Schwefe, G., Pergolizzi, J., Orónska, A., Morlion, B., Mavrocordatos, P., Margarit, C., Mangas, C., Jaksch, W., Huygen, F., Collett, B., Berti, M., Aldington, D., and Ahlbeck, K. "Pharmacological Treatment of Chronic Pain—the Need for Change." *Current Medical Research and Opinion* 26, no. 5 (2010): 1231–45.

CHAPTER 29

Mustafa, M., Bijl, M., and Gans, R. "What Is the Value of Patient-Sought Second Opinions?" *European Journal of Internal Medicine* 13, no. 7 (2002): 445.
Sutherland, L., and Verhoef, M. "Patients Who Seek a Second Opinion: Are They Different from the Typical Referral?" *Journal of Clinical Gastroenterology* 11, no. 3 (1989): 308–13.
Van Dalen, I., Groothoff, J., Stewart, R., Spreeuwenberg, P., Groenewegen, P., and Van Horn, J. "Motives for Seeking a Second Opinion in Orthopaedic Surgery." *Journal of Health Services Research & Policy* 6, no. 4 (2001): 195–201.
Vashitz, G., Davidovitch, N., and Pliskin, J. "Second Medical Opinions" [Hebrew]. *Harefuah* 150, no. 2 (2011): 105–10, 207.
Vashitz, G., Pliskin, J., Parmet, Y., Kosashvili, Y., Ifergane, G., Wientroub, S., and Davidovitch, N. "Do First Opinions Affect Second Opinions?" *Journal of General Internal Medicine* 27, no. 10 (2012): 1265–71.
Wagner, T., and Wagner, L. "Who Gets Second Opinions?" *Health Affairs* 18, no. 5 (1999): 137–45.

CHAPTER 30

Gandhi, W., Becker, S., and Schweinhardt, P. "Pain Increases Motivational Drive to Obtain Reward, but Does Not Affect Associated Hedonic Responses: A Behavioural Study in Healthy Volunteers." *European Journal of Pain* 17, no. 7 (2013): 1093–103.
Jensen, M., Nielson, W., and Kerns, R. "Toward the Development of a Motivational Model of Pain Self-Management." *Journal of Pain* 4, no. 9 (2003): 477–92.
Kendall, N. "Psychosocial Approaches to the Prevention of Chronic Pain: The Low Back Paradigm." *Best Practice & Research Clinical Rheumatology* 13, no. 3 (1999): 545–54.
Kratz, A., Molton, I., Jensen, M., Ehde, D., and Nielson, W. "Further Evaluation of the Motivational Model of Pain Self-Management: Coping with Chronic Pain in Multiple Sclerosis." *Annals of Behavioral Medicine* 41, no. 3 (2011): 391–400.
Krismer, M., Van Tulder, M. "Strategies for Prevention and Management of Musculoskeletal Conditions: Low Back Pain (Non-specific)." *Best Practice & Research Clinical Rheumatology* 21, no. 1 (2007): 77–91.
Rawdin, B., Evans, C., and Rabow, M. "The Relationships among Hope, Pain, Psychological Distress, and Spiritual Well-Being in Oncology Outpatients." *Journal of Palliative Medicine* 16, no. 2 (2013): 167–72.
Thomas, M., Elliott, J., Rao, S., Fahey, K., Paul, S., and Miaskowski, C. "A Randomized Clinical Trial of Education or Motivational-Interviewing-Based Coaching Compared to Usual Care to Improve Cancer Pain Management." *Oncology Nursing Forum* 39, no. 1 (2012): 39–49.
Wright, M., Wren, A., Somers, T., Goetz, M., Fras, A., Huh, B., Rogers, L., and Keefe, F. "Pain Acceptance, Hope, and Optimism: Relationships to Pain and Adjustment in Patients with Chronic Musculoskeletal Pain." *Journal of Pain* 12, no. 11 (2011): 1155–62.

INDEX

5-HT induced protein kinase-C
    activation, 79

α-amino-3hydroxy-5-methyl-4-
    isoxazolepropionic acid receptor
    (AMPA) activation, 79
abdominal aortic aneurysm, 269, 331
abdominal exercises, 250
abstaining from food, 243
Academies and Academic Associations of
    General Practitioners/Family
    Physicians, 123
Academy of Family Physicians of India
    (AFPI), 121, 123, 362n1
ACC synapse, 80
accumulation of toxins, 170
acetylsalicylic acid, 63, 331
active person, 96
acupressure, 302
acupuncture, 61, 213, 330, 331
acute postsurgical pain, 161, 359n11
acute renal failure, 119
addictive drugs, 15
adhesiolysis, 266
adjuvant medications, 279
adolescent medicine, 117, 355n6
adrenaline, 10, 29
adult chronic pain, 41
advanced medical care, 93
alternative ways, 224
amygdalae, 17

aerobics, 253
age, 7, 40–41
age groups, 172
aging process: normal, 199; pain and, xi
alcohol abuse, 13; dependence, 351n10;
    excessive, 202; increased amount of,
    26; influence of, 183; moderate
    amounts, 198; opium and, 46; and
    other drugs, 376n11; and sedatives, 78;
    and smoking problems, 273; tobacco
    and, 101
allergies, 117
allergist-immunologist, 117
allodynia, 165
alternative pain management, 66
Alzheimer's disease, 15, 17, 282, 331
ambulatory care, 89
American Academy of Family Physicians
    (AAFP), 121
American Academy of General Practice
    (AAGP), 121
American Board of Internal Medicine
    (ABIM), 116, 355n3
American Board of Physician Specialties
    (ABPS), 116
American Chronic Pain Association's
    family manual, 294
American Osteopathic Board of Internal
    Medicine (AOBIM), 116, 367n3
The America Pain Society, 55

natural approaches, 223; difference between traditional and, 223–224; benefits and drawbacks of, 227; blending traditional treatments with, 233; herbs and vitamin D for, 229; significance of, 226; three types of, 224–225
natural balance, 233
natural painkillers, 260
neck extension, 247
neck pain, 247
neglected pain, 152
neocerebellum, 13
neocortex, 17
neonatal and infant pain scale (NIPS), 152
nerve, 23; blocking procedure for, 209; growth factor (NGF), 149, 150, 358n9, 383; growth factor beta polypeptide gene (NGFB), 150; hyperexcitability of, 82; root, 246; stimulation of, 274
nervous system: central, 9; as a network, 23; peripheral, 18; structure and function, 23
neural tube, 11
neuroactive peptides, 32
neuroaxial painkillers, 159
neurodegeneration, 83
neuroimaging, 255
neurological occupational pain, 173
neurolysis, 209, 269–270
neuronal loss, 32
neuroplasticity, 81, 84
neurorehabilitation, 128
neuroscience, 9
neurotoxicity, 82
neurotrophic tyrosine kinase receptor Type 1 (NTRK1), 149
New York University School of Medicine, 148
N-methyl-D-aspartate (NMDA) receptors, 79
nociceptors, 35–36, 81–82, 84, 150, 170
nondrug tactics, 159
non-opioid painkiller, 159
nonpharmacological approaches, 131, 142, 226, 263, 275
noradrenaline, 10
norepinephrine: blockage of hormones and, 286; reuptake inhibitors, 376n23;

reuptake of, 284
NSAIDs, 231–233, 279, 283–284, 333, 334
NTRK1 gene mutations, 155
nutrition, 261

obese adults, 236
obesity, 39, 117, 195–196, 200, 206–207, 369n6, 369n7
obsessive compulsive disorder (OCD), 17, 258
occipital: nerve stimulation (ONS), 275, 334, 360n22–360n23; neuralgia, 166, 360n22; seizures, 16
occupational pain, 169; avoidance of, 176–177; disability and, 175; old age and, 199; prevalence of, 172–173; risk of, 171; social characteristics of, 176; type of, 170; workplace and, 174
The Odyssey, 44
olfaction, 10, 17
omega-3, 231, 235, 238, 242, 368n32
opioid: agonist, 284; analgesics, 216–217, 219; induced hyperalgesia, 97; receptor, 80, 279, 285, 369n43
opium, 44–46, 334, 343n8
optical sensors, 89
oral medication, 207–208
orthopedic bed, 246
osteitis pubis, 163
osteoarthritis, 207
osteoporotic spinal fracture, 265
Ottawa Knee Rules, 194
ovarian cyst, 164
overweight, 236
oxygen starvation, 17

Paget's disease, 270
pain, 3, 35, 118, 189, 255, 294; during sex, 108; ladder, 278; of the liver, 243; management, 137; neuropathic, 37; perception, 255; prevalence, 41, 382; proneness, 38; radicular, 37; relief methods, 56; scales, 152; stimuli, 12; supplements, 231; symptoms, 236; therapists, 4; thresholds, 55, 98, 105, 344n2, 364n11; tolerance, 259
painkillers, 65, 89, 130
pain-related neurons, 13

ABOUT THE AUTHORS

Naheed Ali, MD, PhD, began writing professionally in 2005 and has written several books on medical topics and taught at colleges in the United States. Additional information is available at NaheedAli.com.

Moshe Lewis, MD, MPH, is an ivy league-trained pain physician and physiatrist. He currently serves as the chief of physical medicine and rehabilitation at the St. Luke's Campus of the California Pacific Medical Center. He lives in northern California, where he enjoys traveling and writing during his spare time. Visit him online at MosheLewisMD.com.